AF248864

Trichothecene Mycotoxicosis: Pathophysiologic Effects

Volume II

Editor

Val Richard Beasley, Ph.D.

Co-Director
National Animal Poison Control Center
Assistant Professor of Toxicology
College of Veterinary Medicine
University of Illinois
Urbana, Illinois

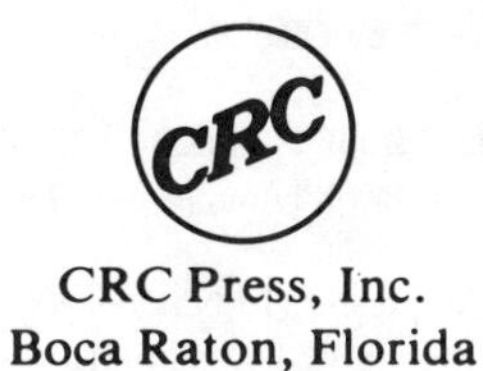

CRC Press, Inc.
Boca Raton, Florida

Library of Congress Cataloging-in-Publication Data

Trichothecene mycotoxicosis : pathophysiologic effects / editor, Val Richard Beasley
   p.   cm.
   Includes bibliographies and index.
   ISBN 0-8493-5088-3 (v. 1). -- ISBN 0-8493-5089-1 (v. 2)
   1. Trichothecenes--Toxicology. 2 Trichothecenes--Physiological effect. 3. Mycotoxicoses. I. Beasley,
Val Richard.
   [DNLM: 1. Mycotoxins--toxicity. 2. Sesquiterpenes--toxicity. QW 630 T823]
RA 1242.T68T75   1989   616.9'69--dc19   88-37491 CIP
DNLM/DLC for Library of Congress

International Standard Book Number 0-8493-5088-3 (v. 1)
International Standard Book Number 0-8493-5089-1 (v. 2)

Library of Congress Card Number 88-37491
Printed in the United States

INTRODUCTION

The mycotoxins, toxins produced by fungi, include compounds of widely varying chemical structure and toxic potential. The differences among mycotoxins are similar to those of plant toxins which also vary widely, but which contain groups of similar compounds that share common mechanisms of action. The trichothecenes are one group of fungal metabolites that occur widely in nature, especially as contaminants of grains and sometimes forages. Although there is evidence that the trichothecenes share common mechanisms of action and similar target organ/systems, differences exist, especially in potency.

The trichothecenes are cytotoxic, but many of their effects are due to secondary processes which are set in motion sometimes by ill-defined mechanisms. This book is arranged to address some of the known primary effects of trichothecene mycotoxins at the biochemical and whole animal levels. It also attempts to review and discuss some of the investigations that have addressed a range of other concerns that pertain to any naturally occurring toxicant that has the potential to contaminate the food supply. For example, information is included on investigations of natural occurrence and of the mutagenic and carcinogenic potential of the toxins. The results of studies of potential preventive and therapeutic approaches are also described.

There are instances of unresolved differences of opinion, as in the case of underlying biochemical mechanisms of action. It has been particularly challenging to interpret the diversity of effects induced by several trichothecenes when studied in various cells, tissues, and organisms, administered by a number of routes of administration, at different doses or concentrations, and at dissimilar intervals. In the hope of shortening the time needed to overcome these difficulties, the authors have sought to discuss a range of observations delineating both areas of agreement and aspects remaining to be clarified.

The final chapter of the volumes is comprised of an effort to integrate the various observations detailed throughout the book. With the continued efforts of not only the many dedicated scientists who served as contributors to these volumes, but also with input from the many other authors cited herein and those to follow, our understanding of these interesting compounds will continue to expand. We have already learned enough to greatly reduce the adverse effects of the trichothecene mycotoxins on humans and other animals.

THE EDITOR

Val Richard Beasley, D.V.M., Ph.D., is Co-Director of the National Animal Poison Control Center and Assistant Professor of Toxicology, College of Veterinary Medicine, University of Illinois, Urbana.

He received his D.V.M. from Purdue University, Lafayette, Indiana, and his Ph.D. from the University of Illinois. Prior to his current position, Dr. Beasley was owner of Old Troy Pike Veterinary Clinic in Dayton, Ohio and a research associate in the University of Illinois College of Veterinary Medicine.

During his career, he has been extremely active in research, publishing, and lecturing. Over 175 publications have been authored, co-authored, or edited by Dr. Beasley, many of which in conjunction with contributors to the present volumes. The research in which he has participated as a principal investigator, investigator, or collaborator has received grant awards in excess of $4.75 million. Under his instruction as a graduate advisor in the College of Veterinary Medicine, two of his students were selected as recipients of the Joseph O. Alberts Award; one of these students was recognized by the American Association of Physiologists and Pharmacologists for best graduate student paper in 1987. Another of his graduate students was presented with an award for best poster presentation at the Midwest Regional Chapter of the Society of Toxicology in 1988. Additionally, Dr. Beasley's expertise in the field of veterinary toxicology has been called upon in EPA hearings and in a civil case pertaining to environmental contamination.

Among his memberships in professional societies are the American Veterinary Medicine Association, the Illinois State Veterinary Medicine Association, Fellow of the American Academy of Veterinary and Comparative Toxicology, and the International Association for Aquatic Animal Medicine. He is a member of Phi Zeta and Sigma Xi and holds veterinary licenses in four states.

*To the most inspiring teacher of science in my life's experience,
John Van Sickle of Westlane Junior High School, Indianapolis, and to my
parents and my beloved family, Victoria, Lelah, and Livia*

CONTRIBUTORS

Val R. Beasley, D.V.M., Ph.D.
Co-Director
National Animal Poison Control Center
Assistant Professor of Toxicology
College of Veterinary Medicine
University of Illinois
Urbana, Illinois

James K. Bubien
Department of Physiology and
 Biophysics
University of Alabama
Birmingham, Alabama

David L. Bunner
Pathophysiology Department
USAMRIID
Fort Detrick
Frederick, Maryland

Giora Feuerstein, M.D.
Department of Neurology
USUHS
Bethesda, Maryland

Robert Fricke
Pathophysiology Division
USAMRIID
Fort Detrick
Frederick, Maryland

Patricia A. Gentry, Ph.D.
Professor
Department of Biomedical Sciences
University of Guelph
Guelph, ON, Canada

Roseanne M. Lorenzana
Veterinary Bioscience Department
University of Illinois
Urbana, Illinois

Gregg Lundeen
Pfizer Central Research
Groton, Connecticut

Victor Fei Pang, Ph.D., D.V.M.
Department of Pathology
Pig Research Institute, Taiwan
Chunan, Taiwan

Robert H. Poppenga
Animal Health Diagnostic Laboratory
College of Veterinary Medicine
Michigan State University
East Lansing, Michigan

H. Bruno Schiefer, Ph.D.
Professor and Director
Toxicology Research Center
University of Saskatchewan
Saskatoon, SK, Canada

Michael J. Taylor, Ph.D.
System Toxicology Branch
NIH, NTP, NIEHS
Research Triangle Park, North Carolina

Charles Templeton
Pathophysiology Division
USAMRIID
Fort Detrick
Frederick, Maryland

W. Thomas Woods, Jr.
Department of Physiology and Biophysics
University of Alabama
Birmingham, Alabama

TABLE OF CONTENTS
Volume I

Volume II

Chapter 1

THE IMMUNOTOXICITY OF TRICHOTHECENE MYCOTOXINS

Michael J. Taylor, Victor F. Pang, and Val R. Beasley

TABLE OF CONTENTS

I. INTRODUCTION

The effects of trichothecene mycotoxins on the immune system of animals have gained much attention recently. Although the trichothecene mycotoxins comprise a large group, only several of its members have been specifically investigated with regard to immunotoxicity. T-2 toxin, fusarenon-X, diacetoxyscirpenol (DAS, anguidine), and deoxynivalenol (DON, vomitoxin) are among those specifically evaluated as immunotoxic compounds. Animal models to date have included poultry, mouse, rat, guinea pig, rabbit, cattle, sheep, swine, cat, and monkey. Much of the information concerning trichothecene-associated immunotoxic effects has been gleaned from studies which include observations on peripheral blood leukocyte counts and histologic changes in lymphoid tissues. Research efforts have also been directed toward understanding both antibody production and cell-mediated immunity following exposure to the toxins. Assessment of mitogenic responses, T-dependent and T-independent antibody production, delayed-type hypersensitivity responses, graft rejection, characterization of cell phenotypes, and the effects of toxin exposure on bacterial, viral, and yeast infections have been investigated. It is clear that the trichothecene mycotoxins suppress the immune network, but the specific functions of various cell type(s) affected by trichothecene mycotoxins have yet to be definitively ascertained. Figure 1 summarizes the possible effects of trichothecene mycotoxin exposure on the immune function.

Reviews to date have focused primarily on results obtained using the mouse as a model.[1,2] Immunologically, the mouse is an appropriate selection. However, the toxicosis induced by trichothecenes has, in fact, affected both man and agricultural animals. In this review, an attempt was made to summarize the effects on both common laboratory animals and other species.

The arrangement of the chapter is as follows: discussion of alimentary toxic aleukia (ATA) and its immunotoxic nature, a brief description of the immune system structure and function, immune-related dermal responses to trichothecene mycotoxins, trichothecene-induced immuno-dysfunction in man, immunological disorders in laboratory and non-laboratory animals and antitrichothecene mycotoxin antibodies. Immunotoxic descriptions include both immunopathologic and immunofunctional information as the two are inseparable aspects of the immune system proper. In closing, proposed mechanisms of trichothecene-induced immunotoxicity have been provided.

A. Alimentary Toxic Aleukia and Its Immunotoxic Nature

Summaries of clinical observations from persons afflicted with ATA have been compiled by Mayer[3] and Joffe.[4] Their summaries, in turn, have made use of the extensive Russian literature.

The name ATA indicates that one of the primary targets of trichothecene mycotoxins is the leukopoietic system. In fact, a leukopenic stage (second stage) has been described for the syndrome. In the first stage of the disease, the total number of peripheral leukocytes either does not change or increases slightly. As the second stage begins, there is a sharp decrease in the absolute number of leukocytes and a relative decrease in the percentage of granulocytes. Throughout much of the second stage, the leukocytes show toxic granulation and vacuolization within the cytoplasm. During the third stage of ATA, a general atrophy of the bone marrow (panmyelophthisis) occurs which is accompanied by impairment of leukocyte-phagocyte and reticuloendothelial functions. Lymph nodes are often swollen with lymphoid depletion and hyperplasia of the reticuloendothelium. Bronchopneumonia, pulmonary hemorrhages, and lung abscesses were frequent complications. Affected persons often died of sepsis.

B. Immune System

Before reviewing the literature pertaining to the trichothecene effects on both mammalian

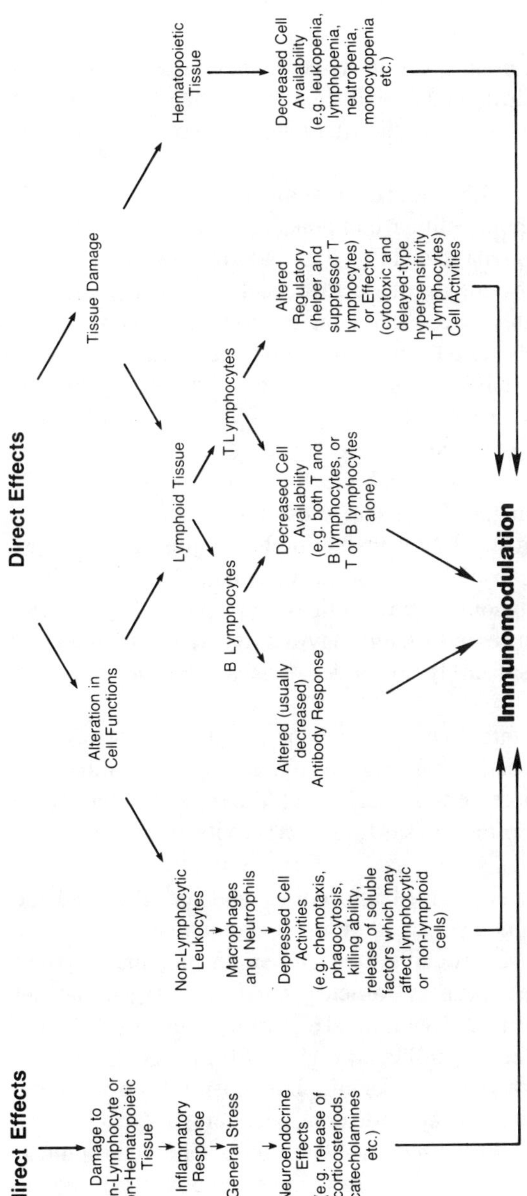

FIGURE 1. The possible effects of exposure to trichothecene mycotoxins on immune function.

and avian immune systems, a short description of the immune system has been provided in an attempt to orient those not familiar with some of the jargon descriptive of the structures and functions of this system.[5-7] Figure 2 summarizes the possible interactions between various cellular components of the immune system.

Functionally, the components of the immune system are involved in many processes such as tissue repair, confinement, removal or killing of infectious organisms, and recognition, killing, or removal of transformed cells. In addition, the immune system may integrate with the nervous and endocrine systems.

The cells of the immune system have been categorized as B, T, natural killer and null cells, granulocytes, macrophages, and dendritic cells. Neither natural killer nor null cells are discussed herein as no information is presently in the literature concerning these cells and the trichothecene mycotoxins.

Structurally, the immune system has both nonlymphoid cellular and primary and secondary lymphoid tissue components. The nonlymphoid cellular components include granulocytes, macrophages, and dendritic cells. The Langerhans cells of the epidermis and the interdigitating reticulum cells of the spleen are examples of dendritic cells. In mammals, the principle postembryonic origin of these immunocytes is the bone marrow. The major classes of leukocytes and lymphoid and myeloid cells arise from distinct progenitor cells. Following differentiation and maturation, the myeloid cells become granulocytes and monocytes. The granulocytes can be further classified as either neutrophils, eosinophils, or basophils. The monocytes become macrophages after leaving blood and entering tissues.

The lymphoid cellular components include both B and T cells. In mammals, mature B cells arise from the bone marrow; in birds, mature B cells arise from the bursa of Fabricius. Although T-cell precursors arise in bone marrow, T cells mature in the thymus. The thymus, bone marrow and bursa of Fabricius are considered as primary lymphoid tissues. Upon immigration (maturation) from primary lymphoid tissues, both B and T cells may take up residence in secondary lymphoid tissues and some of them may recirculate in blood and/or lymph. Secondary lymphoid tissues include spleen, lymph nodes, tonsils and Peyer's patches of the ileum.

Anatomically, the thymus is organized into two main compartments, the cortex and medulla. Differentiation and maturation of T cells (thymocytes) coincide with their migration from the cortex to medulla. The cortex is more densely packed with thymocytes than is the medulla, and as would be expected in a germinal tissue, mitotic activity is higher within the cortex.

Anatomically, the lymph nodes can also be divided into cortex and medulla, and the cortex can be sectioned into the superficial and deep areas. In most mammalian species, the lymphoid nodules or follicles reside in the superficial cortex. When an immune response occurs, the small inactive lymphoid nodules (primary follicles) become enlarged and are transformed into secondary follicles with a central area termed a germinal center containing large proliferating cells, primarily B cells. The interfollicular region of the superficial cortex are primarily composed of T cells. Lymph nodes thus contain T-independent (B cell) and T-dependent (T cell) areas in the superficial and deep cortex, respectively.

Anatomically, the spleen can be divided into the red and white pulp. The white pulp is rich in lymphocytes and, as discussed for lymph nodes, these regions can be further divided into T-dependent and T-independent areas. The T-dependent areas are found immediately surrounding the arterioles and are called the periarteriolar lymphoid sheaths. The T-independent areas surround the T-dependent areas and are the so-called nodular or follicular areas of the spleen.

The B cells, following antigenic activation, are ultimately transformed into antibody-secreting plasma cells. The T cells fill several capacities, generally recognized as either regulators, including helper and suppressor-type T cells, or effectors, including cytolytic and delayed-type hypersensitivity T cells. Most B cells depend on T cells or T-cell products; their functional responses to antigens are termed T-dependent as opposed to T-independent. Thus, B cells (which by definition tend to reside in T-independent areas of lymphoid tissues) may be stimulated by either T-dependent or T-independent mechanisms.

The two principal phagocytic cells in mammals are the macrophages and neutrophils. The macrophages arise from the blood monocytes which originate from the bone marrow. Peripherally circulating blood monocytes then become relatively long-lived tissue macrophages (histiocytes) upon leaving the circulatory system. Resident macrophages are able to produce and secrete nonlysosomal proteins which are called monokines, such as interleukin 1 (a T-lymphocyte-activating factor). Macrophages have been called the antigen-presenting cells and are therefore an early participant in both T- and B-cell responses. Neutrophils are another key cellular component in the inflammatory response, and they may also participate in early signaling to the macrophage since macrophages appear later in inflammatory reactions. The remaining two types of granulocytes, the basophils and eosinophils, are integral components of allergic reactions.

Table 1 summarizes the immunologic tests that have been used to characterize the immunotoxicity of the trichothecene mycotoxins. Results of the tests are discussed within the text. In addition to the parameters listed in Table 1, serum immunoglobulin concentrations (total IgA, IgE, IgG, and IgM), total and differential leukocyte counts for peripheral blood (lymphocytes, granulocytes, and monocytes), and the quantitation of specific categories of lymphocytes (B and T cells) using antibodies directed against membrane-associated determinants have been used to assess immunotoxicity. Pathologic alteration of primary and secondary lymphoid tissues is also an important parameter in assessing immunodysfunction.

II. IMMUNOTOXIC EFFECTS

A. Immune-Related Dermal Responses to Trichothecene Mycotoxins

Janovskij's tenet (cited by Mayer[3]) proposed that the origin of ATA was of an immunological nature and proposed the following progression of an allergic response: (1) local action of the compound, (2) incubation or period of sensitization, (3) anaphylactic changes, followed by (4) convalescence. Perhaps allergic reactions should be studied in greater detail in animals following repeated dermal exposure to the trichothecene mycotoxins. Presently, however, the dermal reaction to trichothecene mycotoxins is described as being an inflammatory response. The ability of trichothecene mycotoxins (extracted from feeds) to induce erythema after topical application has been used as a determinant of trichothecene-contamination. The cutaneous response, to both T-2 toxin and DAS in ethyl acetate, has been studied morphologically and quantitatively using both rats and rabbits.[8] The cutaneous response, described as being inflammatory reactions, are characterized by early accumulations of neutrophils at the luminal margins of venules. Neutrophils were observed throughout the dermis by 12 h and the outer layer of the epidermis by 24 h. The neutrophils were concentrated in and below the epidermis by 48 h; few were observed by 72 h or later.

Although considerable evidence suggests an inflammatory cutaneous response to topically applied trichothecenes, recent information regarding the inhibition of acute phase reactions by parenterally administered T-2 toxin indicates that the toxin may also lessen some nonspecific processes of inflammation.[9] The acute phase response is a dramatic but incompletely understood physiologic reaction to tissue injury and its concomitant inflammation.[9] This response is characterized by a rapid increase in hepatic synthesis of several plasma proteins as diverse as coagulation and complement components. Products of injured tissue, as well as biochemical and cellular constituents of the inflammatory process, are possible mediators of this response, such as interleukin 1. The biological role of the acute phase response is still unclear, but many workers believe that it is a nonspecific and immediate participant in

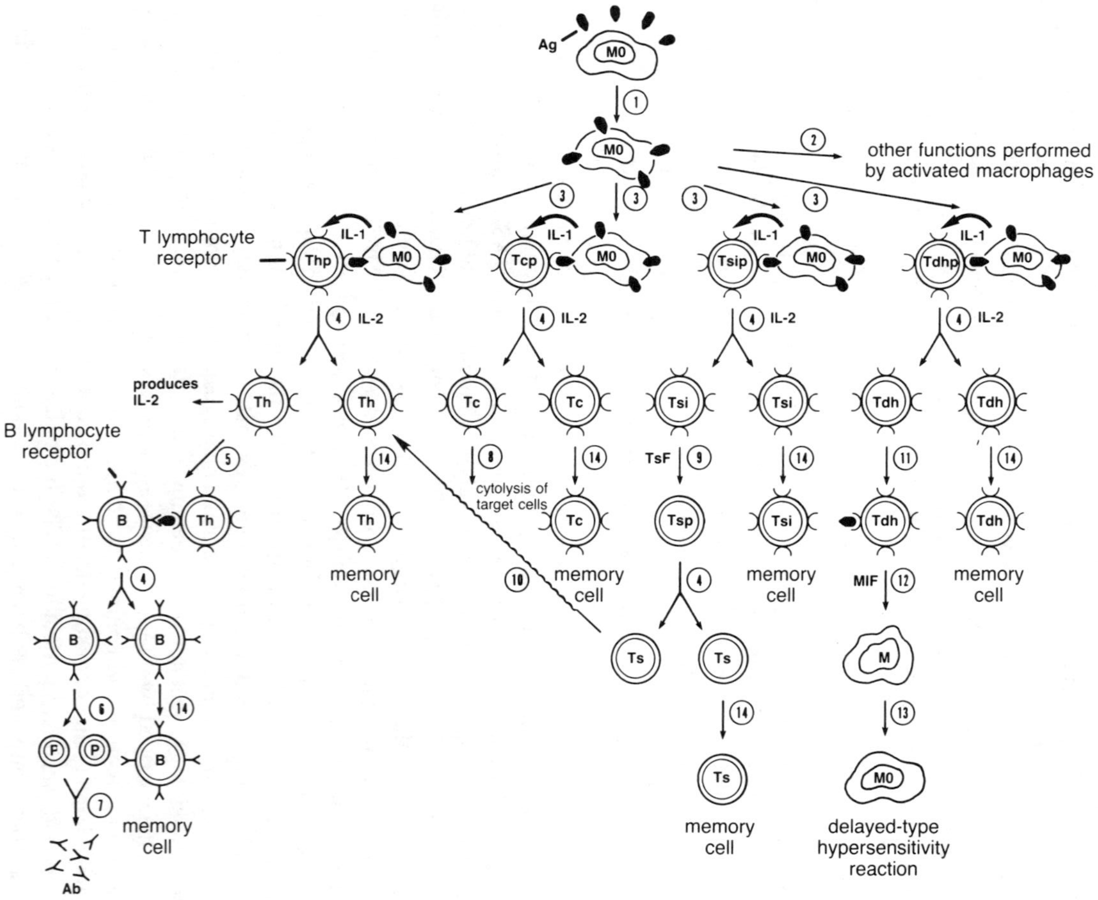

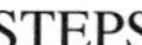

STEPS

1. Antigen contact and internalization by macrophages.
2. Intracellular killing or confinement of microorganisms or particles; killing target cells by cell-to-cell contact; secretion of soluble substances (such as growth factors for a variety of cells, cytotoxic factors, complement components, prostaglandins, etc.).
3. Antigen processing and presentation by activated macrophages.
4. Activation, transformation, and proliferation of precursor cells.
5. Interaction between helper T and B lymphocytes via an antigen bridge.
6. Differentiation of B lymphocytes into plasma cells.
7. Antibody production and secretion.
8. Adhesion of cytotoxic T lymphocyte to target cell.
9. Release of suppressor T lymphocyte activating factor.
10. Inhibition of helper T lymphocyte activities.
11. Antigen encounter.
12. Release of soluble factors, such as macrophage inhibitory factor.
13. Cell transformation and emigration from blood vessels.
14. Memory cell transformation.

FIGURE 2.   Postulated main steps of interaction of subpopulations of T lymphocytes, B lymphocytes, and macrophages responding to a thymus-dependent antigen. The sequence of events can be envisioned as follows: (1) antigens (Ag) are picked up by macrophages (MO) and the macrophages are activated; (2) the activated macrophages can perform some functions without participation of T lymphocytes; (3) the activated macrophages process the ingested antigens and present these processed antigens to the subpopulations of T lymphocytes, such as precursors (lymphoblasts) of helper T lymphocytes (Thp), precursors of cytotoxic T lymphocytes (Tcp), precursors of suppressor T lymphocyte inducers (Tsip), or precursors of delayed-type hypersensitivity T lymphocytes (Tdhp). In addition, the activated macrophages produce a soluble factor, interleukin-1 (IL-1), which acts on the subpopulations of T lymphocytes to stimulate them to produce receptors for another stable factor, interleukin-2 (IL-2); (4) these antigen-stimulated precursors of subpopulations of T lymphocytes are activated and undergo further transformation and proliferation, and become effector cells (more mature lymphocytes), such as helper (Th), cytotoxic (Tc), inducer of suppressor (Tsi), or delayed-type hypersensitivity (Tdh) T lymphocytes. These helper T lymphocytes can also produce IL-2 which acts on the antigen-stimulated precursors of subpopulations of T lymphocytes and helps to convert them into effector cells; (5) helper T lymphocytes interact with B lymphocytes via an antigen bridge and the B lymphocytes are activated and undergo further transformation and proliferation; (6) many of the proliferating B lymphocytes differentiate into plasma cells; (7) antibodies (Ab) are produced and secreted by plasma cells; (8) cytotoxic T lymphocytes adhere to and lyse target cells (such as tumor cells, cells infected by virus, etc.); (9) inducers of suppressor T lymphocytes release a specific suppressor T lymphocyte activating factor (TsF) which acts on precursors of suppressor T lymphocytes to activate them and to stimulate them to undergo further transformation, and proliferation into suppressor T lymphocytes (Ts); (10) the suppressor T lymphocytes in turn inhibit the activities of helper T lymphocytes; (11) delayed-type hypersensitivity T lymphocytes bind antigens in blood vessels (the antigens are probably also presented by macrophages); (12) the restimulated delayed-type hypersensitivity T lymphocytes release soluble factors, the most prominent of which is the macrophage-inhibiting factor (MIF) which stops the flow of monocytes (M) by making them adhere to the endothelium; (13) the adherent monocytes transform into macrophages. While they emigrate from the blood vessel, they release hydrolases attacking the surrounding tissue and inducing the delayed-type hypersensitivity reaction; (14) some of the proliferating B lymphocytes, helper T lymphocytes, cytotoxic T lymphocytes, inducers of suppressor T lymphocytes, suppressor T lymphocytes, or delayed-type hypersensitivity T lymphocytes return to the morphology of small lymphocytes and become memory cells, capable of rapid response to a repeated encounter with the same antigen.

Table 1
SUMMARY OF IMMUNOLOGIC TESTS DISCUSSED IN THE CONTEXT OF TRICHOTHECENE MYCOTOXICOSIS

Immune function assay	Description
1. Mitogen-induced lymphocyte proliferation	*In vitro* culture with mitogen; phytohemagglutinin (PHA), concanavalin A (ConA), lipopolysaccharide (LPS), pokeweed mitogen (PWM), or leukoagglutinin; PHA, ConA-T cell mitogens; PWM, LPS-B cell mitogens (PWM effects on B cells have been described as T-dependent); quantitated by ^{3}H-thymidine incorporation
2. Antibody production	T-dependent response, require T cells or their products (e.g., response to sheep red blood cells, SRBC); T-independent, no requirement for T cells or their products (e.g., dinitrophenyl-bovine serum albumin, DNP-BSA; DNP-ficoll; polyvinylpyrrolidone, PVP; LPS); measured as titer or antibody secreting plaque-forming cells (PFC)
3. Delayed-type hypersensitivity (DTH)	A T-dependent response; local immune reactivity; characterized by T lymphocyte proliferation and monocyte (macrophage) and neutrophil infiltration; no edema; the DTH response is usually initiated by systemic antigen administration followed by a local challenge with the antigen; SRBC are often used as an antigen; swelling or migration of a radiolabeled ligand into the affected area is used to quantitate the response
4. Macrophage and neutrophil function	Phagocytosis, chemiluminescence, chemotaxis, reduction of nitroblue tetrazolium
5. Host resistance to infection	Resistance to bacterial or viral challenge, expulsion of an injected pathogen
6. Adoptive transfer	Injection of immunocompetent cells into immuno-incompetent syngeneic recipients
7. Graft rejection	A T cell-mediated function
8. Compliment factors	Serum proteins activated sequentially by antibody-antigen complexes or by bacterial products; CH_{50} is the 50% lysis endpoint for complement-mediated lysis of antibody-coated red blood cells

inflammation and tissue repair. Although the biological role of some acute phase reactants can be inferred from their known *in vivo* functions (i.e., fibrinogen, C3), the roles of the most dramatic acute phase reactants, C-reactive protein and serum amyloid-A component in man and serum amyloid-P component in the mouse, have been only partially defined.

No acute phase response was observed in mice treated with T-2 toxin (0.01 to 2.0 mg/kg) either subcutaneously (s.c.) or intraperitoneally (i.p.) based on the measurement of the two murine acute phase reactants, serum amyloid-P component and plasma fibronectin.[9] T-2 toxin (0.17 to 1.50 mg/kg, i.p.) was demonstrated to block the acute phase response to s.c. injected $AgNO_3$ in a dose-related fashion. In addition, if T-2 toxin (2.0 mg/kg, i.p.) and $AgNO_3$ (s.c.) together were given to animals, half of them died after 48 h, and the survivors were extremely ill. Mice given the same dose of T-2 toxin along with s.c. injection of buffer, however, appeared well. Since the acute phase is an immediate physiologic reaction to tissue injury and may be a nonspecific participant in the tissue repair, its abrogation by T-2 toxin may contribute to the toxicity of this mycotoxin.

B. Trichothecene-Induced Immunodysfunction in Man

Relatively little information is available concerning the immunotoxicity of trichothecene mycotoxins to the human immune system. Some information has been provided, however, by clinical trials to determine the efficacy of DAS as a therapeutic anticancer agent.[10,11] The selection of DAS as a potential anticancer drug was based on its cytostatic properties and not its modulatory effects on the immune system. Leukopenia and thrombocytopenia were reported in patients given DAS at an i.v. (intravenous push) dose of 4.5 mg/m^2/d (approximately equivalent to 0.12 mg/kg/d on a 5-d schedule. Following DAS exposure, stimulation of peripheral lymphocytes with phytohemagglutinin (PHA), a T-cell mitogen, was evaluated, but the results were not described.[11]

Decreased responses of human peripheral blood lymphocytes to PHA following *in vitro* exposure to T-2 toxin or DAS have been demonstrated.[12] The lymphocytes were first exposed to PHA for a 24-h period after which the toxin was added and incubation continued for another 48 h. The incorporation of ^{3}H-thymidine (^{3}H-TdR) was used as an index of deoxyribonucleic acid (DNA) synthesis and hence a measure of cell proliferation. DAS or T-2 toxin at a concentration of 3.0 ng/ml reduced ^{3}H-TdR incorporation by 80 and 90% respectively. DAS or T-2 toxin also reduced ^{3}H-TdR incorporation in lymphocytes without PHA stimulation; their respective ID$_{50}$ (50% inhibition dose) concentrations were 1.5 and 2.7 ng/ml. Total inhibition of ^{3}H-TdR incorporation was observed with either DAS or T-2 toxin at 8.0 ng/ml.

Not only T-2 toxin but also certain of its metabolites, HT-2, 3'-OH T-2, 3'-OH HT-2, T-2 triol, and T-2 tetraol, were capable of inhibition of mitogen-induced blastogenesis of human peripheral blood lymphocytes *in vitro* at a concentration as low as 1.0 ng/ml.[13] Leukoagglutinin, concanavalin A (ConA), and pokeweed mitogen (PWM) were the selected mitogens. Hydrolysis or hydroxylation of T-2 to HT-2 or 3'-OH T-2, respectively, had only a minimal effect on the toxicity relative to that of T-2 toxin; however, further hydrolysis to the triol and tetraol or hydroxylation to 3'-OH HT-2 resulted in a dramatic reduction in the immunotoxicity.

The incorporation of ^{3}H-TdR into the DNA of PHA stimulated human peripheral blood lymphocytes was also inhibited by both DON and 3-acetyl-DON,[14] with the former being of greater potency. The ID$_{50}$ concentrations were 220 and 1060 ng/ml for DON and 3-acetyl-DON, respectively.

Yarom et al.[15] also studied the effects of T-2 toxin on human leukocytes *in vitro;* viability, chemotaxis, chemiluminescence, and phagocytosis were monitored. The authors reported a difference in the susceptibilities of lymphocytes, monocytes, and neutrophils to T-2 toxin. A dose of 300 μg/10^6 cells caused ultrastructural damage to approximately 40% of the neutrophils, while the lymphocytes and monocytes showed no structural damage. Chemotaxis of peripheral neutrophils was decreased by a dose of 3 μg/10^6 cells; the decrease in chemotaxis was dose related. T-2 toxin (1 to 20 μg/10^6 cells) was also able to reduce the chemiluminescence of neutrophils stimulated with opsonized streptococci. A statistically significant reduction in phagocytic activity was demonstrated for neutrophils following exposure to T-2 toxin.

III. ANIMAL MODELS

Table 2 is offered to permit rapid comparisons between the findings of various studies employing varying toxins, doses, routes and animal models. In addition to summarizing

Table 2
SUMMARY OF THE IMMUNOTOXIC EFFECTS OF TRICHOTHECENE MYCOTOXINS

Species	Toxin	Dose (route)	Exposure time	Additional treatment	Exposure time	Effects(s)	Ref.
Human (cancer patients)	DAS	Varied	From weekly to 5-d courses			Myelosuppression; spacing apart of doses and slower administration may lessen toxicity	106-110
Cat	*F. tricinctum* crude extract, T-2 toxin	0.06 to 0.1 mg/kg (p.o., in capsules)	Every 48 h for 6 to 40 d			Slight leukocytosis but neutropenia early in some, then progressive leukopenia and absolute lymphopenia; neutrophil degeneration; absence of myeloid maturation in marrow; edema, congestion, and lymphoid depletion in all lymphoid tissues; amyloidosis in spleen; cat allowed to recover after 15 doses had no lesions at 1 year	18
Rhesus monkey	T-2	0.5 or 1.0 mg/kg (p.o.)	15 d			Males more susceptible than females and all developed severe leukopenia; decreased spleen weights; died by day 15	16
	T-2	0.1 mg/kg (p.o.)	15 d			Both males and females developed leukopenia; 30% decrease in bacteriocidal activity of neutrophils; 3 died with respiratory infections; cortical lymphoid depletion in nodes; spleen unaffected; PHA responses decreased; IgG and IgM and B cell numbers decreased; recovery by 5 months	17
Guinea pig	T-2	0.5 and 0.75 mg/kg (p.o.)	Days 1 to 21 Days 21 to 42			WBC decreased especially after day 33; lymphocyte counts most reduced after 21 d	40

Animal	Compound	Dose	Duration	Effect	Ref.
	T-2	0.9 mg/kg (p.o.)	Days 1 to 27	WBC, total lymphocyte counts, myeloid:erythroid ratios all decreased; no lesions in lymphoid tissues	40
	DAS	0.6 to 1.6 mg/kg (stomach tube)	Days 1 to 30	No hematology change; no lesions	41
	DAS	1 to 8 mg/kg (stomach tube)	1 dose	Lymphoid necrosis, round cell necrosis in bone marrow	41
Rat	*F. tricinctum* cultures	LD$_{50}$ (p.o.)	1 dose	Neutrophilia, eosinophilia	94
	Fusarenon-X	LD$_{50}$ (i.p.)	1 dose	Degeneration and necrosis in lymph nodes, spleen, and thymus	97
Rabbit	T-2	0.5 mg/kg (i.v.)	1 dose	WBC decreased, especially at 72 h	43
	T-2	2 mg/kg (p.o.)	Days 1 to 4	No effect on WBC	43
Mouse	Fusarenon-X	Lethal and sublethal (i.p.)	3—12 h post-injection	Leukocytosis	95
	Fusarenon-X	3 mg/kg (i.p.)	1 dose	Mesenteric lymph node necrosis especially in germinal centers; thymic cortex changes slower in onset but more progressive	96
	Fusarenon-X	Sublethal injection (i.p. single or repeated)	3—4 d after injection	Leukopenia	95
	Fusarenon-X	10 ppm (diet)	25 d	Leukopenia	95
	Fusarenon-X	3.5 mg/kg (i.p.)	Twice weekly for 12 weeks	Perifollicular amyloidosis in spleen	95

Table 2 (continued)
SUMMARY OF THE IMMUNOTOXIC EFFECTS OF TRICHOTHECENE MYCOTOXINS

Species	Toxin	Dose (route)	Exposure time	Additional treatment	Exposure time	Effects(s)	Ref.
Mouse	*F. tricinctum*	$LD_{50\text{-}70}$ (p.o.)				Enlarged red necrotic lymph nodes; spleen and thymus became smaller; lymphoid depletion in spleens; septicema	98
	Culture filtrates of T-2 producing *Fusarium*	Lethal (i.p.)	1 dose			Karyorrhexis of bone marrow cells	99
	Spleen cells from mice treated 4d previously with SRBC i.v. with or without T-2 toxin on day 2	5×10^7 cells/ mouse	Day 0	SRBC (s.c.)		Decreased delayed-type hypersensitivity in recipient mice given spleen cells from T-2 toxin treated group	
	T-2	3—4 mg/kg (i.p.)	Day 2			Thymus cells depleted and decreased thymus to spleen traffic on day 4	
	F. tricinctum crude extract	$^{1}/_{2}$ and $^{1}/_{4}$ LD_{50} (i.p.)	Days 1, 2			Spleen and especially thymus weights decreased 1 d later; then lymphoid hypertrophy on day 10	55
	F. tricinctum crude extract	$^{1}/_{2}$ and $^{1}/_{4}$ LD_{50} (i.p.)	Days 1, 2			Spleen cells had decreased response to PHA at 3 d, most decreased on day 10; LPS responses increased on day 3, slightly decreased on day 10, but twice normal on day 19	55

						Spleen periarteriolar sheaths (T cells) became atrophic before lymphoid follicles (B cells); thymic cortex (T cells) depleted on day 1 but medulla proliferation; cells in cortex recovered on day 3 but medulla depleted	
	F. tricinctum crude extract	$^{1}/_{2}$ and $^{1}/_{4}$ LD$_{50}$ (i.p.)	Days 1, 2	SRBC (i.p.)	3 or 4 d before being bled	Decreased hemagglutination titers as compared to controls when bled on days 3, 7, and 10, but same as controls by day 26; no bone marrow effect	55
	F. tricinctum crude extract	$^{1}/_{2}$ LD$_{50}$ (i.p.)	Days 1—15	SRBC (i.p.)	Day 10	No difference in spleen or thymus weights as compared to controls receiving sheep red cells; SRBC agglutinin titers reduced; PHA and LPS responses of spleen cells increased	55
Mouse spleen cells and thymocytes	*F. tricinctum* crude	2—10 ppm (*in vitro*)				PHA and LPS responses were inhibited	55

Table 2 (continued)
SUMMARY OF THE IMMUNOTOXIC EFFECTS OF TRICHOTHECENE MYCOTOXINS

Species	Toxin	Dose (route)	Exposure time	Additional treatment	Exposure time	Effects(s)	Ref.
Mouse	DAS	$\frac{1}{4}$ or $\frac{1}{8}$ LD$_{50}$ (i.p.)	Days 5, 6, 7	*Cryptococcus neoformans*	Day 1	Death occurred with combinations, not with either toxin or *Cryptococcus* alone	100
	T-2	0.75 mg/kg (i.p.)	Days 1—7; alternate days until day 20	Skin allograft	Day 8	Delayed graft rejection and diminished mononuclear cell infiltration	53
	T-2	20 ppm (diet)	7—42 days			Lymphoid hypoplasia and lymphopenia did not recover until toxin withdrawn; granulocytopenia recovery in spite of continued toxin; rapid drop in thymus body weight ratio; B cell areas depleted but T cell areas more severely damaged	47
	T-2	20 ppm (diet)	7—28 days	8, 12, or 16% protein diets	Entire study	Neutrophilia, lymphoid depletion; protein level had no effect on lymphopenia, neutropenia, or thymic atrophy induced by T-2 toxin; granulocyte recovery in bone marrow faster with higher protein	47
	F. tricinctum crude extract	$\frac{1}{32}$ LD$_{50}$ (i.p.)	1 week			Decreased thymus weight	51
	T-2	0.75 to 2 mg/ kg (i.p.)	1 week			Dose-related thymus but not spleen weight reduction; essentially maximal effect at 1 mg/kg; thymic cortex but not medulla depleted	51
	F. tricinctum crude extract	$\frac{1}{16}$ LD$_{50}$ (i.p.)	Days 1—7	SRBC (i.p.)	Day 3	Slightly decreased agglutinin titers to SRBC	51

	DAS or T-2	0.5 mg/kg (i.p.)	Days 1—7	SRBC (i.p.)	Day 3	Agglutinin titers reduced by $^1/_3$; thymic atrophy; DAS less potent in both effects	51
	T-2	1.0 mg/kg (i.p.)	Days 1—7	SRBC (i.p.)	Day 3	No agglutinin response	51
	T-2	0.7 mg/kg (i.p.)	Days 1—7	SRBC (i.p.)	Day 3	Agglutinin responses and thymus weights returned to normal by 6 d after T-2 treatment stopped	51
	T-2	0.7 mg/kg (i.p.)	Days 3—4	SRBC (i.p.)	Day 0	Prevented increases in agglutinin titers after T-2 treatment	44
Mouse spleen cells and thymocytes	*F. tricinctum* crude extract	0.05—1 ppm (*in vitro*)				PHA and LPS responses increased	55
Mouse spleen cells	T-2 or DAS	0.1 ppm or > (*in vitro*)				PHA and LPS responses were inhibited; DAS less inhibitory	55
	T-2 or DAS	<0.1 ppm (*in vitro*)				PHA and LPS responses increased with T-2 toxin; no increase at low doses of DAS	55
	Butenolide	20—100 ppm (*in vitro*)				Inhibited PHA and LPS responses, but increased responses at lower doses	55
Mouse thymocytes	T-2 toxin	2—10 ppm (*in vitro*)				PHA response inhibited, but strongly stimulated lymphocytes at lower doses	55
	DAS	0.05—2.0 ppm (*in vitro*)				PHA responses inhibited	55
Mouse	T-2 or DAS	0.5—2.0 mg/kg/d (i.p.)	Days 1—7	Polyvinyl-pyrrolidone or dinitro-phenyl-ficoll	Day 3	Enhanced antibody responses against both	53
		i.v. splenic lymphocytes from mice given T-2 toxin at 0.75	Time 0	SRBC	18 h	50% decrease in anti-SRBC PFU in spleen	53

Table 2 (continued)
SUMMARY OF THE IMMUNOTOXIC EFFECTS OF TRICHOTHECENE MYCOTOXINS

Species	Toxin	Dose (route)	Exposure time	Additional treatment	Exposure time	Effects(s)	Ref.
	T-2	mg/kg for previous 7 d 0.75 mg/kg/d (i.p.)	7 d			50% reduction in splenic T cells	53
	F. tricinctum crude extract	$^1/_2$ and $^1/_4$ LD$_{50}$ (i.p.)	Days 1 and 2			Depressed size of thymus, especially day 3; splenic enlargement on day 10; depressed PHA responses	53
Bovine calves	T-2 or DAS; equivalent toxin in *F. tricinctum* crude extract or whole culture of *F. tricinctum*	0.2 mg/kg; amount to approximate 0.2 or 1.0 mg/kg T-2 (p.o.)	11 d; up to 72 d or up to 78 d, respectively			No gross lesions in any group; leukopenia in whole culture-low dose group	25
Adult cow	T-2	0.44 mg/kg (p.o.)	15 d			Leukopenia, lymphopenia, and neutropenia on day 8; neutrophil count recovered by day 16, but lymphocyte recovery incomplete	103
Newborn	T-2	0.6 mg/kg (esophageal intubation)	11 doses over a 16-d period			No effects on hematology or bone marrow	101
Calves	T-2	0.08—0.3 or 0.6 mg/kg/d (p.o. in capsules)	30, 20 d			No gross or histologic changes in spleen; no changes in WBC	102
Yearling	T-2	0.06—0.12 mg/kg/d (i.m.)	63 d			Abscesses at 1 injection site, fever; hemorrhagic lymph nodes	103

Animal	Toxin	Dose	Duration			Effects	Ref.
Bovine	T-2	0.1 mg/kg/d (i.m.)	65 d			Abscesses at injection sites	104
Calves	T-2	0.1, 0.3, or 0.6 mg/kg/d (p.o., in capsules	42 d			No effects on titer response to *Anaplasma* vaccines; slightly delayed response to IBR challenge; total lymphocyte counts as well as globulin and C3 conc decreased in calves given a dose at 0.6 mg/kg/d at 1—29 but ConA- or PWM-induced blastogenic response reduced on day 29 only; dose-related thymic weight reduction, lymphoid depletion, edema, and thinning of cortex	105
Swine	T-2	0.13—3.2 mg/kg (i.v.)	1 dose			Neither lesions nor changes in WBC or differential counts at 10 d after dosing (survivors)	22
	T-2	0.13—3.2 mg/kg (i.v.)	1 dose			Lymphoid necrosis in lymphoid follicles of nodes, spleen and Peyer's patches of GI (dying pigs)	22
	T-2	1—8 ppm (diet)	56 d	19% protein ration	Entire study	No effects on blood counts or bone marrow	22
Piglets	T-2, DAS, or equivalent toxin in *F. trincinctum* crude extract	0.1 mg/kg (p.o.)	14 to 36 d			No lesions of spleen or intestinal lymphoid tissues	25
Sows	T-2	12 ppm (diet)	Up to 220 d			No effects on bone marrow; no changes in complete blood cell counts	25
	DAS	0.3—0.5 mg/kg (i.v.)	1 dose			Necrosis of germinal centers of mesenteric lymph nodes and splenic white pulp	26
	T-2	1.27 mg/d (diet)	25 d	*Colstridium* vaccine	1 dose	Relative decrease in total leukocyte count; 40 to 50% suppres-	32

Table 2 (continued)
SUMMARY OF THE IMMUNOTOXIC EFFECTS OF TRICHOTHECENE MYCOTOXINS

Species	Toxin	Dose (route)	Exposure time	Additional treatment	Exposure time	Effects(s)	Ref.
						sion of immune responsiveness in antigen-induced blast transformation, immune-rosette-formation, and IF-detectable IgG-positive cell counts; significantly lower neutralizing titers to *Colstridium* vaccine	
	T-2	1.2, 2.4, and 4.8 mg/kg (i.v.)	1 dose			Massive necrosis of all lymphoid tissues, particularly the B cell-dependent areas; inconsistent bone marrow necrosis	27
	T-2	0.6 mg/kg (i.v.)	1 dose			Scattered individual cell necrosis in the cortex of thymus and germinal centers of spleen, tonsil, and lymph nodes	27
	T-2	0.6 and 4.8 mg/kg (i.v.)	1 dose			Early leukocytosis and latter leukopenia due to increase followed by reduction in absolute numbers of both neutrophils and lymphocytes	31
	T-2	15 mg/kg (topical application)	1 dose	SRBC (10^9, s.c.)	Day 0 and 21 d later	Minimal lymphoid necrosis in thymus, tonsil, spleen, lymph nodes, and gut- and bronchus-associated lymphoid tissues; persistent neutrophilia for the first 2 weeks; lower blastogenic responses of enriched peripheral blood lymphocytes to PHA, ConA, and PWM between days 3 and 5 as well as between days 20 and 28; no significant effects on HA titers to SRBC	

| T-2 | 8 mg/kg (inhalation; 20—30% of toxin retained) | 1 dose | SRBC (10^9, s.c.) | Day 0 and 21 d later | Significantly reduced mitogen-induced blastogenic responses of enriched peripheral blood lymphocytes to PHA, ConA, or PWM 1 d after exposure when compared to the predosing values; significantly lower HA titers to SRBC between days 5 and 7 after first immunization | 35 |

much of the following information, the table also contains entries not represented in the following text.

A. Monkey

Rhesus monkeys developed leukopenia after stomach tube administration of T-2 toxin at 0.1 mg/kg/d for 15 d.[16] When greater amounts (1 or 0.5 mg/kg/d) of toxin were given to the animals, leukopenia developed after 1 week, with reductions in neutrophil percentages without noticeable changes in lymphocyte percentages. Spleens and lymph nodes showed the presence of atrophic follicles.

Similarly, when Jagadeesan et al.[17] administered semipurified T-2 toxin per os (p.o.) at 0.1 mg/kg/day for 4 to 5 weeks, total peripheral leukocyte counts were reduced after 4 weeks of treatment, but regeneration occurred since the counts approached normal values by 5 months after cessation of toxin treatment. Histopathologic examination revealed cortical depletion of lymphocytes from the lymph nodes. The bacterial activity of peripheral blood neutrophils, assessed *in vitro* by their ability to phagocytize *E. coli,* was decreased immediately following *in vivo* exposure to T-2 toxin. The number of peripheral blood T and B cells also decreased. In addition, T cell function, investigated using PHA stimulation, decreased in T-2-treated animals. Serum concentrations of immunoglobulin (total IgG and IgM) and hemolytic complement (CH_{50}) were also assessed. Immunoglobulin concentrations decreased, IgG to a greater extent than IgM. Concentrations of hemolytic complement, however, did not change. Most other immunological parameters assessed were reduced by toxin treatment, but increased to near normal values by 5 months after termination of treatment.

B. Cat

The domestic cat has served as a reliable model of ATA in humans. Pancytopenia, bone marrow aplasia, and severe alterations of lymphoid tissues have been observed in cats treated with T-2 toxin.[18-20] Cats given T-2 toxin in capsules p.o. at a dose of 0.08 to 0.1 mg/kg every 48 h exhibited a slight leukocytosis followed by persistent leukopenia. An initial increase in peripheral lymphocytes was accompanied by neutropenia. Subsequently, lymphopenia developed and neutropenia continued. All T-2-treated cats died by the 40th day of treatment. Examination of neutrophils revealed morphologic alterations, including increased size and altered nuclear morphology. Neutrophils from animals in terminal stages of T-2 mycotoxicosis displayed pyknotic nuclei and karyorrhexis. Relative numbers of circulating eosinophils (as compared to other leukocytes) were markedly (as much as 30%) increased. Maturation of the myeloid series was completely absent.

Lymph nodes, especially the mesenteric lymph nodes, were usually enlarged. A loss of typical architectural patterns within lymphoid follicles and hyperplasia of the reticuloendothelial cells were observed. The reticuloendothelial cells were observed to replace cells of the lymphoid compartment. Depletion of lymphocytes from germinal centers of the lymphoid follicles was noted in the spleen.

C. Swine

Pigs developed leukopenia after consuming grains that had caused ATA in people.[21] Massive lymphocytic necrosis, characterized by pyknotic nuclei and karyorrhexis, was present in Peyer's patches of the ileum, lymphoid nodules of the cecum, lymphoid follicles of the spleen, and germinal centers of the mesenteric lymph nodes of pigs that died acutely after being given a single intravascular injection of T-2 toxin at doses ranging from 1.2 to 2.5 mg/kg.[22] However, no changes in leukocyte counts or lesions in lymphoid organs or bone marrow were detected when pigs were killed 1 to 12 d after a single intravascular injection of T-2 toxin at doses ranging from 0.96 to 1.5 mg/kg.[22] Similarly, when DAS was administered i.v. to pigs in a 50% lethal dose (LD$_{50}$) study, there were no effects noted in the bone marrow of survivors.[23] Although bone marrow was not examined from pigs that died, necrosis was consistently observed in germinal centers of mesenteric lymph nodes and spleen white pulp.[23] In contrast, neither T-2 toxin at 1, 2, 4, or 8 ppm nor DAS at 2, 4, 8, or 9 ppm, in 19% protein rations fed to young pigs for 8 weeks, produced effects on the leukocyte counts or morphology of lymphoid tissues.[22,24] Although mild leukopenia developed in 1 piglet given purified T-2 toxin orally at 0.1 mg/kg/d for 36 d, no similar effects or lesions were found in specimens from other pigs given the same dose for 14 d, a similar dose of DAS for 36 d, or an equivalent dose of crude extract of *F. tricinctum* for 14 d.[25]

In an acute study, pigs given DAS in a single intravascular dose of 0.5 or 1.0 mg/kg experienced a marked disruption of granulocyte and lymphocyte kinetics.[26] The initial response, leukocytosis, was accounted for by a marked increase in lymphocytes and followed by neutropenia and lymphopenia from 3 to 5 h after dosing. Thereafter, a rebound leukocytosis, primarily due to neutrophilia, appeared. Immature and often morphologically abnormal granulocytes, metarubricytes, and unidentified pyknotic cells were seen in blood smears 3.5 h after treatment. In this study, edema was noted in some lymph nodes of animals treated with DAS, especially mesenteric lymph nodes of pigs given a 1 mg/kg dose. Microscopically, marked lymphocytic necrosis was seen in the B-cell regions of the peripheral and visceral lymph nodes, tonsil, spleen, Peyer's patches of the ileum, and other tissue-associated lymphoid aggregates. The T-dependent regions were affected to a lesser degree. Thymus was the least affected as compared to other lymphoid tissues. There were moderate to marked amounts of pyknosis, karyorrhexis, and cellular debris in bone marrow of pigs given DAS at a dose of 0.5 or 1.0 mg/kg. The bone marrow of both groups lacked viable hematopoietic elements and had cells with bizarre patterns of fragmented nuclei.

In several independent studies using pigs given T-2 toxin at doses ≥1.2 mg/kg i.v.[27,28] or 2.4 mg/kg p.o.[28] widespread necrosis was observed in B-cell regions of lymphoid tissues, including germinal centers of lymph nodes, palatine tonsil, spleen, Peyer's patches of the ileum, and both gut and bronchial-associated lymphoid tissues. Although necrosis of the T-dependent regions was less prominent in secondary lymphoid organs, a moderate to severe multifocal lymphoid necrosis was evident in the thymus. The lymphocytic necrosis could be observed in sections of secondary lymphoid organs and thymus as early as 1 or 2 h after intravascular administration of T-2 toxin. Cellular necrosis of the bone marrow was noted in pigs given lethal or potentially lethal doses of T-2 toxin, but these lesions were inconsistent, even in some of the animals entering later stages of acute toxicosis. Similarly, extensive lymphocytic necrosis of both B and T cells occurred in pigs that died or were killed in a moribund state afer inhalation exposure to T-2 toxin at a nebulized dose of 9 mg/kg (approximately 20 to 30% of nebulized toxin was retained by the pigs).[29] Minimal to mild individual cell necrosis was occasionally seen in lymphoid tissues of pigs given either a single intravascular sublethal dose of T-2 toxin at 0.6 mg/kg[27] or exposed dermally to a dose of 15 mg/kg.[30]

In a preliminary clinical pathology study, pigs given T-2 toxin i.v. or p.o. at a lethal or potentially lethal dose developed leukocytosis initially, largely attributable to neutrophilia, followed by lymphopenia.[28] Lorenzana et al.[31] reported a similar response in an acute study during which pigs were given i.v. a single lethal (4.8 mg/kg) or sublethal (0.6 mg/kg) dose of T-2 toxin. The initial leukocytosis was followed by leukopenia, due primarily to an absolute neutropenia and secondarily to a lymphopenia.

Rafai and Tuboly[32] found decreased leukocytic counts after 21 d of feeding weanling pigs a ration containing T-2 toxin at 5 ppm (average daily T-2 intake was 1.27 mg/pig). Antigen (*Clostridium perfringens*)-induced blast transformation in the T-2 treated group, as measured by ^{3}H-TdR incorporation and expressed as stimulation index, was approximately 40 to 45% of control. Immunofluorescence detectable (immunoglobulin G positive, IgG$^+$) cell counts were significantly decreased in the T-2 treated group. Although the percentage of rosette forming cells (antigen specific cells that are able to bind sheep red blood cells [SRBC] coated with the ultrasonically disintegrated *bacteria* [*C. perfringens*] in a rosette manner) in the peripheral blood of both T-2-treated and control groups increased, the increases in the T-2-treated group were significantly lower than those of the control group. Toxin-neutralizing titers to *Clostridium* vaccine were also significantly lower in the T-2-treated animals. The relative weights of submaxillary lymph nodes did not differ significantly, but the relative weights of thymus and spleen from T-2-treated pigs were significantly reduced. Interestingly, plasma cortisol concentrations were significantly increased for T-2-treated animals throughout the study. Additionally, the relative adrenal weights of T-2-treated animals were significantly increased. Although a direct effect of T-2 toxin may have played a role, the authors suggested that the increased adrenocortical release of cortisol was attributable to reduced feed consumption. It is known that trichothecene mycotoxins inhibit protein synthesis.[33] The elevated plasma cortisol level in T-2-treated animals may further disrupt protein balance by enhancement of protein degradation via gluconeogenesis. The authors speculated that this dual effect on protein turnover may thereby suppress both cell-mediated and humoral immune responses in growing pigs.

In a sequential immunotoxicity study, T-2 toxin at a single dose of 0 or 15 mg/kg in 0.75 ml absolute dimethylsulfoxide (DMSO) was applied to a 10 × 15 cm clipped area on the back of pigs immunized s.c. with 10^9 SRBC on the same day and again 21 d later.[34] Mitogen-induced blastogenic responses of enriched peripheral blood lymphocytes and hemagglutination (HA) titers to SRBC were evaluated. Significantly lower blastogenic responses to PHA, ConA, and PWM were found in the T-2 toxin-treated group. These lower responses occurred mainly between days 3 and 5 as well as between days 20 and 28 after topical application. In contrast, the blastogenic response to LPS was slightly by significantly higher in T-2-treated animals on day 14. Although between days 10 and 24, mean HA titers for T-2-treated animals were approximately 2-fold greater than control values, these differences were not significant.

Recently, the effects of T-2 toxin on systemic and pulmonary immunity of swine were studied following inhalation exposure.[29,35] In one study, animals were dosed with 0 or 8 mg/kg of nebulized T-2 toxin in absolute ethanol.[35] Approximately 20 to 30% of the nebulized toxin was retained by the pigs. The small volume of ethanol was dried off by the addition of dry, filtered dilution air leaving crystals with a mass medium aerodynamic diameter of 1.5 μm. The pigs were then immediately immunized s.c. with 10^9 SRBC and challenged 21 d later. The blastogenic responses to mitogens (PHA, ConA, PWM) were significantly reduced in the T-2-treated group at 1 d after treatment when compared to their predosing values, but blastogenesis then returned to normal values. Significantly lower HA titers were also found in the T-2-treated pigs between 5 and 7 d after primary immunization with SRBC.

In a separate study, pigs were dosed with 0 or 9 mg/kg nebulized T-2 toxin in absolute ethanol (similar retention) and both systemic and local pulmonary immunity were evaluated.[29] Effects on systemic immunity were measured by mitogen-induced blastogenic responses performed on enriched peripheral blood lymphocytes. Effects on local pulmonary immunity were measured by monitoring bacterial phagocytosis by alveolar macrophages and mitogen-induced blastogenic responses of enriched pulmonary lymphocytes. Alveolar macrophages and enriched pulmonary lymphocytes were obtained by bronchoalveolar lavage. A few pigs died or were killed in a moribund state shortly (8 to 10 h) after inhalation of T-2 toxin. Other pigs which survived exposure were killed on days 1, 3, or 7. No effects were noted in the T-2-treated group with regard to the mitogen-induced blastogenic responses of enriched peripheral blood lymphocytes. The capacity of alveolar macrophages to phagocytize bacteria was significantly decreased in the T-2-treated animals dying 8 to 10 h or killed 1 or 3 d after exposure. No effects on phagocytosis were noted on day 7. The mitogen (PHA, ConA, or PWM)-induced blastogenic responses of enriched pulmonary lymphocytes were significantly lower in the T-2-treated animals than controls at 1 or 3 d after exposure.

These studies indicated that exposure of pigs via inhalation or topical application to a sufficient amount of T-2 toxin may result in adverse effects on local pulmonary or systemic immunity, particularly cellular immune responses.

D. Cattle

Recently, the effects of T-2 toxin on cellular immune responses of calves were studied.[36] When treated p.o. (by capsule) with either 0.3 mg/kg/d for 56 d or 0.5 mg/kg/d for 28 d, the animals at the lower dose displayed reduced neutrophil function as quantitated via nitroblue tetrazolium reduction. The numbers of peripheral blood B cells, identified as immunoglobulin positive (Ig$^+$) cells, were reduced. The numbers of T cells, identified as peanut agglutinin positive cells, however, were slightly elevated above control values on days 7, 35, and 42. In animals exposed to T-2 toxin at 0.5 mg/kg/d, the numbers of Ig$^+$ cells initially fell below control values, then increased between days 7 and 19, and decreased thereafter. T-cell numbers did not vary greatly between treated and control animals.

The response to PHA of both unseparated peripheral blood mononuclear cells and a T-cell enriched (nylon wool nonadherent) population was decreased after the animals were treated with T-2 toxin at 0.5 mg/kg/d for 19 d.[36] Similarly, PHA responses of lymphocytes from calves exposed to T-2 toxin at 0.6 mg/kg/d for a total of 43 d were decreased on days 1, 8, and 29.[37] In addition, the lymphocyte responses to ConA and PWM were also decreased on day 29. When calves were immunized with *Anaplasma* vaccine on days 1 and 21,[37] lymphocyte responses to *Anaplasma* antigen *in vitro* (used similarly to mitogens) did not differ between treated animals and controls. In addition, neutrophil function, with regard to random migration under agarose, nitroblue tetrazolium reduction, or glucose uptake, was unchanged during exposure to T-2 toxin, but chemotaxis was depressed.

In vitro treatment of bovine lymphocytes with varying concentrations of T-2 toxin and either PHA, PWM, or ConA demonstrated the suppressive effects of the toxin on ^{3}H-TdR incorporation.[36] Cell responses to ConA were inhibited 50% by T-2 toxin at 2.0 ng/ml. Nylon wool separated cells, both adherent (B-cell enriched) and nonadherent (T-cell enriched), were more sensitive to the effects of *in vitro* T-2 toxin treatment than the unseparated cells. A 50% reduction of the lymphoblastic response to mitogens occurred in both populations by T-2 toxin in concentrations as low as 1.4 ng/ml.

Mann et al.[38] observed reductions of total serum globulin of calves treated orally with T-2 toxin at 0.6 mg/kg/d for 43 d. IgM, IgA, and complement factor 3 (C3) concentrations were decreased, but the IgG concentration did not change.

These studies indicated that a persistent exposure of calves to T-2 toxin p.o at doses of 0.3 to 0.6 mg/kg could result in adverse effects on both humoral and cellular immunity.

E. Sheep

Leukopenia was evident on day 7 for sheep administered T-2 toxin in capsule at 0.6 mg/kg/d.[39] Recovery from the depression in total leukocyte counts, however, was apparent by day 21 of T-2 treatment. Lymphopenia was also observed on days 7 and 14. Several microscopic changes in lymphoid tissue cellularity were also recorded. There was a decrease in the cellularity of spleen white pulp in which germinal centers of the lymphoid follicles were more affected than periarteriolar lymphoid sheaths. Cortical areas of mesenteric lymph nodes were depleted (depletion was not evident in medullary regions), and lymphocytes from all areas of the mesenteric lymph nodes were markedly depleted with numerous pyknotic cells. An increased myeloid:erythroid ratio was observed. Responses to the B cell mitogen, lipopolysaccharide (LPS), were reduced in treated animals on days 7, 14, and 21. ConA responses, reduced on day 7, were comparable to control values on days 14 and 21. The results of mitogen-induced blastogenic responses suggest that in sheep the effect of T-2 treatment on T-cell function appeared transitory; however, the effect on B-cell function persisted throughout the study.

F. Guinea Pig

Guinea pigs treated with a single dose of T-2 toxin (2.5 or 5.0 mg/kg p.o.) developed necrotic lesions of lymphoid tissue.[40] Such lesions were observed in the cortical follicles of mesenteric lymph nodes, Peyer's patches of the ileum, peribronchiolar lymphoid follicles, and palpebral lymphoid follicles. The necrosis within mesenteric iymph nodes was characterized by pyknosis, karyorrhexis, and karyolysis. Necrosis was less evident in the thymus and minimal in the spleen. Lower doses, 0.5 and 0.75 mg/kg p.o., given daily for 21 days produced no observable microscopic lesions. However, moderate leukopenia was recorded by day 33 and both lymphopenia and neutrophilia were observed by day 21. A higher daily dose (0.9 mg/kg) for 27 d similarly produced moderate leukopenia, however, lymphopenia was less severe and neutrophilia was not observed. Within the bone marrow of the T-2 dosed group, the myeloid:erythroid ratio and the number of lymphocytes were reduced.

When guinea pigs were dosed with DAS at 0.6 to 1.6 mg/kg daily for 30 d, no effects on hematology were detected, and no lesions were found.[41] However, in an LD_{50} study, guinea pigs, dying from single oral doses of 1 to 8 mg/kg had necrosis of lymphoid organs. Dying animals, and to a lesser extent survivors, had necrosis of round cells in bone marrow.

Daily treatment for 5 d with T-2 toxin at 0.5 mg/kg depressed the anti-DNP-BSA (dinitrophenyl-bovine serum albumin) antibody response of guinea pigs.[42] In contrast, a similar treatment regimen with fusarenon-X (0.75 mg/kg) did not affect the anti-DNP-BSA antibody response. T-2 toxin was also considerably more potent than fusarenon-X in the *in vitro* suppression of mitogenic responses of spleen cells to either LPS or ConA.

G. Rabbit

After rabbits had been given a single intravascular dose of T-2 toxin at 0.5 mg/kg, there was a rapid and significant decrease in the numbers of circulating total white blood cells.[43] The decline was greatest at 66% of normal on the 3rd day and then gradually returned toward normal. Differential counts were not performed. However, during and after daily administration of T-2 toxin orally (2 mg/kg for 4 consecutive days), no changes were observed in total white blood cell counts, total serum protein, or albumin. Neither p.o. nor intravascular administration of T-2 toxin produced any changes in rectal temperature of the rabbits.

H. Rat

In-depth studies of T-2 toxin-induced alterations in the morphology and functional capacity of rat alveolar macrophages were recently described in two reports.[44,45] The alveolar macrophages were isolated by tracheal lavage; toxin treatment was then performed *in vitro* for a total exposure time of 20 h. Effective concentrations of T-2 toxin which reduced cell viability, cell number, and viability index by 50% were 8.93, 0.33, and 0.89 μM, respectively, which are equivalent to 4.134, 0.153, and 0.412 ppm T-2 toxin. The viability index reflected the number of viable cells as a percentage of control. Mean cell volume also decreased in a dose-related fashion; cells treated with 0.1 μM (0.0463 ppm) T-2 toxin were reduced in size by a factor of as great as 19% when compared to controls. Chromium release from preloaded cells increased in a dose-related manner in the presence of T-2 toxin. Scanning electron microscopy (SEM) revealed several alterations of alveolar macrophage surface following the 20-h exposure to T-2 toxin. Most cells completely lost their surface processes and developed bleb-like structures and an appearance of being broken open.

Leucine incorporation immediately ceased in cultures of alveolar macrophage upon addition of 0.1 μM (0.0463 ppm) T-2 toxin and terminated after a 2-h incubation in cultures containing 0.01 μM (0.00463 ppm) T-2 toxin. The toxin also effectively reduced phago-cytosis of serum-opsonized yeast cells. Concentrations of 0.01 (0.00463 ppm) and 0.05 μM (0.0231 ppm) reduced the phagocytic activity of alveolar macrophages by approximately 25 and 85% respectively. It was determined that the binding of yeast cells to the surface of alveolar macrophages was not impaired. The effect of T-2 toxin on the activation of alveolar macrophages by endotoxin or lymphokines (supernatants from ConA- or PHA-stimulated spleen cell cultures) was assessed by macrophage uptake of [^{14}C]-glucosamine. This param-eter of macrophage function was decreased by 0.01 to 0.10 μM T-2 toxin.

Yarom et al.[15] investigated the effects of T-2 toxin on the cellularity of peripheral blood and bone marrow in rats dosed i.p. at 0.5 mg/kg/d for 1, 2, or 3 d. Peripheral leukocyte counts decreased daily. Differential counts indicated an initial increase in granulocytes on day 1 followed by granulocytopenia on days 2 and 3. The numbers of circulating lymphocytes increased on days 2 and 3. Differential counts for the bone marrow revealed a decrease in myeloid cells and an increase in lymphoid cells on days 1, 2, and 3. The total number of nucleated cells within the bone marrow decreased drastically on days 1, 2, and 3. Impaired inflammatory cellular responses, such as those of neutrophils and macrophages, to local bacterial inoculation were also observed in the T-2-treated rats.[15] In normal rats, intramus-cular (i.m.) injection of *Staphylococcus aureus* was typically followed by massive infiltration of the area by neutrophils and a later immigration of macrophages. In rats given 5 daily i.m. doses of T-2 toxin (0.5 mg/kg), however, there was much local edema and some myofiber necrosis, but the cellular elements were few in number.

Saito et al.[46] reported on the incidence of tumors found in animals following chronic exposure to fusarenon-X. The toxin was incorporated into diet at 7 and 3.5 ppm, and the animals were treated for 1 to 2 years. Treated animals were often afflicted with pulmonary infections. Moreover, chronic bronchopneumonia with acute exacerbation and abscess for-mation was the major cause of death in the 7 ppm treatment group. One case of leukemia was present in a toxin-treated animal; no cases were observed in controls. The authors noted no histologic alterations of the thymus, spleen, or bone marrow. Although atrophy of these organs was apparent in animals that succumbed to pneumonia, it may have been secondary to exhaustion of cellularity as a result of chronic infection.

Both DON and 3-acetyl-DON caused dose-dependent reductions in ^{3}H-TdR uptake in PHA-stimulated peripheral blood lymphocytes.[14] DON was more effective than 3-acetyl-DON. The ID$_{50}$ concentrations for ^{3}H-TdR incorporation were 90 and 450 ng/ml for DON and 3-acetyl-DON, respectively, indicating a degree of sensitivity similar to that described above for human lymphocytes.

I. Mouse

The mouse model has been used more often than any other in the study of trichothecene mycotoxin immunotoxicity. As a result of these efforts, the mechanisms by which trichoth-ecenes exert their effects on immunological function have been best characterized in this species. The following discussion, therefore, attempts to describe the impact of trichothecene mycotoxins on the murine immune system with regard to its structure and function, and a union of the two is attempted in the discussion of *in vitro* cellular reconstitution experiments. Lastly, resistance to infection is discussed.

1. Immunopathology

Hayes et al.[47] continuously provided mice with a diet containing 20 ppm T-2 toxin and monitored hematologic and pathologic events after 1, 2, 3, 4, and 6 weeks. Peripheral blood leukocyte counts were reduced after 1 week and remained lower than controls for the entire treatment period. Absolute neutrophilia was apparent with a concomitant reduction in the number of peripheral blood eosinophils. The spleen weights of treated mice initially decreased in size and then increased and surpassed control values by 4 weeks. The thymus decreased in size and became atrophic as did Peyer's patches. Macroscopically, the white pulp of the spleen diminished and was no longer visible after 3 weeks. The red pulp was also atrophied, turning pale then tan, and being greatly reduced in size by days 7 and 14. The splenomegaly mentioned earlier was observed by day 28 and was due to proliferation of a grayish-red homogenous tissue throughout the red pulp. By day 41, splenomegaly was observed in 3 out of 4 mice, and the red pulp had resumed its normal dark color. Microscopically, cortical depletion of lymphocytes from the thymus was observable on day 7, and there was an infiltration of neutrophils and eosinophils into the medulla and some areas of the depleted cortex. The follicles in lymph nodes and spleen virtually disappeared. T-dependent regions, including periarteriolar sheaths in the spleen, paracortical regions of lymph nodes, and intraepithelial lymphocytes of the small intestine, were depleted. T-independent (B-cell) regions in the intestinal lamina propria, medullary cords of lymph nodes, and splenic follicles also decreased in all mice consuming T-2 toxin. Neutrophilic myelopoiesis, however, appeared hyperplastic from days 21 through 28.

Other investigators have observed decreases in the weights of the spleen[47-54] and/or thymus of animals exposed to T-2 toxin or DAS.[51,53,55,56] These reductions in weights of both thymus and spleen were reversible.[55] Thymic weight was more sensitive than that of the spleen for both DAS and T-2 toxin.[50,51] Peripheral blood total leukocyte and lymphocyte counts increased following a single i.p. injection of T-2 toxin; the increases were not accompanied by changes in numbers of neutrophils.[54] The increases occurred by 3 h and were followed by decreases in both total leukocytes and lymphocytes. Decreased leukocyte counts have been reported for mice given T-2 toxin at 3.0 mg/kg i.p.[50] Histologic alterations of lymphoid tissues following short-term treatment of animals with *Fusarium* extracts by i.p. injection, consisting of one injection of 1/2 LD_{50} and a second with 1/4 LD_{50} 24 h later were reported by LaFarge-Frayssinet et al.[55] In the spleen, atrophy of T-dependent areas (periarteriolar sheaths) was observed before T-independent areas (lymphoid follicles). In the thymus, rapid depletion of cortical areas occurred with proliferation in the medulla. Rosenstein et al.[51] reported similar cortical depletion of thymic lymphocytes with the medulla remaining proliferative. Using Parodi's alkaline elution test, LaFarge-Frayssinet et al.[57] found the lymphoid tissues of mice to be more sensitive than the liver to the adverse effects of T-2 toxin on DNA.

Radiomimetic effects of *Fusarium nivale* extracts on tissues containing actively dividing cells such as lymphoid tissues were described by Saito et al.[58] The authors reported a loss of reaction against stimulation of the skin but did not describe the type of stimulation and reaction. Necrosis with karyorrhexis developed in the germinal centers of lymphoid follicles and the thymic cortex. In bone marrow, atrophy of the pulp and dilation of the sinus, followed by karyorrhexis of hematopoietic cells, were observed. One fraction of the extract caused an increase in leukocytes and percentage of neutrophils at 3 h. Increased numbers of immature neutrophils were present at both 24 and 96 h.

Counts of B and T cells in lymphoid tissues of mice have been performed after treatment with T-2 toxin or fusarenon-X. Numbers of T cells, identified by the antigenic phenotype Thy-1.2, were decreased by approximately 50% in spleens of mice treated daily for 7 d with T-2 toxin at 0.75 mg/kg i.p.[53] The usual increase in spleen T-cell numbers which follows the injection of control mice with SRBC did not occur in mice treated with a single i.p. dose of T-2 toxin at 3 mg/kg. Counts of Ig^+ cells (B cells) within the spleen, however, were not affected.[59] Masuda et al.[60] also reported a decrease in spleen T cells in mice treated i.p. with fusarenon-X at 50 μg/d for 7 d; again, no changes in numbers of B cells were observed. Interestingly, the total number of cells within the spleen increased by approximately 50%; the increase was probably caused by elevations in the numbers of myeloblasts, erythroblasts, and other nonlymphocytic cells. Similarly, no statistically significant changes were observed in spleen B- or T-cell numbers (though T cells were reduced) after mice were treated with 5, 10, 25, or 50 μg fusarenon-X i.p. daily for 7 d. As described above, however, the total number of cells residing in the spleen did increase.[61]

2. Lymphocyte Proliferation

Mitogens have often been used as stimuli to evaluate the blastogenic responsiveness of lymphocytes isolated from animals treated with toxin or lymphocytes treated directly with a toxin in culture. Reports of mitogenic responses of lymphocytes obtained from mice exposed to T-2 toxin are, nevertheless, limited.

Responses to ConA were clearly decreased in mice fed a diet supplemented with T-2 toxin at 20 ppm for 1 to 4 weeks.[52] The responses to ConA, however, were comparable to control values after 6 weeks of toxin treatment. A similar phenomenon was observed for the responses to LPS. Taylor et al.[62] observed a decreased response to PHA after a 2-week treatment with T-2 toxin at 2.5 mg/kg p.o. every 3rd day. T-cell responses were comparable to control values after 4 weeks. In contrast, the responses to PWM were increased at both 2 and 4 weeks for animals treated with 2.5 mg/kg T-2 toxin.

Intraperitoneal treatment of mice with crude *Fusarium* extracts on days 0 and 1 resulted in an increased LPS response together with a decreased PHA response.[55] The initial increase in the LPS response occurred on day 3 and was followed by a decreased response on day 10 and a second increase on day 19. After day 1, the PHA response continued its decline, reaching a minimum on day 10, but it returned to normal by day 19. Similar results were obtained with lymphocytes, isolated from mice treated with crude *Fusarium* extracts (i.p.) and stimulated with PHA.[53] *In vivo* exposure of mice to fusarenon-X at 25 μg/d (i.p.) resulted in a slight enhancement of both PHA and ConA responses and a clear decrease in LPS response of lymphocytes.[60]

Experiments involving exposures of murine lymphocytes to trichothecene mycotoxins *in vitro* have yielded similar findings. When lymphocytes were exposed to T-2 toxin *in vitro* and simultaneously exposed to PHA, the toxin at 0.1 ng/ml caused an increased uptake of ³H-TdR; however, there was a decrease in uptake with increasing toxin concentrations.[63] ConA-stimulated lymphocytes simultaneously exposed to T-2 toxin at concentrations ⩾12.5 ng/ml exhibited a decreased proliferative response.[64] Stimulation of both LPS and PHA responses was observed for spleen cells treated with T-2 toxin at 0.05 to 1.0 ng/ml; again, inhibition occurred with greater concentrations.[55] No stimulation was observed with DAS and the inhibitory effect of DAS was less severe than that of T-2 toxin. In the same study, the response of thymic cells to T-2 toxin and PHA in culture was greatly enhanced when the toxin concentration was less than 2.0 ng/ml, but greater concentrations resulted in a depressed response. Results obtained in our (MJT) laboratory suggest that an inverse time-dependent relationship exists with regard to the mitogen responsiveness of T- and B-cell populations isolated from the spleen.[65] With *in vitro* exposure of cells to T-2 toxin, the decreased PWM and LPS responses were correlated with increased PHA and ConA responses and vice-versa, depending on the time of toxin exposure. A slight stimulation of all mitogen (ConA, PHA, LPS) responses was observed when spleen cells were pretreated with fusarenon-X at 0.001 μg/ml for 24 h; however, the 24-h pretreated of spleen cells with fusarenon-X at higher concentrations ranging from 0.05 to 10 μg/ml, prior to mitogen addition, resulted in greater degree of inhibition of T-cell responses to both PHA and ConA than was observed for B-cell responses to LPS.[60]

3. Antibody Production

Rosenstein et al.[51,53] studied the effects of both T-2 toxin and DAS on T-dependent and -independent antibody production and found that both trichothecenes suppressed the T-dependent production of anti-sheep red blood cell (α-SRBC) antibodies. A daily i.p. injection of T-2 toxin at a dose >0.75 mg/kg for 7 d completely suppressed antibody production. A slightly higher dose of 2.0 mg/kg DAS, however, was required to completely stop antibody production. Both toxins exerted their influences in a dose-related manner. The effective range for T-2 toxin was much narrower than that observed for DAS. T-2 toxin given i.p. for 7 d at doses of 0.5 to 2.5 mg/kg also suppressed the number of plaque-forming cells (PFC) per spleen, indicating that conversion to antibody production status was inhibited. The evolution of antibody production toward SRBC was immediately reduced after toxin exposure but regained a value comparable to controls by 12 d posttoxin treatment. If T-2 toxin (0.75 mg/kg) was administered during the development of an α-SRBC response, the associated antibody response failed to attain the normal level. Intermittent oral administration of T-2 toxin at 2.5 mg/kg also caused a depression in the number of α-SRBC PFC.[62]

In contrast to the inhibition of T-dependent antibody response, the T-independent antibody responses to both DNP-ficoll and polyvinylpyrrolidone (PVP) were increased above control values for mice treated i.p. with T-2 toxin at doses of 0.75 mg/kg for 14 d or at 0.5 to 2 mg/kg for 7 d.[53] DAS given i.p. at doses of 0.75 to 2 mg/kg for 7 d also caused an increased DNP-ficoll response.[53]

Although, as described above, the T-dependent α-SRBC antibody response was reduced by T-2 treatment,[51,53] elevated α-SRBC titers have also been reported following T-2 treatment. Sheep red blood cell sensitized mice given a single 3 mg/kg i.p. injection of T-2 toxin at 2 d after antigen sensitization developed higher titers than nontoxin-treated controls.[59] The α-SRBC titers (measured 8 or 15 d after SRBC sensitization) were also elevated in mice dosed i.p. with T-2 toxin at 3 mg/kg either 2 d before or on the same day as the SRBC sensitization.[66] However, as described above, with regard to repeated dosing of T-2 or DAS, the α-SRBC responses of mice treated p.o. with DAS at ≥0.75 mg/kg for 5 weeks were lower than control values; the PFC response was also depressed.[67] In addition, when fusarenon-X was given to mice at 50 μg/d for 7 d prior to antigenic challenge with the T-independent antigen DNP-OVA (ovalbumin), the IgE and IgG1 (immunoglobulin G subclass 1) class titers were depressed. In contrast, the IgE antibody response appeared to be elevated above control values by lower doses of fusarenon-X at 14 and 21 d after immunization. The effect of fusarenon-X on antibody response was diminished with increasing temporal separation of antigen sensitization and subsequent toxin exposure.

Overall, the complexity of the effects of trichothecenes on antibody production remains difficult to interpret. The dose, frequency of exposure, and time of exposure appear to play an important role. Although T-dependent antibody production often tends to decrease and T-independent antibody production often increases as a response to a repeated lower dose of trichothecenes, a single explanation cannot be assuredly provided. Possible mechanisms for the reduction in T-dependent antibody production include a direct toxic effect on B cells or helper T cells, or an enhanced function of a particular population of suppressor T cells. In addition, the function of macrophages, such as presenting antigens to T cells and secreting T cell-activating factor (interleukin 1), may be adversely affected.

The differing response (the increase) in antibody production by T-independent B cells may be explained in part by the fact that these are cells of a distinct population with differing susceptibility to trichothecenes from those of the T-dependent B cells.

At sufficient doses, however, toxic effects may occur in populations of B cells and perhaps also T cells. Because of the interplay between these cells *in vivo*, identifying the specific site(s) of action for any one effect is not a simple matter.

4. Delayed-Type Hypersensitivity

T-2 toxin is capable of enhancing the development of a delayed-type hypersensitivity (DTH) reaction, a T cell-mediated event.[66] Mice were first sensitized to SRBC and subsequently challenged on day 7 or 14 with SRBC in the foot pad to elicit the swelling (measured at 24 h) typical of a DTH reaction. If T-2 toxin was given as a single dose (3 mg/kg, i.p.) 2 or 3 d after the first injection of SRBC, then the DTH responses on days 7 and 14 were increased above control values. Support for the above phenomenon was given by Otokawa et al.[59] The authors looked at the effects of T-2 toxin in mice made tolerant to a subsequent SRBC response by supraoptimal antigen sensitization. Such mice normally do not respond to challenge with SRBC. If mice were injected with T-2 toxin 1 or 2 d after the supraoptimal dose of SRBC, however, a subsequent DTH reaction occurred. In effect, the mechanism whereby tolerance manifests itself (induction of the suppressor T cells which then inhibit this DTH reaction) was blocked by the trichothecene. Thus, the T-2 treated mice had a DTH response because of suppressed induction of tolerance to the DTH response. These observations have been interpreted to be a result of a T-2 toxin associated preferential inhibition of the particular subset of suppressor T cells which participate in the DTH response.[66] In contrast, repeated treatment with T-2 toxin ($\geqslant$0.1 mg/kg, p.o., every 3rd day) was observed to decrease a DTH response.[62]

5. Graft Rejection

Mice given daily i.p. injections of T-2 toxin at 0.75 mg/kg for 7 d prior to receiving allografts, and continuously treated with the same dose 2 to 4 times a week for 20 d after the graft, had an increased time to tissue rejection as compared to control rejection times.[51] Graft rejection is typically a T-cell function. Thus, this delayed graft rejection suggests that T-2 treatment may cause impairment of T-cell function.

6. Adoptive Transfer

Otokawa et al.[59] used spleen cells from mice injected with 10^9 SRBC (i.v.) as a source of DTH suppressor cells. The suppressor cells were collected 4 d after SRBC injection and transferred (i.v.) to syngeneic recipients pretreated with cyclophosphamide. When the suppressor cells were obtained from mice pretreated i.p. with T-2 toxin at 3 or 4 mg/kg, the DTH resposne of recipients was decreased, but the reduction in the DTH response was significantly less than that observed for animals given cells from control animals. Thus, this experiment demonstrated a negative effect of T-2 toxin on the generation of suppressor cells participating in the DTH response. This is in agreement with those findings in the DTH studies described previously.

In a similar experiment, Rosenstein et al.[53] evaluated the effects of spleen cells from T-2 treated animals on the generation of α-SRBC PFCs. Animals were treated with 0.75 mg/kg/d i.p. for 7 d, and their spleen cells were injected into syngeneic recipients. Spleen cell recipients were immunized with SRBC and their PFC responses were enumerated 5 d later. There was a reduced PFC response in recipients following the injection of spleen cells from animals that had been treated with T-2 toxin. Treatment of mice with T-2 toxin alone increased the suppressor cell activity for PFC response within the spleen.

The results of the preceding two experiments may appear contradictory. In the first, T-2 toxin decreased the activity of suppressor cells and in the latter, suppressor cell activity was enhanced. The suppressor cells involved in DTH and PFC responses, however, have been reported to be two distinct populations of cells.[68] In a recent review, Ozer[69] discussed various positive and negative effects on different regulatory (helper and suppressor) T cell functions being affected by cyclophosphamide.

7. In Vitro *Cellular Reconstitution Experiments*

Masuda et al.[60,61] separated membrane Ig^+ and Ig^- cells from the spleens of mice pretreated with fusarenon-X at 50 μg i.p. daily for 7 d. Membrane Ig^+ cells are normally transformed into intracytoplasmic Ig^+ cells (plasma cells) following stimulation with B cell mitogens LPS or PWM. Culturing various combinations of Ig^+ and Ig^- cells from fusarenon-X-treated and -nontreated animals revealed that Ig$^-$ fusarenon-X-treated cells decreased the number of intracytoplasmic Ig$^+$ cells (plasma cells) formed in the presence of PWM or LPS. It was determined that the suppressive Ig$^-$ cells were best characterized as nonlymphocytic cells.[61] This observation was supported by the finding that the addition of T cells from fusarenon-X-treated animals did not disrupt the formation of intracytoplasmic Ig$^+$ cells. The implicated nonlymphocytic Ig$^-$ cells were mainly composed of both nongranular (macrophage) and granular (neutrophil) cells. Furthermore, by virtue of their phagocytic activity, these suppressive nonlymphocytic cells could be depleted from spleen cells by using iron filings and a magnet so that they adhered to the culture disk.[61] It was, therefore, suggested that fusarenon-X could induce nonlymphocytic suppressor cells having features in common with activated macrophages in the spleen of treated mice.[61]

8. Resistance to Infection

Kanai and Kondo[49] described a decrease in resistance to infection in mice treated with T-2 toxin. The animals were dosed orally with T-2 toxin (0.1 mg) both before and after infection with either a kanamycin resistant strain of tubercle bacilli (H37vR-km) or *Mycobacterium bovis*. Toxin was given 1 d before infection and continued at 1-d intervals for 8 to 12 d. Counts of vital tubercle bacilli per spleen were increased above controls in animals treated with T-2 toxin. The spleen weights of infected mice, not treated with T-2 toxin, increased as expected. The spleen weights of T-2 treated infected mice, however, changed very little and eventually decreased. The effect of T-2 toxin on the infection of BCG (bacillus Calmette-Guerin) vaccinated mice was also assessed. Toxin-treatment impaired the immunity stimulated by vaccination as evidenced by increased bacillus counts of the spleen and lung and by decreased survival times when a milder exposure schedule was established at 0.1 mg every other day for a total of six doses. The average survival period for mice infected with *M. bovis* was decreased from 35 to 19 d as a result of the T-2 treatment.

Friend et al.[52] examined mice for the reactivation of a latent infection of Herpes Simplex virus-1 (HSV-1, KOS strain) after treatment with T-2 toxin. The mice had been infected with HSV-1 (6.0 × 10^7 PFU/ml) via application to scarified lips. Human anti-HSV-1 antibody was given to the infected animals at 3, 48, and 95 h postinfection in an effort to minimize mouse immunity to HSV-1 but resulted in the development of latency. In spite of T-2 treatment (5, 10, or 20 ppm in the feed) begun 10 weeks after HSV-1 infection, no reactivation of herpesvirus infections was observed.

Intraperitoneal treatment with DAS at either 1.12 or 2.25 mg/kg resulted in increased mortality of mice treated with *Candida albicans*.[56] Inoculation with *C. albicans* was done on day 0 followed by DAS injections on days 3, 4, 7, 8, and 9. At either dose of DAS, mortality was greater than that of controls.

J. Poultry

The negative effects of T-2 toxin on tissue components of the avian immune system have been realized for several years. Wyatt et al.[70] reported decreased weights of the bursa of Fabricius or spleen when broiler chickens were fed diets containing T-2 toxin at 8 or 4 ppm, respectively. Similar effects were not observed for turkey poults maintained on a 10 ppm T-2 toxin diet for 4 weeks, although the thymus was reduced in size.[71] Additionally, microscopic evaluation of thymic tissue revealed cortical depletion of lymphocytes with accumulations of macrophages in the depleted areas. The medullary regions of the thymus were characterized by loss of large lymphocytes and proliferation of epithelial and reticular cells. In the same study, birds (both chicks and turkey poults) were immunized with *Pasteurella multocida* on day 11 and their antibody titers evaluated at the end of the 4-week treatment. The authors reported no significant differences in titers between T-2 treated and control animals; however, the mean and maximum titer values of turkey poults treated with

T-2 toxin were greater than the control values. Electrophoresis of serum proteins revealed increased concentrations of total protein, albumin, total globulin, and α-, β-, and γ-globulins in T-2 treated turkey poults.

Lymphoid necrosis and depletion of lymphocytes from the spleen, bursa of Fabricius, cecal tonsil, thymus, and ectopic lymphoid foci were reported for chickens fed diets containing ≥50 ppm T-2 toxin or DAS for a total of 7 d.[72] Daily dosing of chickens for 14 d with T-2 toxin (1.5, 2.0, 2.5, or 3.0 mg/kg) or DAS (2.5, 3.0, or 3.5 mg/kg) produced histologic changes similar to those reported above.[73] Dose-related reductions were observed in the weights of spleen and bursa of Fabricius. The authors concluded that as compared to DAS, T-2 toxin was more harmful to the lymphoid tissues of chickens.

The effects of T-2 toxin and DAS have been reported as rapid in onset but transient for chickens given a single dose of either toxin.[74] Necrosis of lymphoid tissues and bone marrow was observed 1 h after a single treatment with T-2 toxin (2.5 mg/kg) p.o. by crop gavage, but complete restoration of typical lymphoid tissue cellularity was seen 72 h after dosing. As stated above, the authors reported that the lesions induced by the two toxins were similar, but T-2 toxin was more potent than DAS in the disruption of lymphoid tissues.

Boonchuvit et al.[75] infected T-2 treated (16 μg/g feed for 3 weeks) chickens with pathogenic *Salmonella* sp. and observed an increase in mortality as compared to controls not treated with T-2 toxin. Neither factor alone caused mortality, but in combination, there was a significant mortality in all groups. The increased mortality was not associated with differences in specific antibacterial antibody titers. T-2 toxin alone decreased the weights of the spleen and bursa. The spleens of birds infected with *Salmonella* alone or treated with T-2 toxin and infected with bacteria, however, were increased in weight. This phenomenon was not observed for the bursa of Fabricius.

Mallard ducks exhibited changes in lymphoid tissues similar to those of chickens and turkeys, including generalized atrophy of all lymphoid tissues.[76] When fed diets containing 20 to 30 ppm T-2 toxin for 2 to 3 weeks, cortical depletion of lymphocytes was seen in the thymus, and the bursa of Fabricius was atrophic with marked depletion of follicular lymphoblasts and mature lymphocytes. Lymphocytes in spleen white pulp were also depleted.

Detailed microscopic investigations on the independent effects of T-2 toxin, fusarenon-X, and nivalenol on the bursa of Fabricius (dissected from day-old chicks) were conducted by Terao et al.[77] The toxins were injected into the residual yolk sac at a dose of 5 mg/kg. Histologic changes were monitored over time using both light and transmission electron microscopy techniques. Both fusarenon-X and nivalenol were less potent than T-2 toxin. Within 15 min after injecting T-2 toxin, pinocytotic vesicles within follicle-associated deck epithelial cells had increased in size and number. Considerable cellular disruption was observable after 30 to 60 min in the central portion of deck epithelium. Large cytoplasmic autophagic vacuoles were seen to contain cellular debris. By 30 min, lipid droplets were noted in the cytoplasm of lymphoid cells adjacent to the degenerated deck epithelial cells. The disk-like formations on the deck epithelial cells had completely disappeared by 6 h after injection of T-2 toxin. Macrophages, containing cell remnants, were occasionally seen. The surface epithelium of the bursa of Fabricius was relatively insensitive. No pathologic changes were observed in the reticular epithelial cells juxtaposed with affected lymphoid cells. The authors concluded that these trichothecene toxins were 40 times more toxic to bursal lymphoid cells than was cyclophosphamide.

IV. ANTITRICHOTHECENE MYCOTOXIN ANTIBODIES

It is doubtful that antitrichothecene antibodies are produced *in vivo* as a result of exposure to the powerful cytotoxic agents. The capacity of trichothecene mycotoxins to inhibit macromolecular synthesis is well documented. In addition, T-2 itself functions as a hapten, which by definition has only one antigenic determinant and is too small to induce immune response by itself. Facilitation of the normally nonimmunogenic T-2 toxin hapten by conjugating it to ethylene diamine-modified bovine serum albumin (BSA), functioning as a protein carrier, has been demonstrated.[78] Indeed, Chu et al.[79] also produced an anti-T-2 toxin antibody using a BSA-T-2 hemisuccinate conjugate. Subsequently, Hunter et al.[80] employed a concentration of the hapten-carrier used in standard immunizing regimens to demonstrate the toxicity of conjugated T-2 toxin-BSA to human B lymphoblastoid cells; this was probably due to the release of T-2 toxin from the protein carrier. Free T-2 toxin at concentrations as low as 10 ng/ml caused profound inhibition of protein synthesis in these cells. The major significance of the production of anti-T-2 toxin antibodies, however, is their utility as a tool for the detection and localization of T-2 toxin in the body.[81,82]

V. PROPOSED MECHANISMS OF IMMUNOTOXICITY

With both *in vivo* and *in vitro* systems, several trichothecene mycotoxins have been demonstrated to be immunomodulatory compounds; both stimulatory and inhibitory effects have been observed. The disparity of effects appears to be related to the dose, frequency of exposure, and time of exposure. This can be explained by the fact that the response of the immune system to an antigenic stimulation is a premeditated event in which various types of cells participate in a programmed sequence and that the sensitivities of these cells to trichothecene mycotoxins are different. Many investigations have pursued the T cell regulatory mechanism as the target of trichothecene mycotoxins, and more specifically, suppressor T cells may be particularly sensitive. One could speculate, based on studies in mice, that a particularly trichothecene-sensitive subpopulation of suppressor T cells may exist and that when these cells are damaged, at a dose sparing other lymphocytes, an increase in particular T and B cell responses may occur. This possible explanation seems to hold true primarily with single large dose administrations. In contrast, repeated administrations of T-2 toxin at a lower dose have been associated with reduced T-dependent (T cell, B cell, or macrophage) responses, which may be accounted for by stimulation of suppressor T cells or harmful effect(s) on helper T cells, B cells, or macrophages. The increased T-independent responses may be accounted for by a stimulation of B cells. These possible explanations remain to be investigated. In addition, trichothecene mycotoxins may cause other adverse effects, morphologically or functionally, on other T cells and neutrophils.

While trichothecene mycotoxins are known to be immunotoxic by direct cytocidal effect or by inhibition of macromolecular synthesis, particularly protein and DNA syntheses,[44,45,63] hormone-mediated reductions in immunoresponsiveness should also be considered to be potentially contributing. Elevation in serum concentrations of cortisol[32] as well as epinephrine and norepinephrine[83] have been reported in T-2 treated pigs. These hormones individually or together, even at physiologic concentrations, can reduce mitogen-induced T cell blastogenesis, inhibit interleukin 2 production by T cells, or inhibit the expression of Ia antigens and interleukin 1 production by macrophages.[84-87]

Trichothecene mycotoxins are known to be able to induce inflammatory responses in a variety of animal species. Some inflammatory mediators, such as prostaglandins, histamine, etc., may also play a role in regulating immune responses since prostaglandins and histamine, at physiologic concentrations, can induce a profound inhibition of lymphocyte response to mitogens.[88-90] Studies to date have shown elevations in plasma concentrations of certain prostaglandins in pigs, rats, and guinea pigs in response to trichothecene treatment.[83,91] In spite of the evidence of mast cell degranulation in T-2 treated rats,[92] no increases in plasma histamine were observed in T-2 treated pigs[83] and no benefit from antihistamine was observed in fusarenon-X treated rats.[50] Endotoxins, known for their stimulatory effects on spleen progenitor cells,[93] are another factor that should be considered. Gastroenteritis is commonly observed in animals following sufficient exposure to trichothecene mycotoxins, and disruption of the gut mucosa would facilitate the absorption of endotoxins.

Trichothecene mycotoxins appear to have both direct and indirect actions on the immune system. The trichothecene mycotoxins are distinctively immunotoxic, but their induction of immunotoxicity is clearly a multifaceted event. The exact role(s) of hormones, inflammatory mediators, or endotoxins in the trichothecene mycotoxin-induced immunotoxicity remains to be established.

VI. CONCLUSION

Trichothecene mycotoxins are potentially immunotoxic to animals. Known chronic exposures of man to the toxins via contaminated food sources have been associated with a substantially increased incidence of bacterial infections. Long-term exposure to concentrations which fail to produce overt primary toxic effects may have far-reaching ramifications for both man and animals. Because of the importance of the immune system in surveillance for neoplastically transformed cells, chronic depression of immunocompetence may indeed exert effects not realized for many years after exposure, although at least for most adult animals significant recovery of function after termination of exposure is apparent. Often, debilitating effects may not be directly correlated with mycotoxin exposure since immunosuppression associated with trichothecene exposure may be inappropriately diagnosed as a primary problem of microbial infection.

REFERENCES

1. **Otokawa, M.,** Immunological disorders, in *Trichothecenes, Chemical, Biological and Toxicological Aspects, Developments in Food Science,* Vol. 3, Ueno, Y., Ed., Elsevier, New York, 1983, 163.
2. **Ueno, Y.,** Toxicological evaluation of trichothecene mycotoxins, in *Natural Toxins,* Eaker, D. and Wadstrom, T., Eds., Pergamon Press, Oxford, 1980, 663.
3. **Mayer, C. F.,** Endemic panmyelotoxicosis in the Russian grain belt, *Milit. Surg.,* 113, 173, 1953.
4. **Joffe, A. Z.,** *Fusarium poae* and *F. sporotrichioides* as principle causal agents of alimentary toxic aleukia, in *Mycotoxic Fungi, Mycotoxins, Mycotoxicoses An Encyclopedic Handbook,* Vol. 3, Wyllie, T. D. and Morehouse, L. G., Eds., Marcel Dekker, New York, 1978, 21.
5. **Paul, W. E.,** The immune system: an introduction, in *Fundamental Immunology,* Paul, W. E., Ed., Raven Press, New York, 1984, chap. 1.
6. **Butcher, E. C. and Weissman, I. L.,** Lymphoid tissues and organs, in *Fundamental Immunology,* Paul, W. E., Ed., Raven Press, New York, 1984, chap. 6.
7. **Benacerraf, B. and Unanue, E. R.,** *Textbook of Immunology,* Williams & Wilkins, Baltimore, 1979, 298.
8. **Hayes, M. A. and Schiefer, H. B.,** Quanitative and morphological aspects of cutaneous irritation by trichothecene mycotoxins, *Food Cosmet. Toxicol.,* 17, 611, 1979.
9. **Dyck, R. F., Issa, M. I. C., Roger, S. L., Murphy, F., and Khachatourians, G. G.** The effects of T-2 toxin on the acute phase reaction in mice, *J. Am. Coll. Toxicol.,* 4, 71, 1985.
10. **Goodwin, J. W., Bottomley, R. H., Vaughn, C. B., Frank, J., and Pugh, R. P.,** Phase II evaluation of anguidine in central nervous system tumors: a southwest oncology group study, *Can. Treat. Rep.,* 67, 285, 1983.
11. **Goodwin, W., Haas, C. D., Fabian, C., Heller-Bettinger, I., and Hoogstraten, B.,** Phase I evaluation of Anguidine (Diacetoxyscripenol, NSC-141537), *Cancer,* 42, 23, 1978.
12. **Cooray, R.,** Effects of some mycotoxins on mitogen-induced blastogenesis and SCE frequency in human lymphocytes, *Food Chem. Toxicol.,* 22, 529, 1984.
13. **Forsell, J. H., Kateley, J. R., Yoshizawa, T., and Pestka, J. J.,** Inhibition of mitogen-induced blastogenesis in human lymphocytes by T-2 toxin and its metabolites, *Appl. Environ. Microbiol.,* 49, 1523, 1985.
14. **Atkinson, H. A. C. and Miller, K.,** Inhibitory effect of deoxynivalenol, 3-acetyldeoxynivalenol and zearalenone on induction of rat and human lymphocyte proliferation, *Toxicol. Lett.,* 23, 215, 1984.

15. **Yarom, R., Sherman, Y., More, R., Ginsburg, I., Borinski, R., and Yagen, B.,** T-2 toxin effect on bacterial infection and leukocyte functions, *Toxicol. Appl. Pharmacol.,* 75, 60, 1984.

16. **Rukmini, C., Prasad, J. S., and Rao, K.,** Effects of feeding T-2 toxin to rats and monkeys, *Food Cosmet. Toxicol.,* 18, 267, 1980.

17. **Jagadeesan, V., Rukmini, C., Vijayaraghavan, M., and Tulpule, P. G.,** Immune studies with T-2 toxin; effect of feeding and withdrawal in monkeys, *Food Chem. Toxicol.,* 20, 83, 1982.

18. **Lutsky, I., Mor, N., Yagen, B., and Joffe, A. Z.,** The role of T-2 toxin in experimental alimentary toxic aleukia: a toxicity study in cats, *Toxicol. Appl. Pharmacol.,* 43, 111, 1978.

19. **Lutsky, I. and Mor, N.,** Experimental alimentary toxic aleukia in cats, *Lab. Anim. Sci.,* 31, 43, 1981.

20. **Lutsky, I. and Mor, N.,** Human model of human diseases. Alimentary toxic aleukia (septic angina, endemic panmyelotoxicosis, alimentary hemorrhagic aleukia). T-2 toxin induced intoxication of cats, *Am. J. Pathol.,* 104, 189, 1981.

21. **Forgacs, J. and Carll, W. J.,** Mycotoxicosis, *Adv. Vet. Sci.,* 7, 273, 1962.

22. **Weaver, G. A., Kurtz, H. J., Bates, F. Y., Chi, M. S., Mirocha, C. J., Behrens, J. C., and Robison, T. S.,** Acute and chronic toxicity of T-2 mycotoxin in swine, *Vet. Rec.,* 103, 531, 1978.

23. **Weaver, G. A., Kurtz, H. J., Mirocha, C. J., Bates, F. Y., and Behrens, J. C.,** Acute toxicity of the mycotoxin diacetoxyscripenol in swine, *Can. Vet. J.,* 19, 267, 1978.

24. **Weaver, G. A., Kurtz, H. J., and Bates, F. Y.,** Diacetoxyscirpenol toxicity in pigs, *Res. Vet. Sci.,* 31, 131, 1981.

25. **Patterson, D. S. P., Matthews, J. G., Shreeve, B. J., Roberts, B. A., McDonald, S. M., and Hayes, A. W.,** The failure of trichothecene mycotoxin and whole cultures of *Fusarium tricinctum* to cause experimental hemorrhagic syndromes in calves and pigs, *Vet. Rec.,* 105, 252, 1979.

26. **Coppock, R. W.,** Studies on the Pharmacokinetics and Toxicopathy of Diacetoxycyscripenol and Deoxynivalenol in Swine, Cattle and Dogs, Ph.D. thesis, University of Illinois, Chicago, 1984.

27. **Pang, V. F., Lorenzana, R. M., Beasley, V. R., Buck, W. B., and Haschek, W. M.,** Experimental T-2 toxicosis in swine. III. Morphologic changes following intravascular administration of T-2 toxin, *Fund. Appl. Toxicol.,* 8, 298, 1987.

28. **Beasley, V. R.,** The Toxicokinetics and Toxicodynamics of T-2 Toxicosis in Swine and Cattle, Ph.D. thesis, University of Illinois, Chicago, 1983.

29. **Pang, V. F., Lambert, R. J., Felsburg, P. J., Beasley, V. R., Buck, W. B., and Haschek, W. M.,** Experimental T-2 toxicosis in swine following inhalation exposure: effects on pulmonary and systemic immunity, and morphologic changes, *Toxicol. Pathol.,* 15, 308, 1987.

30. **Pang, V. F., Swanson, S. P., Beasley, V. R., Buck, W. B., and Haschek, W. M.,** The toxicity of T-2 toxin in swine following topical application: clinical signs, pathology and residual concentrations, *Fund. Appl. Toxicol.,* 9, 41, 1987.

31. **Lorenzana, R. M., Beasley, V. R., Buck, W. B., and Ghent, A. W.,** Experimental T-2 toxicosis in swine. II. Effect of intravascular T-2 toxin on serum enzymes and biochemistry, blood coagulation, and hematology, *Fundam. Appl. Toxicol.,* 5, 893, 1985.

32. **Rafai, P. and Tuboly, S.,** Effect of T-2 toxin on adrenocortical function and immune response in growing pigs, *Zentralbl. Vet. Med.,* 29, 558, 1982.

33. **Ueno, Y. and Shimada, A.,** Reconfirmation of the specific nature of reticulocytes bioassay system to the trichothecene mycotoxins of *Fusarium, Chem. Pharm. Bull. Suppl.,* 22, 2744, 1974.

34. **Pang, V. F., Felsburg, P. J., Beasley, V. R., Buck, W. B., and Haschek, W. M.,** The toxicity of T-2 toxin in swine following topical application: effects on hematology, serum biochemistry and immune response, *Fund. Appl. Toxicol.,* 9, 50, 1987.

35. **Pang, V. F., Lambert, R. J., Felsburg, P. J., Beasley, V. R., Buck, W. B., and Haschek, W. M.,** Effects on pulmonary and systemic immunity, and morphologic changes, *Toxicol. Pathol.,* 15, 308, 1987.

36. **Mann, D. D., Buening, G. M., Osweiler, G. D., and Hook, B. S.,** Effect of subclinical levels of T-2 toxin on the bovine cellular immune system, *Can. J. Comp. Med.,* 48, 308, 1984.

37. **Buening, G. M., Mann, D. D., Hook, B., and Osweiler, G. D.,** The effect of T-2 toxin on the bovine immune system: cellular factors, *Vet. Immun. Immunopathol.,* 3, 411, 1982.

38. **Mann, D. D., Buening, G. M., Hook, B. S., and Osweiler, G. D.,** Effect of T-2 toxin on the bovine immune system: humoral factors, *Infect. Immun.,* 36, 1249, 1982.

39. **Friend, S. C. E., Hancock, D. S., Schiefer, H. B., and Babiuk, L. A.,** Experimental T-2 toxicosis in sheep, *Can. J. Comp. Med.,* 47, 219, 1983.

40. **DeNicola, D. B., Rebar, A. H., and Carlton, W. W.,** T-2 toxin mycotoxicosis in the guinea-pig, *Food Cosmet. Toxicol.,* 16, 601, 1978.

41. **Kriegleder, H.,** Morphological findings in guinea pigs after acute and subacute intoxication with diacetoxyscripenol, *Zentralbl. Vet. Med.,* 28, 165, 1981.

42. **Hiromichi, R., Watanabe, K., and Koyama, J.,** The immunosuppressive effects of trichothecenes and cyclochorotine on the antibody responses in guinea pigs, *J. Pharm. Dyn.,* 5, 403, 1982.

43. **Gentry, P. A. and Cooper, M. L.,** Effects of *Fusarium* T-2 toxin on hematological and biochemical parameters of the rabbit, *Can. J. Comp. Med.,* 45, 400, 1981.
44. **Gerberick, G. F. and Sorenson, W. G.,** Toxicity of T-2 toxin, a *Fusarium* mycotoxin, to alveolar macrophages *in vitro, Environ. Res.,* 32, 269, 1983.
45. **Gerberick, G. F., Sorenson, W. G., and Lewis, D. M.,** The effects of T-2 toxin on alveolar macrophage function *in vitro, Environ. Res.,* 33, 246, 1984.
46. **Saito, M., Horiuchi, T., Ohtsubo, K., Hatanaka, Y., and Ueno, Y.,** Low tumor incidence in rats with long-term feeding of fusarenon-X, a cytotoxic trichothecene produced by *Fusarium nivale, Jpn. J. Exp. Med.,* 50, 293, 1980.
47. **Hayes, M. A., Bellamy, J. E. C., and Schiefer, H. B.,** Subacute toxicity of dietary T-2 toxin in mice: morphological and hematological effects, *Can. J. Comp. Med.,* 44, 203, 1980.
48. **Friend, S. C. E., Schiefer, H. B., and Babiuk, L. A.,** The effects of dietary T-2 toxin on acute Herpes Simplex Virus type 1 infection in mice, *Vet. Pathol.,* 20, 737, 1983.
49. **Kanai, K. and Kondo, E.,** Decreased resistance to mycobacterial infection in mice fed a trichothecene compound (T-2 toxin), *Jpn. J. Med. Sci. Biol.,* 37, 97, 1984.
50. **Ueno, Y.,** Toxicological features of T-2 toxin and related trichothecenes, *Fundam. Appl. Toxicol.,* 4, S124, 1984.
51. **Rosenstein, Y., LaFarge-Frayssinet, C., Lespinats, G., Loisillier, F., Lafont, P., and Frayssinet, C.,** Immunosuppressive activity of *Fusarium* toxins: effects on antibody synthesis and skin grafts of crude extracts, T-2 toxin and diacetoxyscripenol, *Immunology,* 36, 111, 1979.
52. **Friend, S. C. E., Babiuk, L. A., and Schiefer, H. B.,** The effects of dietary T-2 toxin on the immunological function and Herpes Simplex reactivation in Swiss mice, *Toxicol. Appl. Pharmacol.,* 69, 234, 1983.
53. **Rosenstein, Y., Kretschmer, R. R., and LaFarge-Frayssinet, C.,** Effect of *Fusarium* toxins, T-2 toxin and diacetoxyscripenol on murine T-independent immune responses, *Immunology,* 44, 555, 1981.
54. **Lafont, P., LaFarge-Frayssinet, C., Lafont, J., Bertin, G., and Frayssinet, C.,** Metabolite toxiques de *Fusarium* agents de L'alevemie Toxique Alimentaire, *Ann. Microbiol. (Inst. Pasteur),* 128B, 215, 1977.
55. **LaFarge-Frayssinet, C., Lespinats, G., Lafont, P., Loisillier, F., Mousset, S., Rosenstein, Y., and Frayssinet, C.,** Immunosuppressive effects of *Fusarium* extracts and trichothecenes: blastogenic response of murine splenic and thymic cells to mitogens, *Proc. Soc. Exp. Biol. Med.,* 160, 302, 1979.
56. **Formentin, H., Salazar-Mejicanos, S., and Mariat, F.,** Pouvoir pathogene de *Canidia albicans* pour la souris normale ou deprimee par une mycotoxine: le Diacetoxyscirepnol, *Ann. Microbiol. (Inst. Pasteur),* 131B, 39, 1980.
57. **LaFarge-Frayssinet, C., Decloitre, F., Mousset, S., Martin, M., and Frayssinet, C.,** Induction of DNA single-strand breaks by T-2 toxin, a trichothecene metabolite of *Fusarium*. Effect on lymphoid organs and liver, *Mutat. Res.,* 88, 115, 1981.
58. **Saito, M., Enomoto, M., and Tatsuno, T.,** Radiomimetic biological properties of the new scirpene metabolites of *Fusarium nivale, Gann,* 60, 599, 1969.
59. **Otokawa, M., Shibahara,Y., and Egashira, Y.,** The inhibitory effect of T-2 toxin on tolerance induction of delayed-type hypersensitivity in mice, *Jpn. J. Med. Sci. Biol.,* 32, 37, 1979.
60. **Masuda, E., Takemoto, T., Tatsuno, T., and Obara, T.,** Immunosuppressive effect of a trichothecene mycotoxin, fusarenon-X, in mice, *Immunology,* 45, 743, 1982.
61. **Masuda, E., Takemoto, T., Tatsuno, T., and Obara, T.,** Induction of suppressor macrophages in mice by fusarenon-X, *Immunology,* 47, 701, 1982.
62. **Taylor, M. J., Reddy, R. V., and Sharma, R. P.,** Immunotoxicity of repeated low level exposure to T-2 toxin, a trichothecene mycotoxin, in CD-1 mice, *Mycotoxin Res.,* 1, 57, 1985.
63. **Rosenstein, Y. and LaFarge-Frayssinet, C.** Inhibitory effect of *Fusarium* T-2 toxin on lymphoid DNA and protein synthesis, *Toxicol. Appl. Pharmacol.,* 70, 283, 1983.
64. **Gyongyossy, M. I. C. and Khachatourians, G. G.,** Interaction of T-2 toxin and murine lymphocytes and the demonstration of a threshold effect on macromolecular synthesis, *Biochem. Biophys. Acta,* 844, 167, 1985.
65. **Taylor, M. J., Hughes, B. J., and Sharma, R. P.,** Dose and time related effects of T-2 toxin on mitogenic response of murine splenic cells *in vitro, Int. J. Immunopharmacol.,* 9, 107, 1987.
66. **Masuko, H., Ueno, Y., Otokawa, M., and Yaginuma, K.,** The enhancing effect of T-2 toxin on delayed hypersensitivity in mice, *Jpn. J. Med. Sci. Biol.,* 30, 159, 1977.
67. **Tryphonas, H., O'Grady, L., Arnold, D. L., McGuire, P. F., Karpinski, K., and Vesonder, R. F.,** Effect of Deoxynivalenol (Vomitoxin) on the humoral immunity in mice, *Toxicol. Lett.,* 23, 17, 1984.
68. **Whistler, R. L. and Stobo, J. D.,** Suppression of humoral and delayed hypersensitivity responses by distinct T cell subpopulations, *J. Immunol.,* 121, 539, 1978.
69. **Ozer, H.,** Effects of alkylating agents on immunoregulatory mechanisms, in *Biological Responses in Cancer,* Vol. 3, Mihich, E. and Sakurai, Y., Eds., Plenum Press, New York, 1985, chap. 4.
70. **Wyatt, R. D., Hamilton, P. B., and Burmeister, H. R.,** The effects of T-2 toxin in broiler chickens, *Poult. Sci.,* 52, 1853, 1973.

71. **Richard, J. L., Cysewski, S. J., Pier, A. C., and Booth, G. D.,** Comparison of effects of dietary T-2 toxin on growth, immunogenic organs, antibody formation, and pathlogic changes in turkeys and chickens, *Am. J. Vet. Res.,* 39, 1674, 1978.

72. **Hoerr, F. J., Carlton, W. W., Yagen, B., and Joffe, A. Z.,** Mycotoxicosis caused by either T-2 toxin or diacetoxyscirpenol in the diet of broiler chickens, *Fundam. Appl. Toxicol.,* 2, 121, 1982.

73. **Hoerr, F. J., Carlton, W. W., Yagen, B., and Joffe, A. Z.,** Mycotoxicosis produced in broiler chickens by multiple doses of either T-2 toxin or diacetoxyscirpenol, *Avian Pathol.,* 11, 369, 1982.

74. **Hoerr, F. J., Carlton, W. W., and Yagen, B.,** Mycotoxicosis caused by a single dose of T-2 toxin or diacetoxyscirpenol in broiler chickens, *Vet. Pathol.,* 18, 652, 1981.

75. **Boonchuvit, B., Hamilton, P. B., and Burmeister, H. R.,** Interaction of T-2 toxin with *Salmonella* infections of chickens, *Poult. Sci.,* 54, 1693, 1975.

76. **Hayes, M. A. and Wobeser, G. A.,** Subacute toxic effects of dietary T-2 toxin in young mallard ducks, *Can. J. Comp. Med.,* 47, 180, 1983.

77. **Terao, K., Kera, K., and Yazima, T.,** The effects of trichothecene toxins on the bursa of Fabricius in day-old chicks, *Virchows Arch.,* 27, 359, 1978.

78. **Chu, F. S., Lau, H. P., Fan, T. S., and Zhang, G. S.,** Ethylenediamine modified bovine serum albumin as protein carrier in the production of antibody against mycotoxins, *J. Immunol. Methods,* 55, 73, 1982.

79. **Chu, F. S., Grossman, R., Wei, D., and Mirocha, C. J.,** Production of antibody against T-2 toxin, *Appl. Environ. Microbiol.,* 37, 104, 1979.

80. **Hunter, K. W., Jr., Brimfield, A. A., Miller, M., Finkelman, F. D., and Chu, F. S.,** Preparation and characterization of monoclonal antibodies to the trichothecene mycotoxin T-2, *Appl. Environ. Microbiol.,* 49, 168, 1985.

81. **Peters, H., Dietrich, M. P., and Dose, K.,** Enzyme-linked immunosorbent assay for detection of T-2 toxin, *Hoppe-Seyler's Z. Physiol. Chem.,* 363, 1437, 1982.

82. **Fontelo, P. A., Beheler, J., Bunner, D. L., and Chu, F. S.,** Detection of T-2 toxin by an improved radioimmunoassay, *Appl. Environ. Microbiol.,* 45, 640, 1983.

83. **Lorenzana, R. M., Beasley, V. R., Buck, W. B., Ghent, A. W., Lundeen, G. R., and Poppenga, R. H.,** Experimental T-2 toxicosis in swine. I. Changes in cardiac output, aortic mean pressure, catecholamines, 6-keto-PGF$_{1\alpha}$, thromboxane B$_2$ and acid-base parameters, *Fundam. Appl. Toxicol.,* 5, 879, 1985.

84. **Cray, B., Borysenko, M., Sutherland, D. C., Kutz, I., Borysenko, J. Z., and Benson, H.,** Decrease in mitogen responsiveness of mononuclear cells from peripheral blood after epinephrine administration in humans, *J. Immunol.,* 130, 694, 1983.

85. **Gills, S., Crabtree, G. R., and Smith, K. A.,** Glucocorticoid-induced inhibition of T cell growth factor production. I. The effect on mitogen-induced lymphocyte proliferation, *J. Immunol.,* 123, 1624, 1979.

86. **Snyder, D. S. and Unanue, E. R.,** Corticosteroids inhibit murine macrophage Ia expression and interleukin 1 production, *J. Immunol.,* 128, 1803, 1982.

87. **Westley, H. J. and Kelley, K. W.,** Physiologic concentrations of cortisol suppress cell-mediated immune events in the domestic pig, *Proc. Soc. Exp. Biol. Med.,* 177, 156, 1984.

88. **Chouaib, S., Welte, K., Mertelsmann, R., and Dupont, B.,** Prostaglandin E$_2$ acts at two distinct pathways of T-lymphocyte activation: inhibition of interleukin 2 production and down-regulation of transferrin receptor expression, *J. Immunol.,* 135, 1172, 1985.

89. **Suzuki, S. and Huchet, R.,** Mechanism of histamine-induced inhibition of lymphocyte response to mitogens in mice, *Cell. Immunol.,* 62, 396, 1981.

90. **Al-Imara, L. J. and Dale, M. M.,** The inhibitory effect of histamine on lymphoid tissue proliferation in mice, *Cell. Immunol.,* 91, 284, 1985.

91. **Feuerstein, G., Goldstein, D. S., Ramwell, P. W., Zerbe, R. L., Lux, W. E., Faden, A. I., and Bayorh, M. A.,** Cardiorespiratory, sympathetic and biochemical responses to T-2 toxin in the guinea pig and rat, *J. Pharm. Exp.,* 232, 786, 1985.

92. **Yarom, R., Bergmann, F., and Yagen, B.,** Cutaneous injury by tropical T-2 toxin: involvement of microvessels and mast cells, submitted.

93. **Burgess, A. and Nicola, N.,** *Growth Factors and Stem Cells,* Academic Press, New York, 1983, 96.

94. **Kosuri, N. R., Smalley, E. B., and Nichols, R. E.,** Toxicologic studies of *Fusarium tricinctum* (Corda) Synder et Hansen from moldy corn, *Am. J. Vet. Res.,* 32, 1843, 1971.

95. **Ohtsubo, K.,** Pathology of trichothecene toxicosis, *Proc. Jpn. Assoc. Mycotoxiol.,* 13, 19, 1981.

96. **Shimizu, T., Nakano, N., Matsui, T., and Aibara, K.,** Hypoglycemia in mice administered with fusarenon-X, *Jpn. J. Med. Sci. Biol.,* 32, 189, 1979.

97. **Ueno, Y., Ueno, I., Iitoi, Y., Tsunoda, H., Enomoto, M., and Ohtsubo, K.,** Toxicological approaches to the metabolites of *Fusaria.* III. Acute toxicity of fusarenon-X, *Jpn. J. Exp. Med.,* 41, 521, 1971.

98. **Schoental, R. and Joffe, A. Z.,** Lesions induced in rodents by extracts from cultures of *Fusarium poae* and *F. sporotrichioides, J. Pathol.,* 112, 37, 1974.

99. **Ueno, Y., Ishii, K., Sakai, K., Kanaeda, S., Tsunoda, H., Tanaka, T., and Enomoto, M.,** Toxicological approaches to the metabolites of *Fusaria*. IV. Microbial survey "bean-hulls poisoning of horses" with the isolation of toxic trichothecenes, neosolaniol and T-2 toxin of *Fusarium solani* M-1-1, *Jpn. J. Exp. Med.,* 42, 187, 1972.
100. **Fromentin, H., Salazar-Mejicanos, S., and Mariat, F.,** Experimental cryptococcosis in mice treated with diacetoxyscirpenol, a mycotoxin of *Fusarium, Sabouraudia,* 19, 311, 1981.
101. **Weaver, G. A., Kurtz, H. J., Mirocha, C. J., Bates, F. J., Behrens, J. C., Robison, T. S., and Swanson, S. P.,** The failure of purified T-2 mycotoxin to produce hemorrhaging in dairy cattle, *Can. Vet. J.,* 21, 210, 1980.
102. **Pier, A. C., Cysewski, S. J., Richard, J. L., Baetz, A. L., and Mitchell, L.,** Experimental mycotoxicoses in calves with aflatoxin, ochratoxin, rubratoxin, and T-2 toxin, *Proc. U.S. Anim. Health* Assoc., 80, 130, 1976.
103. **Kosuri, N. R., Grove, M. D., Yates, S. G., Tallent, W. H., Ellis, J. J., Wolff, I. A., and Nichols, R. E.,** Response of cattle to mycotoxins of *Fusarium tricinctum* isolated from corn and fescue, *J. Am. Vet. Med. Assoc.,* 157, 938, 1970.
104. **Grove, M. D., Yates, S. G., Tallent, W. H., Ellis, J. J., Wolff, I. A., Kosuri, N. R., and Nichols, R. E.,** Mycotoxins produced by *Fusarium tricinctum* as possible causes of cattle diseases, *J. Agric. Food Chem.,* 18, 734, 1970.
105. **Osweiler, G. D., Hook, B. S., Mann, D. D., Buening, G. M., and Rottinghaus, G. E.,** Effects of T-2 toxin in cattle, *Proc. U.S. Anim. Health Assoc.,* 85, 214, 1981.
106. **Yap, H. Y., Murphy, W. K., DiStefano, A., Blumenschein, G. R., and Bodey, G. P.,** Phase II study of anguidine in advanced breast cancer, *Cancer Treat. Rep.,* 63, 789, 1979.
107. **Murphy, W. K., Burgess, M. A., Valdivieso, M., Livingston, R. B., Bodey, G. P., and Freireich, E. J.,** Phase I clinical evaluation of anguidine, *Cancer Treat. Rep.,* 62, 1497, 1978.
108. **DeSimone, P. A., Greco, F. A., and Lessner, H. F.,** Phase I evaluation of a weekly schedule of anguidine, *Cancer Treat. Rep.,* 63, 2015, 1979.
109. **Thigpen, T. Vaughn, C., and Stuckey, W. J.,** Phase II trial of anguidine in patients with sarcomas unresponsive to prior chemotherapy: a southwest oncology group study, *Cancer Treat. Rep.,* 65, 9, 1981.
110. **Belt, R. J., Hass, C. D., Joseph, U., Goodwin, W., Moore, D., and Hoogstraten, B.,** Phase I study of anguidine administered weekly, *Cancer Treat. Rep.,* 63, 1993, 1979.

Chapter 2

EFFECTS ON HEMOSTASIS AND RED CELL PRODUCTION

P. A. Gentry

TABLE OF CONTENTS

I. INTRODUCTION

Coagulopathies induced by the ingestion of moldy feeds and characterized by the development of clinical hemorrhagic conditions have classically been associated with trichothecene mycotoxicosis. Indeed, in one of the earliest reviews of the clinical problems associated with stachybotryotoxicosis in horses, moldy corn toxicosis in pigs, hemorrhagic syndrome in poultry, and alimentary toxic aleukia in man, hematological and hemostatic abnormalities, either separately or in combination, were among the most consistent findings.[1]

For the hemostatic mechanism to function normally, it is essential that the integrity of each of the components of the system be maintained. The components involved in hemostasis include the coagulation proteins, the cellular components including blood platelets and red blood cells (RBC) and blood vessels, which are discussed in the chapter "Effects on the Circulatory System". The effects of trichothecenes on white blood cells (WBC) are discussed in the chapter "The Immunotoxicity of Trichothecene Mycotoxins"; reference is made below only to some of the concomitant effects of the mycotoxins on WBC. In this chapter, hemorrhage is discussed specifically in relation to the hemostatic mechanism. Hemorrhage is also mentioned in the chapters "Effects on the Digestive System" and "Effects on the Circulatory System".

In different species, wide variations exist in the sensitivity of the response of the hemostatic components to trichothecene mycotoxin exposure. The responses of the various components also appear to vary within a species depending on the route of toxin administration and the dose and duration of exposure to the toxin. In this chapter, effects of trichothecene mycotoxins on blood cell production are considered first, then effects on coagulation are discussed.

The sequence of events involved in the hemostatic mechanism can be briefly summarized as follows. Blood platelets are attracted to and adhere to a site of damage on a blood vessel wall, undergo a shape change, and release their granular contents. The released chemicals promote the accumulation and aggregation of additional platelets and accelerate the rate of fibrin formation around the damaged area. While the platelet reactions are proceeding, specific coagulation proteins, referred to as "factors" and which normally circulate as inactive precursors, interact sequentially to form active proteolytic enzymes. The process culminates in the formation of thrombin, which acts on fibrinogen and factor XIII to produce an insoluble fibrin clot. Red blood cells trapped in the fibrin mesh can release adenosine diphosphate (ADP) which also enhances the formation of platelet aggregates. In both mammals and birds the coagulation proteins are synthesized by the liver and adequate hepatic concentrations of the reduced form of vitamin K (vit K) are essential for the production of the biologically active form of factors V, VII, IX, X, and prothrombin. In mammals, quantitative rather than qualitative differences exist in the hemostatic mechanism of different species.

Factors XII, XI, and IX are involved in the initial stages of the "intrinsic blood coagulation pathway". Fish and birds lack factors XI and XII, and the level of factor IX appears to be variable. Perhaps to compensate for the reduction in activity of this coagulation pathway, tissue thromboplastin, the initiating protein of the "extrinsic pathway" appears more potent in birds than in mammals.[2] Mammalian erythrocytes and platelets are anuclear while in birds the red cell is nucleated. The thrombocytes (platelets) of birds are larger than mammalian platelets.[3,4]

There are several laboratory methods for the evaluation of blood coagulation. The whole blood clotting time (WBCT) is subject to such wide variation due to extraneous factors that the activated partial thromboplastin time (APTT) and the prothrombin time (PT) assays are generally used for the overall evaluation of the coagulation profile. The APTT assay measures the "intrinsic coagulation pathway" and will detect abnormalities of factors XII, XI, IX, VIII, X, prothrombin, and fibrinogen. The PT assay estimates the competency of the "extrinsic pathway'' and will detect abnormalities of factors V, VII, X, prothrombin, and fibrinogen. Platelet function can be evaluated by estimating the rate of whole blood clot retraction but this procedure, like the WBCT, is subject to many extraneous variables. Platelet function is more satisfactorily evaluated by aggregometry procedures.[2]

II. RED BLOOD CELL AND PLATELET PRODUCTION

A. Fish

A dose-dependent decrease in hematocrit values was recorded in fingerling rainbow trout (*Salmo gairdneri*) fed diets containing purified T-2 toxin at 5.0 to 15.0 mg/kg feed for 16 weeks.[5] The hematocrit values of control fish were 37.6 ± 4.0% compared to 28.9 ± 1.1% for the fish fed 5.0 mg T-2 toxin per kilogram of feed. Lower doses of the toxin had no significant effect on the hematocrit. Blood loss may have contributed to the reduced hematocrit since, at necropsy, hemorrhagic intestinal tracts and focal hemorrhages in muscle tissue were found in the trout given the ration containing T-2 toxin at 15 mg/kg feed.[5]

B. Birds
1. Ducks

A significant ($p < 0.01$) reduction in both hematocrit and hemoglobin values was observed in young male and female Mallard ducks fed T-2 toxin at 20 or 30 ppm for 14 d.[6] The hematocrit decreased from an initial mean value of 41.4 ± 2.0% to 35.2 ± 3.0% and 37.6 ± 3.3% and the hemoglobin concentration declined from 13.5 ± 0.5 g/dl to 11.8 ± 0.7 g/dl and 12.5 ± 1.0 g/dl for the 20 and 30 ppm treatment groups, respectively. Despite the changes in the hematologic profile, normal hematopoietic activity was evident in bone marrow sections after 21 d of T-2 toxin ingestion. In contrast to the absence of effects on bone marrow of repeated exposure to T-2 toxin, fusarenon-X, administered to Peking ducklings as a single oral dose of 5.0 mg/kg body weight or given as a single subcutaneous (s.c.) injection at doses ranging from 0.5 to 5.0 mg/kg body weight, produced unspecified cytotoxic changes in bone marrow.[7]

2. Broiler Chicks

The hematopoietic system of growing broiler chickens appears to be more sensitive to the effects of T-2 toxin than that of laying hens. In broiler chickens the observed changes in hematocrit, hemoglobin, and RBC counts are seemingly dependent on the dosage of T-2 toxin, the route of administration, the duration of toxin exposure, and the time interval following toxin administration at which hematologic parameters are evaluated.

No changes were detected in the hematocrit values following the feeding of purified T-2 toxin at as high as 16 mg/kg feed to day-old male broiler chickens for 3 weeks.[8] Similarly, no changes were recorded in either hematocrit or hemoglobin values for broiler chickens fed rations containing up to 4.0 ppm T-2 toxin from 1 d to 9 weeks of age, or for 8-week-old chickens given a single oral dose of up to 5.5 mg/kg body weight.[9,10] However, single oral doses of 6.0 and 6.5 mg T-2 toxin per kilogram of body weight produced transient dose-related reductions in hematocrit, hemoglobin, and RBC counts at 10 d posttreatment. All values had returned to normal by 30 d posttreatment.[9] No pathologic changes in either blood smears or in the bone marrow were noted following any of these treatment schedules.[9,10] In contrast to these results, a transient increase in both hemoglobin and hematocrit values was found in 4-week-old broiler chickens given a single oral dose of 2.5 mg T-2 toxin per kilogram body weight.[11] Within 24 h of toxin administration, the mean hematocrit value was 28.0 ± 0.8% compared to 25.2 ± 1.9% in control birds and the hemoglobin concentration had increased to 9.43 ± 0.47 g/dl compared to the control value of 8.30 ± 0.41 g/dl. Although this dose of T-2 toxin produced a significant decline in the WBC count 24 h after administration, no changes were observed in the RBC counts. It was suggested that the increased hematocrit and hemoglobin values, coupled with the decreased WBC count, may have been a result of stress induced in the chickens by the oral dosing of T-2 toxin.[11] Contrary to the increase in hematocrit observed at 24 h after dosing, a dose-related decrease in hematocrit was recorded after 14 d during which young male broiler chickens had been treated orally with 1.5 to 3.0 mg T-2 toxin per kilogram per day.[12] In this study, reductions in hematocrit values appeared to correlate with the necrosis and reduction in hematopoietic cellularity found in the bone marrow.

Broiler chickens appear to be more sensitive to the effects of T-2 toxin than to diacetoxyscirpenol (DAS). In comparative studies in which day-old male broiler chickens were treated for 7 d with doses of 2.0 or 2.5 mg T-2 toxin per kilogram body weight or with 2.7 mg DAS, similar evidence of necrosis and cell depletion in bone marrow tissue was found, but the lesions were more severe in the T-2 toxin-treated birds.[13]

3. Laying Hens

No changes in hematocrit, hemoglobin, or RBC counts were produced when 30-week-old laying hens were fed pure T-2 toxin at 20 mg/kg feed for 3 weeks, although this treatment did induce a leukopenia and a decrease in total plasma protein and plasma lipid content.[14] A single oral administration of purified T-2 toxin to 24-week-old laying hens, at doses ranging from 3.0 to 6.5 mg toxin per kilogram body weight, produced no significant changes in hematocrit or hemoglobin values. Nevertheless, a marked increase in RBC count was noted at a dose of 6.5 mg/kg on posttreatment day 10 but not on day 30.[9] No changes in hematocrit or hemoglobin values were detected in white Leghorn laying hens fed for 28 d on diets containing either 2.5 or 5.0% of corn contaminated by *Fusarium tricinctum* and containing 8 and 16 ppm T-2 toxin, respectively, or when 4 to 16 ppm of purified T-2 toxin were included in the feed.[15] In this study, however, the group of hens which were fed for 28 d on corn contaminated with *F. roseum*, containing up to 50 ppm monoacetoxyscirpenol, developed an increase in both hematocrit and hemoglobin values.[15]

C. Mice

Crude extracts of both *F. tricinctum* and *F. sporotrichioides* cultures were lethal to mice when administered intraperitoneally (i.p.) at 50 mg/kg body weight and caused severe damage, including mitotic injury and karyorrhexis, in the actively dividing cells in the small intestine, spleen, thymus, and bone marrow.[7] The presence of T-2 toxin, HT-2 toxin, and neosolaniol, but not fusarenon-X or nivalenol, were detected by chemical analysis of the crude extract.

The susceptibility of mouse hematopoietic tissue to trichothecene mycotoxins has also been documented in a number of studies with pure toxin preparations. A single oral dose of T-2 toxin at 5.0 mg/kg body weight administered to 6-week-old male ddYS mice caused a transient increase in the platelet count 1 h after dosing followed by a continuous and significant decline between 6 and 48 h later.[16] The RBC count was not affected by this treatment. When the duration of exposure to the toxin was increased, similar results were obtained. Mice treated with a daily oral dose of 3.0 mg T-2 toxin per kilogram body weight for up to 5 d developed thrombocytopenia and leukopenia, but not anemia. After 5 d of treatment, the platelet count was reduced from $770 \pm 90 \times 10^3/\mu l$ to $160 \pm 60 \times 10^3/\mu l$ and the WBC count had fallen from $3.2 \pm 0.8 \times 10^3/\mu l$ to $0.7 \pm 0.5 \times 10^3/\mu l$, while the RBC count, the hematocrit, and hemoglobin values were unaffected.[16] Since the depression in circulating numbers of WBC, platelets, and RBC could be correlated with the circulating half-lives of each cell type, it was concluded that T-2 toxin could induce a disorder of the hematopoietic system. This conclusion was confirmed in another study in which male weanling Swiss mice, weighing 16 g, were fed purified T-2 toxin at 20 mg/kg dry feed for 41 d.[17] The mice progressively developed normochromic normocytic anemia. Initially the anemia was not regenerative, with less than 0.1% reticulocytes detectable in the circulation, but by day 41, reticulocytes had returned to the circulation. In the T-2 toxin-treated mice, the RBC count declined from $9.1 \pm 0.4 \times 10^6/\mu l$ on day 0 to $3.3 \pm 1.2 \times 10^6$ μl on day 41, the hematocrit progressively declined from $41.5 \pm 1.9\%$ on day 0 to $16.7 \pm 7.0\%$ on day 41, and the hemoglobin concentration fell from 13.8 ± 0.3 g/dl to 6.0 ± 2.2 g/dl. During the first 3 weeks of the study, the lymphoid tissues, bone marrow, and splenic red pulp became hypoplastic but during the subsequent 3 weeks, despite continued exposure to the toxin, hematopoietic cells regenerated in both bone marrow and splenic red pulp and these tissues became hyperplastic. The megakaryocyte population in the bone marrow was moderately reduced during the first 2 weeks of treatment but thereafter returned to near normal values.[17] The hematologic and morphologic changes in hematopoietic tissues do not appear to be related to the reduced food intake which occurs in mice exposed to T-2 toxin. Similar hematologic changes were produced in young, male Swiss mice fed T-2 toxin at 20 mg/kg of dry feed for up to 4 weeks irrespective of the inclusion of 0, 8, 12, or 16% protein in the diet;[18] however, juvenile mice are more susceptible to hematopoietic suppression induced by T-2 toxin than are adult mice.[19] The feeding of purified T-2 toxin at 20 ppm for 28 d produced erythroid hypoplasia and anemia in the young mice, but not in the adult mice. After 28 d of ingesting toxin the RBC count in the juvenile mice was $6.2 \pm 0.6 \times 10^6/\mu l$ compared to $8.4 \pm 0.3 \times 10^6/\mu l$ in the toxin-treated adult mice and $10.3 \pm 0.1 \times 10^6/\mu l$ in the juvenile control groups.[19]

Trichothecene mycotoxins other than T-2 toxin can also affect hematologic parameters in mice. The single i.p. infusion of 11.0 mg neosolaniol per kilogram body weight to 6-week-old male ddYS mice produced an increase in the circulating reticulocyte count within 30 min of administration.[16] The reticulocyte count remained elevated until 6 h posttreatment when it began to fall and by 72 h it had declined to approximately 50% of pretreatment values. Although no changes in the RBC counts or plasma protein concentrations were noted following a single i.p. administration of 2.5 mg Fusarenon-X per kilogram body weight, a reduction in platelet count was recorded between 1 and 24 h after treatment.[16] In studies with weanling mice it has been demonstrated that 3-acetyldeoxynivalenol (3-AcDON) is less toxic than T-2 toxin, but affects the dividing cells of the body in a manner characteristic of trichothecenes.[20] Between 4 and 96 h after gavage administration of 3-AcDON at 20 and 40 mg/kg body weight, multifocal necrosis characterized by nuclear pyknosis and karyorrhexis occurred in the spleen.[20] No pathologic lesions or hematologic changes were detected in weanling mice fed 3-AcDON for 48 d at up to 20 ppm in a semipurified diet.[21]

D. Rats

The daily i.p. administration of T-2 toxin at 0.5 mg/kg body weight to male albino rats for 1 to 5 d produced a dose-related decrease in both the circulating RBC and platelet counts.[22] The RBC count fell from an initial value of $7.0 \pm 1.2 \times 10^6/\mu l$ to $6.5 \pm 0.9 \times 10^6/\mu l$ by day 5, while the platelet count declined from a pretreatment value of $672 \pm 283 \times 10^3/\mu l$ to $487 \pm 242 \times 10^3/\mu l$. Over the same time period, the decreases in total WBC count and the percentage of circulating granulocytes were more pronounced than the effects of the toxin on either the circulating RBC or platelet counts. T-2 toxin induced a more severe reduction in the bone marrow cell count (from $117 \pm 15 \times 10^6$ nucleated cells per femur to $26 \pm 18 \times 10^6$ cells after 3 d of treatment) than in the blood cell count. The decline in myeloid cells in the bone marrow was also more dramatic than the decline in the erythroid cells, a result which correlates with the pattern of change in the circulating blood.[22] The daily intramuscular (i.m.) injection of T-2 toxin to rats at 0.2 mg/kg body weight also produced a decrease in hematocrit values.[23] Within 2 d of receiving toxin, the mean hematocrit value was $39.3 \pm 1.8\%$ compared to $44.7 \pm 2.2\%$ in control animals. The hematocrit values remained lower in the toxin-treated group throughout the 10-d treatment period. In rats, the route of exposure to T-2 toxin may significantly influence the hematologic damage induced in the animals since no alteration in RBC counts was observed in adult male rats fed purified T-2 toxin at 20 ppm for 28 d.[19] In this study, adult rats appeared to be less sensitive to the ingestion of T-2 toxin than either adult or juvenile mice.[19]

In addition to suppressing RBC production in the bone marrow, T-2 toxin may impair hemoglobin synthesis.[24] Rats given T-2 toxin intragastrically at 3.0 mg/kg body weight, an approximate LD_{50} dose, exhibited a 5-fold increase in urinary coproporphyrin excretion. The excretion increased progressively, peaking at day 4 posttreatment, and subsequently declined to approximately pretreatment values. When the administration of the toxin was repeated, the urinary excretion of porphyrin increased in a similar fashion. Increased porphyrin excretion generally indicates inhibition of heme formation, especially at the stage of insertion of the metal iron. It has not been determined how T-2 toxin impairs heme formation.[24] T-2 toxin also has hemolytic properties since it can cause essentially complete hemolysis when added to suspensions of washed rat erythrocytes.[25] The hemolysis occurs in a two-step process; the first phase is reversible during which the toxin can be washed off the erythrocytes, while in the second phase osmotic swelling followed by irreversible damage to the erythrocyte membrane and cell rupture occur. The length of the first phase is inversely proportional and the severity of the second phase is directly proportional to the concentration of T-2 toxin within the range of 12 to 350 μg/ml. Based on the similarities of the effects of T-2 toxin and those of saponins, H_2O_2, and polyoxyethylene surfactants, it was suggested that T-2 toxin may act on the rat erythrocyte membrane through a free radical mechanism.[25] The disruption of rat erythrocyte membranes does not appear to be a universal property of trichothecenes. No evidence of hemolysis was found in rat erythrocyte suspensions incubated at 37°C for 24 h in the presence of fusarenon-X at concentrations of 10 and 100 μm/ml.[26] Like T-2 toxin, however, fusarenon-X can produce a reduction in the hematopoietic cells in the bone marrow of rats orally exposed to the toxin.[7,27] Atrophy of the bone marrow and spleen were usually observed in male Donryu rats which survived after being fed fusarenon-X at 50 μg/d for 2 years or 105 μg/d for 1 year.[28]

E. Guinea Pigs

Intragastric administration of purified T-2 toxin to adult male Hartley strain guinea pigs at 0.5 mg/kg body weight for 21 d followed by 0.75 mg/kg for an additional 21 d caused essentially no change in the total RBC count, hematocrit, hemoglobin concentration, or circulating platelet count, although a marked decrease occurred in the total WBC count.[29] When the dosage was increased to 0.9 mg/kg/d for 27 d, the RBC count decreased from an initial value of $5.5 \pm 0.6 \times 10^6$/ml to $4.2 \pm 1.0 \times 10^6$/ml, and the platelet count decreased from $630.7 \pm 127.2 \times 10^3$/ml to $537.1 \pm 140.3 \times 10^3$/ml, while the hematocrit and the hemoglobin concentration remained essentially unchanged.[29] Marked differences were noted in the RBC morphology in the T-2 toxin-treated guinea pigs. The RBC had basophilic stippling, fragmentation, increased polychromasia, anisocytosis, and increased nuclear forms. These abnormalities increased during the experimental period. The morphological alteration of the peripheral RBC, together with the hypercellularity and reduction in the myeloid to erythroid ratio of the bone marrow, suggested that T-2 toxin could produce a hyperplastic reaction in the erythroid compartment of the bone marrow.

The single i.m. injection of T-2 toxin to adult Hartley strain guinea pigs at a dose of 1 mg/kg body weight, a dose which was lethal within 24 h to approximately 50% of the animals, also produced alterations in platelet and WBC counts and hematocrit values in surviving animals.[30] A transient increase in the hematocrit at 6 h postinjection was followed by a decrease at 24 h and a return to pretreatment values by 48 h. The platelet count remained unchanged for the first 24 h, showed a marked decrease at 48 h and returned to initial values moglobin, and with both treatments the total WBC count was more severely depressed than WBC counts of the animals decreased throughout the remaining 66 h of the experimental period.

Guinea pig erythrocytes, like rat erythrocytes, can be lysed *in vitro* in a dose-dependent manner by T-2 toxin. The lysis of guinea pig RBC suspensions was essentially complete 4 to 6 h after 20 μg T-2 toxin had been incubated with 5×10^6 cells at 37°C.[31] The physiologic significance of this observation is uncertain since lower concentrations of T-2 toxin were considerably less effective at inducing hemolysis.

The bone marrow tissue of newborn guinea pigs appears to be more affected by the systemic administration of fusarenon-X than is that of the adult.[7] Degeneration of bone marrow cells was observed in newborn guinea pigs which died within 18 h after the s.c. injection of 0.1 or 1.0 mg fusarenon-X per kilogram body weight. No abnormalities were found in the bone marrow of adult guinea pigs which died 8 to 11 h following the i.p. injection of 5.0 mg fusarenon-X per kilogram body weight.

F. Rabbits

Although oral administration of T-2 toxin to New Zealand white rabbits at 2.0 mg/kg/d for 4 d caused no change in hematocrit values, the single i.v. injection of 0.5 mg/kg body weight did produce a significant ($p < 0.05$) decrease in this parameter.[32] The maximum decrease in the hematocrit was observed 4 d posttreatment when the mean hematocrit was $28.0 \pm 1.0\%$ compared to the pretreatment mean of $32.8 \pm 2.0\%$. Hematocrit values were also depressed within 2 d after rabbits had received i.m. injections of T-2 toxin at 0.2 mg/kg/d and the hematocrit remained depressed throughout the 10-d treatment period.[23] Although platelet counts were unaffected by a single i.v. injection of 0.5 mg T-2 toxin per kilogram body weight,[33] a reduction in the WBC was observed.[32]

G. Dogs

The effect of DAS on the hematopoietic system in dogs appears to be generally dose related. Beagle dogs given toxic doses of DAS of either 5 mg/m² as a single dose or daily doses of 2.5 mg/m²/d for 5 d developed anemia and mild thrombocytopenia.[34] The presence of nucleated RBC in the circulation was also noted. These dosages of DAS correspond to approximately 0.23 and 0.12 mg/kg body weight, respectively. As had been found in other species, the hematologic abnormalities produced by the toxin were reversible.

No changes in the hematocrit, hemoglobin, RBC count, and red cell indices were detected up to 8 h posttreatment following the i.v. administration of DAS to male and female dogs at 0.5 mg/kg.[35] However, within 3 h after toxin administration, a linear increase in the nucleated RBC count in peripheral blood smears was noted. The nucleated RBC count peaked at 7 h before beginning to decline. The bone marrow of the dogs was void of cellular elements at 8 h following DAS exposure.[35]

H. Cats

Similar marked abnormalities in the hematologic profile developed in cats exposed either to crude extracts of *F. solani* containing 4% T-2 toxin and 1% neosolaniol, or to purified T-2 toxin.[36] The s.c. injection of the crude toxin to cats weighing 2 to 3 kg, at 1 mg/kg/week for 5 weeks followed by a daily oral dose of 15 mg per animal for 17 d, produced a 26% reduction in RBC count, a 31% reduction in hemoglobin concentration, and a 24% reduction in the hematocrit. The s.c. injection of the purified T-2 toxin to a male and a female adult cat, at 0.1 and 0.05 mg/kg, respectively, at 1 to 11 day intervals for 24 d, produced an approximately 25% reduction in RBC count, hemoglobin concentration, and hematocrit values by the end of the treatment period. Neither the crude nor purified toxin produced any significant alteration in mean corpuscular volume or mean corpuscular he-by 72 h posttreatment. Following a transient increase at 6 h after toxin administration, the the RBC count.[36] Post mortem histologic study showed that the purified toxin had produced atrophy of hematopoietic tissues.

Marked abnormalities in the hematologic profile of mature male and female short-haired domestic cats were also induced by crude extracts of *F. sporotrichioides* containing T-2 toxin and by T-2 toxin purified from this source.[37] Reductions in the hematocrit and hemoglobin concentrations were consistent observations. Thrombocytopenia developed in all cats and macrocytic anemia was frequently observed following either; the oral administration, every 48 h, 6 to 12 times, of the crude extract at 0.06 or 0.076 mg/kg body weight; or the oral administration of purified T-2 toxin, 3 to 12 times per os, at dosages of 0.08 or 0.1 mg/kg. As the number of circulating platelets decreased, bizarre forms, including giant platelets, were seen on blood smears. Nucleated RBC (15/100 WBC) were also seen in the peripheral blood of a cat which had received 19 doses of crude extract. Changes in the RBC also included anisocytosis, poikilocytosis, and macrocytosis. Bone marrow samples taken at necropsy were usually hemorrhagic, hypocellular, and contained very few marrow spicules. Megakaryocytes were reduced in number, and in some cases completely absent, while necrotic erythroblasts were found in all bone marrow preparations. Despite these cytotoxic effects of T-2 toxin, in cats with the longer survival times regeneration of erythroid cells was observed despite continued dosing with the toxin. In these cats, megakaryocytes with well-defined granular cytoplasm, but with no platelet formation visible in the margins, were present in normal or increased numbers.[37] In cats given T-2 toxin orally at 0.08 mg/kg body weight a marked increase in erythrocyte sedimentation rate was observed in addition to the other hematologic changes.

I. Pigs

When healthy crossbred weanling pigs were given a single i.v. injection of 0.13 to 3.20 mg T-2 toxin per kilogram body weight as part of an acute LD_{50} study or were fed 0 to 8 ppm T-2 toxin daily for 8 weeks as part of a chronic study, no abnormalities were observed in the hematologic profile or in the bone marrow smears of animals which survived the treatments.[38] Similar results were found when white, crossbred female swine were given a single i.v. dose of T-2 toxin at 0.6 mg/kg body weight.[39] However, when the dosage of toxin was increased to 4.8 mg/kg, significant elevations occurred in hematocrit, RBC count, and hemoglobin concentration between predosing and 7 h postdosing.[39] The hematocrit increased from 33.4 ± 2.1% to 38.5 ± 2.1%, the RBC count increased from 7.6 ± 0.6 × $10^6/\mu l$ to 9.0 ± 0.7 × $10^6/\mu l$ and the hemoglobin increased from 10.9 ± 0.6 g/dl to 12.8 ± 0.9 g/dl. In this study, nucleated RBC were seen in peripheral blood smears in both the high and low dose T-2 toxin treatment groups, but the presence of the nucleated cells was only transient in the low dose group.

Three sows in the third trimester of pregnancy aborted 48 h after a single i.v. injection of 0.41 mg T-2 toxin per kilogram body weight but experienced no significant changes in hematologic parameters between 3 and 14 d posttreatment.[40] Similarly, no hematologic abnormalities or changes in bone marrow smears were produced in sows which were fed 12 ppm T-2 toxin per day for up to 220 d.[41] No clinical signs or alterations in hematology were observed in weanling Landrace pigs fed crude extracts of *F. tricinctum* at a level which exposed the animals to 1.0 mg T-2 toxin per kilogram daily for 14 d.[42] The Landrace pigs were also fed purified T-2 toxin or DAS at 0.2 mg/kg/d for up to 36 d and the only abnormality observed was a leukopenia which developed in the T-2 toxin-treated animals.[42] The absence of change in the hematologic profile in response to DAS did not appear to be increased by a longer duration of exposure to the toxin since no changes in hematologic parameters or in bone marrow smears were induced in weanling male crossbred pigs fed up to 10 ppm DAS per day for 9 weeks.[43] Similarly, the i.v. administration of DAS to male of 4.5 mg DAS/m²/d by 4 h i.v. infusions every 5 d, myelosuppression was the most significant adverse effect.[55] The platelet count dropped from the normal range of >100 × counts, or hemoglobin concentration.[35] In the higher dose group, a marked increase in nucleated RBC was evident in peripheral blood smears by 4 h posttreatment and there was a distinct lack of viable hemopoietic elements in the bone marrow by 8 h postdosing.[35]

J. Sheep

Male crossbred lambs fed 0.6 mg T-2 toxin per kilogram per day for 21 d became lymphopenic within 7 d of the start of treatment and remained lymphopenic throughout the experimental period.[44] The animals did not develop anemia and no alteration was observed in the circulating platelet count. At the end of the 21-d feeding trial, an increase in the myeloid to erythroid ratio in the bone marrow was found and the bone marrow appeared hypocellular with degenerating cells, pyknotic nuclei, and cellular debris present. In contrast to the effect of T-2 toxin in lambs, the single oral administration of T-2 toxin to mature sheep at doses of 0.5 to 8.0 mg/kg body weight caused an increase in hemoglobin values, in RBC count, and leukocytosis.[45]

K. Cows

Hematologic parameters in cattle, like those of swine, appear to be relatively insensitive to the influence of trichothecene mycotoxins. No alterations in hematocrit, hemoglobin concentration, or RBC count were induced in a cow intubated with 0.44 mg T-2 toxin per kilogram per day for 15 d.[46] Similarly, after a calf was intubated with a total of 26.2 mg T-2 toxin over a period of 16 d, the hematocrit and hemoglobin values and the RBC count remained within the normal range.[46] When T-2 toxin was injected as a single i.v. dose of 0.25 mg/kg to healthy male Holstein calves, the platelet count remained unchanged, although a 10% reduction in hematocrit was observed 48 to 96 h after dosing.[47] The lack of response in circulating RBC and platelet numbers has also been noted in various studies in cattle employing concentrations of T-2 toxin which can induce a depression of circulating WBC counts,[47] the impairment of lymphocyte and neutrophil function,[48,49] and significant alterations in both the immunoglobulin and coagulation proteins.[50,51]

Cattle appear to be less sensitive to the effects of DAS than swine. No change in hematocrit, RBC counts, or hemoglobin concentration were observed in calves given a single i.v. injection of purified DAS at 0.5 mg/kg and only a few nucleated RBC were detected in peripheral blood smears 4 h postdosing.[35]

L. Monkeys

A slight decrease in hematocrit values was observed in adult male and female Rhesus monkeys receiving 0.1 mg T-2 toxin per kilogram per day orally for up to 35 d, and although the RBC remained unchanged, a marked decrease in the WBC occurred.[52,53] When 3 male and 2 female adult Rhesus monkeys were orally dosed with 1 mg T-2 toxin per kilogram per day for 5 d followed by 0.5 mg/kg/d for an additional 10 d, all the males died between days 8 and 15 of the treatment while in the surviving females, by day 15, the hematocrit values had declined by 34%, the hemoglobin concentration had decreased approximately 20% and the platelet count had decreased by approximately 13%.[52] In contrast to the effects of the oral administration of T-2 toxin in Rhesus monkeys, a single i.v. infusion of pure T-2 toxin to cynomolgus monkeys at a dose of 0.65 mg/kg produced no changes in either hematocrit values or circulating platelet numbers although the total WBC count showed a significant transient increase at 6 h posttreatment.[54]

M. Man

The trichothecene DAS (anguidine) has been evaluated as a possible anticancer drug in a number of studies in human cancer patients. In 25 patients treated for 21 d with an average and female pigs at doses of 0.5 or 1.0 mg/kg induced no alterations in hematocrit, RBC $10^3/\mu l$ to a mean of $55 \times 10^3/\mu l$ in 6 of the patients and a decrease in WBC count occurred in 14 of the patients. In patients receiving up to 5.0 mg T-2 toxin per square meter per day for up to 5 d, the nadir of the reduction in both WBC and platelet count occurred between 19 and 26 d from the onset of treatment.[56,57] In other anticancer trials only occasional mild thrombocytopenia was observed in patients treated with DAS at up to 5 mg/m²/d for 5 d every 3 weeks.[34,58] In these studies the thrombocytopenia was minimal compared to the other toxic effects such as nausea, vomiting, hypotension, skin erythema, and somnolence.[34,58] No reduction in either platelet or WBC counts were observed in a group of 29 cancer patients treated at weekly intervals with DAS at up to 7.5 mg/m² by 3 h i.v. infusions.[59]

The variability in platelet response may be related to prior or concomitant drug therapy which the patients received along with DAS. Thrombocytopenia developed in 14 out of 30 cancer patients treated with a combination of 300 to 350 mg 5-fluorouracil and 2.5 to 3.0 mg/m² DAS given as 4 h i.v. infusions daily for 5 d.[60] In another study, 5 out of 7 patients given up to 6.0 mg DAS/m² over an 8 h i.v. infusion exhibited a reduced platelet count. The authors[61] suggested that exposure to nitrosourea prior to DAS treatment had predisposed the patients to developing thrombocytopenia. The same conclusion was reached in a study in which thrombocytopenia developed in 5 out of 10 patients given 2.0 to 3.5 mg DAS/m²/week, but only in 3 of 23 patients given higher doses.[62]

III. BLOOD COAGULATION

A. Fish

Although hemorrhages in the intestinal tract and in muscle tissue were observed in 300 g trout fed pure T-2 toxin at 15 mg/kg body weight for 16 weeks,[5] this does not appear to be a uniform response of fish to the feeding of trichothecenes. No hemorrhages were found in rainbow trout exposed to 200 and 400 ppm T-2 toxin for 12 months[63] or in fingerling rainbow trout fed diets containing deoxynivalenol (DON) at up to 109.6 ppm for 4 weeks.[64]

B. Birds

Hemorrhagic enteritis and microscopic hemorrhages in the liver and heart muscle were found in geese fed 3 ppm purified T-2 toxin,[65] but no evidence of hemorrhage was found in ducks or geese following the ingestion of barley contaminated with T-2 toxin in a natural outbreak of mycotoxicosis.[66,67] Similarly, no signs of hemorrhage were found at the end of a 9-week period during which chickens were given rations containing up to 4 ppm T-2 toxin,[10] but in chickens exposed to higher doses of the toxin, hemorrhagic lesions were produced.[15,68] In 5 of 10 male 6-week-old chickens given T-2 toxin at 0.75 mg/kg body weight by i.m. injection, hemorrhagic lesions of the liver were present at 96 h after toxin treatment.[68] The hemorrhagic lesions induced by T-2 toxin appear to be reversible. In male broiler chicks given T-2 toxin orally at 2.0 or 2.5 mg/kg body weight for 7 d and killed at intervals up to 168 h after treatment, the most severe lesions in the liver, involving multiple foci of hemorrhage in areas of necrosis, were observed during the first 24 h after treatment. By 168 h the livers appeared normal.[13]

The single oral administration of DAS at 3.5 mg/kg body weight produced transient focal hemorrhagic necrosis throughout the liver.[13] Extensive ecchymotic hemorrhages throughout the intestinal tract, liver, and musculature were produced by DON when it was administered to day-old male broiler chicks by crop intubation at dosages from 140 to 1120 mg/kg.[69] The hemorrhaging was so extensive and intensive that the carcass was described as ''burgundy colored''.

The blood coagulation profile, evaluated with the prothrombin time (PT) assay, was unaltered after white Leghorn laying hens were fed either balanced rations containing 2.5 or 5.0% of corn containing 8 or 16 ppm T-2 toxin due to contamination with *F. tricinctum* for 28 d or when the hens were fed pure T-2 toxin at 4, 8, or 16 ppm for 21 d.[15] In 1-day-old, male broiler chickens fed purified T-2 toxin at up to 16 ppm in the diet for 21 d, no significant change was observed in the WBCT but an increase in the PT assay was observed with diets containing growth inhibitory doses of T-2 toxin of 8 and 16 ppm.[70] The lack of apparent response in the parameters which evaluate the overall integrity of the hemostatic mechanism may reflect the insensitivity of the methodology since individual coagulation proteins appear relatively sensitive to the effects of T-2 toxin. In day-old, male broiler chickens fed a diet in which T-2 toxin was incorporated at 0 to 16 ppm for 21 d, a dose-dependent reduction in the biological activity of coagulation factors V, VII, X, pro-thrombin, and fibrinogen was observed.[71] When the concentration of T-2 toxin in the feed was 16 ppm, the coagulant activities of prothrombin and factor VII were reduced approximately 45%, the activities of factors V and X were reduced approximately 20 and 15% respectively, and the concentration of plasma fibrinogen was reduced 42%. Of the coagulation proteins, factor VII appeared most sensitive to T-2 toxin since its activity was reduced at concentrations as low as 4 ppm in the feed. Factor X, prothrombin, and fibrinogen were affected only by the highest concentration of toxin. The clot retraction time was increased in the chickens fed T-2 toxin at 16 ppm in the diet which may correlate with the reduced fibrinogen levels recorded in this treatment group. Although no change in total plasma lipids was observed, a reduction in the lipid component of tissue thromboplastin was found in the birds fed T-2 toxin at 16 ppm.[71]

C. Mice

Marked bleeding in the small intestine was reported for mice injected i.p. with lethal doses (50 mg/kg body weight) of crude extracts of *F. tricinctum* and *F. sporotrichiodes* containing T-2 toxin, HT-2 toxin, and neosolaniol;[72] but evidence of hemorrhage has not been a frequent observation in mice exposed to pure trichothecene mycotoxins. Nevertheless, as has been found in other species, it would appear that T-2 toxin can reduce the efficiency of blood clot formation in mice. The coagulation profile of young male ddYS mice, treated with oral doses of T-2 toxin at 3.0 mg/d for up to 5 d was evaluated with a thromboelas-tograph. The thromboelastograph monitors the rate of clot formation and the strength or size of the fibrin clot. After 5 d of T-2 toxin treatment all of these parameters were significantly reduced.[16] The single oral administration of pure T-2 toxin at 3.0 mg/kg body weight to CD-1 mice on days 7, 8, 10, 11, or 12 of pregnancy resulted in 17% mortality which peaked 48 h after treatment.[73] In some instances vaginal hemorrhage preceded death. Necropsy revealed that in those female mice that died, the reproductive tract was filled with unclotted blood; however, no histologic lesions were observed in any of the fetuses.

Crude extracts of *F. nivale*, as well as fusarenon-X isolated from the extracts, produced hemorrhages in the intestines and heart muscle in male ddS mice.[74] Lethal doses of the crude extract (0.1 to 0.3 g/kg body weight) and of the purified toxin (8.0 mg/kg body weight administered i.p.) were required to produce these effects.

D. Rat

Rats orally dosed with crude extracts of *F. tricinctum* containing T-2 toxin developed hemorrhages of the urinary tract and ecchymotic hemorrhages on the serosal surfaces of the large and small intestines.[75] Local cytotoxic effects of the toxin probably contributed to the hemorrhagic condition since the extracts produced only transient changes in the blood co-agulation profile. The mean WBCT increased from 60 to 76 s and the mean PT increased from 15 to 26 s in rats orally dosed with crude T-2 toxin at 150 mg/kg body weight.[75] The maximum increase in the WBCT occurred at 8 h after dosing and the WBCT returned to near normal values by 24 h.[75] Likewise, in rats exposed to a single i.p. injection of crude T-2 toxin at 1 mg/kg body weight, the maximum increase in the mean PT assay was observed at 8 h posttreatment and thereafter, the PT results gradually returned toward pretreatment values.[76] When the rats were pretreated with phenobarbital to activate hepatic microsomal enzymes, no significant alteration in the effect of the toxin on the prolongation of the PT assay was observed.[75] Rats given crude T-2 toxin at 1 mg/kg body weight by i.p. injection had PT values of 29 s compared to 15 to 20 s in control animals. There was some evidence that T-2 toxin might function as a vit K antagonist. The WBCT and PT were prolonged despite the lack of alteration of plasma fibrinogen concentration and the pretreatment of rats with vit K partially alleviated the prolongation of the PT assay caused by the toxin. In rats injected i.p. with 0.1 mg vit K 1 h before toxin administration, the PT averaged 19 s compared to 28 s for both the rats not given vit K and those rats pretreated orally with 2 g calcium gluconate per kilogram before T-2 toxin administration.[75] Although dexamethasone, given i.v. at 1.6 mg/kg to white male Sprague Dawley rats, protected the animals from lung edema and diarrhea produced by an i.v. dose of T-2 toxin at 0.75 mg/kg, the incidence of gastrointestinal hemorrhages was increased in these animals compared to rats which were not pretreated with dexamethasone.[77]

Crude cultures from a number of *Fusarium* spp. including *F. tricinctum*, *F. poae*, *F. sporotrichiodes*, and *F. moniliforme* apparently caused congestion and fatal hemorrhage in rats following the feeding for 5 d of 1:1 contaminated rice and ground complete rat chow.[78]

E. Guinea Pig

Intragastric and cecal hemorrhages developed in adult male Hartley strain guinea pigs exposed to a single dose of T-2 toxin at 2.5 or 5.0 mg/kg body weight by gastric intubation.[29] In contrast, guinea pigs given a single i.m. injection of T-2 toxin at 1 mg/kg body weight displayed marked alterations in blood coagulation parameters without any clinical evidence of hemorrhage.[30] Within 6 h of toxin administration both the PT and APTT assays were prolonged, with the maximum increases occurring at 48 and 24 h posttreatment, respectively. The prolongation of these coagulation screening tests could be attributed to a significant decrease ($p < 0.01$) in the circulating activity of a number of specific coagulation proteins. Within 6 h of toxin administration, a decrease was observed in the activity of factors V, VII, VIII, IX, X, XI, XII, and prothrombin.[30] The maximum decrease in prothrombin activity occurred at 48 h while the maximum decrease in the activities of the other coagulation proteins occurred at 24 h. Unlike the results reported for rats, pretreatment of the guinea pigs with vit K at 0.3 or 3.0 mg/kg by i.m. injection 2 h before the i.m. injection of the toxin produced no alleviation in the depression of the biological activity of the coagulation factors. Unlike the PT and APTT assays, the thrombin time was shortened at both 24 and 48 h after toxin administration. This shortening of the thrombin time correlated with the marked increase in plasma fibrinogen concentration between 24 and 72 h posttreatment. T-2 toxin also depressed platelet function in the guinea pigs.[30] Platelet aggregation in whole blood in response to the aggregating agents ADP and collagen was depressed in blood samples obtained from T-2 toxin-treated animals. The effect of the toxin on ADP-induced aggregation was more pronounced than the effect on collagen-induced aggregation. The toxin appeared to be without effect when platelet aggregation was studied in platelet-rich plasma. The *in vitro* addition of T-2 toxin to normal pooled guinea pig plasma at 1 μg/ml had no effect on either coagulation factor activity or on platelet aggregation.[30]

F. Rabbit

As has been found for guinea pigs, T-2 toxin can produce a marked depression in the plasma coagulation competency in rabbits without inducing clinical signs of hemorrhage.[33] The single i.v. injection of purified T-2 toxin at 0.5 mg/kg body weight to New Zealand white rabbits resulted in the prolongation of both the PT and APTT assays. The APTT assay became prolonged within 6 h of toxin administration and reached a maximum between 24 and 30 h posttreatment before showing a gradual return to pretreatment values. The PT assay showed a gradual prolongation throughout the 96 h observation period, but did not become significantly longer ($p <0.05$) than pretreatment values until 54 h posttreatment.[33] These prolongations of the plasma clotting times correlated with the observed reductions in the plasma activity of specific coagulation factors. Within 6 h of T-2 toxin administration, the activity of each of the factors VII, VIII, IX, X, and XI had decreased from pretreatment values of 1.0 U/ml plasma to approximately 0.6 U/ml plasma. The activity of factors VII and X appeared to be the least sensitive to the effects of the toxin, exhibiting only a transient depression at the 6 and 24 h postinjection period followed by a gradual increase to above pretreatment values for the remainder of the 96 h experimental period. The apparent insensitivity of factor VII in rabbits to the effects of T-2 toxin is in marked contrast to the sensitivity of this protein in chickens and cattle. In the rabbits the activity of factors VIII, IX, and XI remained depressed for 24 h following toxin administration before returning to or exceeding pretreatment values. These results were confirmed in a separate study which also demonstrated that thrombin clotting times were unchanged despite a prolongation in the APTT assay. Also, the biological activity of factor XII declined 6 h after toxin administration along with the other specific coagulation proteins.[79] In agreement with the results reported for guinea pigs, the administration of vit K to the rabbits by s.c. injection at 0.5 mg/kg/d for 5 d before toxin administration and throughout the 4 d observation period had no effect on the T-2 toxin-induced depression of the coagulation protein activity.[33] This result, together with the observation that non-vit K dependent proteins (factors VIII and XI) are equally or more sensitive to the toxin than are the vit K dependent proteins (factors VII and X), indicate that T-2 toxin does not function as a vit K antagonist in the rabbit.[33] In contrast to the depression in the activities of the other coagulation factors, plasma fibrinogen concentrations increased almost 2-fold within 2 h of toxin administration and the fibrinogen values remained elevated. The similar responses of plasma fibrinogen in rabbits and guinea pigs may reflect a stress reaction due to the injection of T-2 toxin.

Unlike the response to T-2 toxin, fusarenon-X administered orally to rabbits twice a week for 4 weeks at 5 mg/kg body weight produced subarachinoidal hemorrhages which were implicated as the cause of death.[74] This response may be similar to the brain hemorrhages observed in cats chronically exposed to T-2 toxin.[36]

G. Dog and Cat

Beagle dogs exposed to DAS in a single dose of 0.23 mg/kg body weight or daily doses of 0.12 mg/kg for 5 d developed hemorrhages of Peyer's patches of the colon and lymph node hemorrhages.[34]

In two cats given T-2 toxin by s.c. injection at doses of either 0.1 or 0.05 mg/kg at intervals up to 24 d, marked meningeal hemorrhage of the brain and extensive bleeding in the lung were found at post mortem.[36] In mature male domestic short-haired cats treated with T-2 toxin at 0.08/kg per os, 3 to 16 times at 48 h intervals, post-mortem observations included hemorrhagic lymph nodes, multiple hemorrhagic erosions on the gastric and intestinal mucosae, and petechial hemorrhages and ecchymoses on the myocardium.[80] Defective hemostasis was also observed in laboratory tests determined in four of the cats during the treatment period. The bleeding time increased from an initial mean value of 2.8 min to a mean of 12.3 min. The WBCT showed a similar prolongation, increasing from an initial value of 2.3 min to a mean of 15.5 min.[80]

H. Pig

In natural outbreaks of mycotoxicosis, hemorrhagic bowel syndrome has been associated with swine feeds contaminated with DAS at 380 and 500 μg/kg feed.[81] Hemorrhagic lesions of the stomach, heart, intestines, lungs, urinary bladder, and kidneys have been observed in pigs following the ingestion of moldy corn contaminated with T-2 toxin at 2 mg/kg dry corn.[82] Hemorrhagic lesions have also been reported in piglets given T-2 toxin at 0.2 mg/kg body weight by mouth or by i.m. injection[83] and in female swine given T-2 toxin by inhalation or by i.v. injection.[84,85] Pigs exposed to T-2 toxin at approximately 2 to 3 mg/kg body weight by inhalation and killed 8 to 10 h after dosing had extensive necrosis, congestion, edema, areas of hemorrhage, and fibrinoid degeneration of the vascular wall of the stomach.[84] In some animals, focal subepicardial hemorrhages were found in the left atrium, although no evidence of hemorrhage was found in the lungs. A single i.v. injection of T-2 toxin at 4.8 mg/kg body weight produced hemorrhagic lesions in the heart, stomach, adrenal glands, pancreas, and lymph nodes.[85] Despite this clinical evidence of hemorrhage, no changes were detected in the blood coagulation profile assessed by PT and APTT assays, activated coagulation time, fibrin degradation products, and platelet counts.[39] In pigs, the hemorrhagic response to T-2 toxin may be dose related since, not only was the evidence of hemorrhage less widespread and less severe in pigs given a single i.v. injection of T-2 toxin at 0.6 mg/kg body weight compared to animals which received 4.8 mg/kg, but also no clinical or pathologic evidence of hemorrhage was observed in studies in which pigs were treated i.v. with T-2 toxin at doses lower than 0.6 mg/kg body weight.[38,40]

A similar dose-related hemorrhagic response of pigs to DAS administration appears to exist.[35,42,43] Both male and female adult pigs given a single i.v. injection of DAS at 0.5 or 1.0 mg/kg body weight had evidence of severe hemorrhagic gastritis and hemorrhagic enteritis was also observed over the Peyer's patches in the intestinal tract.[35] Hemorrhagic lesions were also observed in the adrenal cortex, renal cortex, brain, and gall bladder. In contrast, piglets fed pure DAS at 0.1 mg/kg body weight for 36 days[42] or adult crossbred pigs fed a diet containing DAS up to 10 ppm for up to 9 weeks failed to develop an experimental hemorrhagic syndrome.[43] Similarly, no evidence of hemorrhage occurred in piglets fed diets containing DON at up to 43 ppm for 21 d[86] and the APTT and PT assays remained unchanged throughout the 21 d period.[87]

I. Sheep

Natural outbreaks of stachybotryotoxicosis in sheep have been characterized by clinical hemorrhagic problems.[88-90] In ewes that died after feeding on hay and straw contaminated with *Stachybotrys alternans*, nasal hemorrhages and hemorrhagic enteritis were consistent findings.[88] Following the consumption of wheat, barley, and rye straw contaminated with *S. chartarum*, ewes developed epitaxis and intermittent hemorrhagic diarrhea in the first phase of the disease.[89] In the second phase, the hemorrhage became less severe and anemia became the most predominant clinical sign. Hemorrhage was also one of the major autopsy findings in sheep that died following the ingestion of straw contaminated with *S. atra*.[90] Satratoxins G and H were isolated from this contaminated straw. The oral dosing of Romney sheep with cytotoxic cultures of *Myrothecium roridum* and *M. verrucaria* at lethal doses produced subepithelial hemorrhages in the omasal folds and submucosal hemorrhages in the abomasum.[91]

Post-mortem examination of mature sheep which had been given a single oral dose of T-2 toxin at dosages of 2.0 to 8.0 mg/kg body weight revealed multiple hemorrhages in s.c. tissue, myocardium, spleen and liver, and catarrhal hemorrhagic gastroenteritis.[45] In crossbred lambs fed T-2 toxin at 0.6 mg/kg/d, the PT assays became significantly prolonged within 7 d increasing to 12.8 ± 0.4 s compared to 11.4 ± 0.4 s in control animals.[44] The APTT assay was, however, unaffected by the inclusion of the toxin in the diet and no evidence of hemorrhage was observed in the lambs. The aggregation of ovine platelets suspended in homologous plasma and stimulated with either collagen, ADP, serotonin, or arachidonic acid as aggregating agents is significantly reduced when T-2 toxin is present in the platelet suspension at concentrations of 25 to 100 μg/ml.[92] Because of the levels of toxin required to inhibit platelet function *in vitro*, the contribution of platelet dysfunction to the hemorrhagic condition remains to be clarified.

J. Cow

Compared to other species, the hemostatic mechanism of cattle appears sensitive to impairment by trichothecenes ingested in moldy feed. The principle lesions observed in 7 lactating cows that died following the chronic ingestion of moldy corn, containing at least 2 ppm T-2 toxin, were extensive hemorrhages on the serosal surfaces of all internal viscera.[93] Bloody stools have been associated with the ingestion of mixed feed containing 76 μg T-2 toxin.[81] In a herd of Hereford cattle, hemorrhagic diarrhea and epitaxis occurred in addition to excessive hemorrhage following castration and dehorning of the 220 kg feeder calves.[94] In two of the adult cows that died, extensive serosal, mucosal, and s.c. hemorrhages were found and unclotted blood could be collected from the carotid artery. The PT was prolonged in affected animals. Analysis of feed samples by thin-layer chromatography (TLC) indicated that T-2 toxin or a T-2 toxin-like toxin was present; however, no other confirmatory tests were performed on the feed. In another commercial feed lot operation, uncontrolled bleeding occurred in 200 kg beef calves following dehorning and castration and the only effective therapy appeared to be whole blood transfusions.[95] The most obvious changes in the coagulation profile were a prolongation of the WBCT and a reduction in the activity of factor VII. The administration of vit K was followed by an increase in factor VII activity, but presumably the contaminated feed was also withdrawn from the diet. In this incident *F. tricinctum* was isolated from the feed and a T-2 toxin-like mycotoxin was identified using a biological assay. The major clinical features in an outbreak of mycotoxicosis, which resulted in the deaths of 9 of 115 dairy cows, were bloody diarrhea and multiple petechial hemorrhages of the mucous membranes.[96] Although *F. tricinctum* was not cultured from any of the feed samples, TLC revealed the presence of T-2 toxin.

In outbreaks of stachybotryotoxicosis in young cattle, caused by straw and hay contaminated with *Stachybotrys alternans*, post-mortem examination revealed large hemorrhages in the musculature, s.c. connective tissue, and both serous and mucous membranes.[97] In a 114 kg calf given 2.5 kg of straw contaminated with *S. atra* for 14 d, the WBCT increased from 9 to 19 min and a pronounced increase was observed in the clot retraction time.[98]

Despite the severe hemorrhagic syndromes induced by natural outbreaks of mycotoxicosis, attempts to duplicate the syndrome in experimental studies have produced only mixed results. Following the daily i.m. injection of pure T-2 toxin at 0.1 mg/kg body weight to a 295 kg steer for 64 d, the animal developed a thin bloody discharge from both nostrils, and by the 65th day the animal developed bloody feces and died.[99] A clotting time taken 12 h before death was 6 to 7 times normal. On postmortem examination, petechial and ecchymotic hemorrhages of the epicardium, endocardium, and small intestine were observed. Similar results were produced in a 300 kg heifer treated daily with 0.06 to 0.24 but usually 0.12 mg T-2 toxin per kilogram for 2 months.[100] Toward the end of the treatment period, the PT had markedly increased from 55 to 200 s. In a separate study, bloody feces developed in a Jersey calf treated orally with T-2 toxin at 0.64 mg/kg/d for 20 d and in a second calf treated with 0.32 mg toxin/kg/d for 30 d. In both calves the clinicopathological changes were restricted to increased plasma PT results.[101]

The development of the hemorrhagic syndrome may depend on both the dose and duration of exposure of cattle to T-2 toxin since, in a number of studies, no evidence of hemorrhage has been produced under conditions in which T-2 toxin has caused changes in blood parameters, including the coagulation profile.[42,46,48,51] The APTT assay was consistently prolonged and the PT assay frequently prolonged in Friesian calves dosed orally with T-2 toxin at 0.2 mg/kg/d either in whole culture extracts of *F. tricinctum* for 78 d or in purified form for

11 d.[42] The calves treated with purified toxin developed clinical signs of weakness and inappetance before death. The APTT assay was increased from a mean of 55.6 ± 5.7 to 89.6 ± 16.3 s, while the mean PT result was increased only to 23.3 ± 1.7 s from an initial value of 17.8 ± 12.5 s. In this study, the administration of pure DAS at 0.2 mg/kg body weight daily for 11 d produced no alteration in the coagulation parameters of the calves. Similarly, the single i.v. administration of T-2 toxin at 0.25 mg/kg body weight to 2- to 3-week-old calves produced only transient, small increases in the APTT and PT results.[51] Despite the lack of alteration in these assays, the biological activity of specific coagulation factors was significantly depressed by the toxin treatment. Between 6 and 24 h after the toxin injection the plasma activity of factors VII, IX, X, and XI was reduced by at least 40%, while plasma fibrinogen fell from an initial value of 4.8 ± 1.1 g/l to 3.7 ± 1.3 g/l. Factor VIII was the only coagulant protein measured which did not appear to be affected by the toxin.

It therefore seems that the lack of clinical hemorrhage in many trichothecene exposed cattle may be related to the limited extent of the increase in the clotting times. Since calves receiving oral doses of 25 mg vit K per kilogram prior to and during toxin treatment developed identical changes in the coagulation parameters as was found in the calves with no vit K supplement, it was concluded that as suggested for the guinea pig and rabbit, T-2 toxin does not act as a vit K antagonist in the bovine species.[51] It was also concluded that the action of T-2 toxin was not mediated through direct impairment of protein synthesis in the liver because there is normally a wide variation in the biological half-lives of the coagulation proteins while there was marked uniformity in the response of the activity of these proteins to T-2 toxin.

The addition of T-2 toxin, HT-2 toxin, DAS, or DON to bovine platelet rich plasma *in vitro* produces a dose-dependent decrease in the ability of the platelets to aggregate in response to the aggregating agents ADP, collagen, and platelet activating factor.[102,103] Although T-2 toxin inhibits thromboxane B_2 release from both ADP and collagen stimulated platelets this does not appear to be the primary inhibitory mechanism in bovine platelets.[104] While aggregation induced by platelet activating factor appears most sensitive to impairment, as was discussed for ovine platelets, the concentrations of T-2 toxin and HT-2 toxin are sufficiently high (15 and 8 μg/ml, respectively) that the relevance of these results in relation to the mycotoxin exposure of the intact animal has yet to be resolved.

K. Monkeys

Although clinical signs of toxicosis developed in both male and female Rhesus monkeys given T-2 toxin at 1 mg/kg for 5 d, only the males developed petechial hemorrhages of the face.[52] The administration of pure T-2 toxin as a single i.m. injection to adult male cynomolgus monkeys at 0.65 mg/kg body weight produced a progressive increase in both PT and APTT assays which reached a maximum 24 h after treatment.[54] A concomitant transient decrease in the biological activities of specific coagulation proteins, factors V, VII, VIII, IX, X, XI, XII, and prothrombin and in fibrinogen values was observed with a nadir occurring 24 h postinfusion. Of the 9 monkeys in the study, 3 died after receiving T-2 toxin, and although none had clinical evidence of hemorrhage, at necropsy mild petechial hemorrhages involving the colon and heart were present.[54]

L. Man

In man, the disorder alimentary toxic aleukia (ATA), has been documented following the ingestion of overwintered moldy grain or its by-products likely to have been contaminated with trichothecenes produced by *F. sporotrichioides*.[1,105] The clinical features of ATA can be divided into four stages and hematologic and hemorrhagic abnormalities appear during the second and third stages. During the second stage, a decrease in RBC, platelets, and hemoglobin occurs along with progressive leukopenia and the decrease continues into the third stage when the RBC may drop to $\leq 1.0 \times 10^3/\mu l$, the hemoglobin may be as low as 10 g/dl, and the platelet count may drop to $25 \times 10^3/ml$, although counts as low as 3.0 to $5.0 \times 10^3/ml$ have been found. A return of bone marrow function characterizes the beginning of the fourth or convalescent stage. The WBC count rises first, followed by platelets and RBC, and over a 2-month period all of the parameters slowly return to normal. The development of petechial hemorrhages on the skin and mucous membranes occurs during the transition from the second to the third stage of the disease. Increased capillary fragility is believed to result in hematoma development from the slightest trauma. As in the animal studies, the hemorrhagic condition is not reflected by marked alterations in the coagulation profile. The bleeding and clotting times are not excessively prolonged with the PT, ranging from 23 to 56 s. A deficiency of plasma fibrinogen has been reported in severely affected individuals. The hemorrhagic problems are resolved within 2 weeks of the withdrawal of the contaminated products from the diet.[1] Many of the effects of ATA in man have been duplicated in cats following administration of T-2 toxin.[106]

During the late 1970s and early 1980s, there have been reports from Southeast Asia of people becoming ill and developing various clinical signs, including skin irritation, dizziness, nausea, vomiting of blood, diarrhea, and hemorrhaging following exposure to a "yellow-rain"-like material.[107-110] The trichothecene mycotoxins, T-2 toxin, DAS, and DON have been identified in some samples of the yellow-rain material.[111,112] It has also been shown that isolates of six *Fusarium* spp. collected in Southeast Asia from plant and soil samples can produce T-2 toxin, HT-2 toxin, neosolaniol, DAS, monoacetoxyscirpenol, and fusarenon-X in various combinations and amounts when grown in liquid cultures or on rice;[113] however, the causative agent(s) for the mycotoxicosis reported among the human population have not been fully elucidated. While some of the clinical signs are similar to those of ATA[105-110] and are similar to those induced experimentally by T-2 toxin and DAS in swine,[35,83,84,114] the clinical signs are also consistent with stachybotryotoxicosis, a disease caused by macrocyclic trichothecenes.[108]

When human platelets are incubated *in vitro* with T-2 toxin at 37°C for 15 min, a dose-dependent inhibition of aggregation induced by epinephrine, arachidonic acid, and collagen occurs with toxin at above $50 \ \mu g/10^9$ platelets suspended in plasma.[115] Platelet aggregation is slightly enhanced by T-2 toxin in amounts ranging from 10 to $150 \ \mu g/10^9$ platelets; however, aggregation is inhibited or abolished by all aggregating agents when the T-2 toxin concentration is increased to $\geq 300 \ \mu g/10^9$ platelets. Histologic examination of the T-2 toxin-treated human platelets indicated that the toxin induced an alteration in membrane permeability and a dose-related release of dense bodies consisting mainly of serotonin-containing granules. The microtubules or cytoskeleton of the platelets were unaffected by the toxin treatment.[115]

IV. SUMMARY

Investigations of the effects of trichothecene mycotoxins on hematologic and coagulation parameters have been mainly concerned with T-2 toxin. In poultry, laboratory animals, dogs, and cats, the general hematologic response to T-2 toxin is a reduction in RBC and platelet counts which is usually less than the reduction in total WBC counts. Both hematologic and coagulation parameters of chickens are sensitive to T-2 toxin. The effects of T-2 toxin on bone marrow in mice, rats, and cats are reversible — so much so that recovery of RBC and platelet production can occur while the animals are still ingesting toxin. In both man and Rhesus monkeys thrombocytopenia is a consistent observation after exposure to DAS and T-2 toxin, respectively, while RBC counts are relatively unaffected. RBC and platelet production in pigs and cattle appear to be relatively insensitive to the effects of T-2 toxin;

however, the hemostatic mechanism of cattle seems to be subject to impairment by T-2 toxin. The biological activity of specific coagulation factors are markedly depressed by T-2 toxin in calves, monkeys, rabbits, and guinea pigs, but the amount of T-2 toxin required to produce the effects in calves is 50% of that required in rabbits, 40% of that required in monkeys, and 25% of that required in guinea pigs. Overall it can be concluded that T-2 toxin does not act as a vit K antagonist. In all species, the depression of coagulant activity induced by the toxin in experimental studies is inadequate to explain the hemorrhagic syndrome observed in natural outbreaks of trichothecene mycotoxicosis. Despite the variation in responses of different species to experimental trichothecene exposures, the hemorrhagic problems associated with natural routes of intoxication are among the most consistent clinical and pathologic findings in all species. The possibility of interaction between various trichothecenes and other related and unrelated metabolites in mold-infested foodstuffs may therefore deserve further study.

REFERENCES

1. **Forgacs, J. and Carll, W. T.,** Mycotoxicoses, *Adv. Vet. Sci.,* 7, 273, 1962.
2. **Gentry, P. A. and Downie, H. G.,** Blood Coagulation, in *Duke's Physiology of Domestic Animals,* 10th ed., Swenson, M. J., Ed., Cornell University Press, Ithaca, NY, 1984, chap. 3.
3. **Schalm, O. W., Jain, N. C., and Carroll, E. J.,** *Veterinary Hematology,* Lea & Febiger, Philadelphia, 1975, chap. 3.
4. **Mitruka, B. M. and Rawnsley, H. M.,** *Clinical Biochemical and Hematological Reference Values in Normal Experimental Animals,* Masson, New York, 1977, 71.
5. **Poston, H. A., Coffin, J. L., and Combs, G. F.,** Biological effects of dietary T-2 toxin on rainbow trout, *Salmo Gairdneri, Aquat. Toxicol.,* 2, 79, 1982.
6. **Hayes, M. A. and Wobeser, G. A.,** Subacute toxic effects of dietary T-2 toxin in young Mallard ducks, *Can. J. Comp. Med.,* 47, 180, 1983.
7. **Ueno, Y., Ueno, I., Iitoi, Y., Tsunoda, H., Enomoto, M., and Ohtsubo, K.,** Toxicological approaches to the metabolites of *Fusaria.* III. Acute toxicity of Fusarenon-X, *Jpn. J. Exp. Med.,* 41, 521, 1971.
8. **Wyatt, R. D., Hamilton, P. B., and Burmeister, H. R.,** The effects of T-2 toxin in broiler chickens, *Poult. Sci.,* 52, 1853, 1973.
9. **Chi, M. S., Mirocha, C. J., Kurtz, H. J., Weaver, G., Bates, F., Shimoda, W., and Burmeister, H. R.,** Acute toxicity of T-2 toxin in broiler chicks and laying hens, *Poult. Sci.,* 56, 103, 1977.
10. **Chi, M. S., Mirocha, C. J., Kurtz, H. J., Weaver, G., Bates, F., and Shimoda, W.,** Subacute toxicity of T-2 toxin in broiler chicks, *Poult. Sci.,* 56, 306, 1977.
11. **Chi, M. S., El-Halawani, M. E., Waibel, P. E., and Mirocha, C. J.,** Effects of T-2 toxin on brain catecholamines and selected blood components in growing chickens, *Poult. Sci.,* 60, 137, 1981.
12. **Hoerr, F. J., Carlton, W. W., Yagen, B., and Joffe, A. Z.,** Mycotoxicosis produced in broiler chickens by multiple doses of either T-2 toxin or diacetoxyscirpenol, *Avian Pathol.,* 11, 369, 1982.
13. **Hoerr, F. J., Carlton, W. W., and Yagen, B.,** Mycotoxicosis caused by a single dose of T-2 toxin or diacetoxyscirpenol in broiler chickens, *Vet. Pathol.,* 18, 652, 1981.
14. **Wyatt, R. D., Doerr, J. A., Hamilton, P. B., and Burmeister, H. R.,** Egg production, shell thickness, and other physiological parameters of laying hens affected by T-2 toxin, *Appl. Microbiol.,* 29, 641, 1975.
15. **Speers, G. M., Mirocha, C. J., Christensen, C. M., and Behrens, J. C.,** Effects on laying hens of feeding corn invaded by two species of *Fusarium* and pure T-2 mycotoxin, *Poult. Sci.,* 56, 98, 1977.
16. **Saito, N., Ito, T., Kumada, H., Ueno, Y., Asano, K., Saito, M., Ohtsubo, K., Ueno, I., and Hatanaka, Y.,** Toxicological approaches to the metabolites of Fusaria. XIII. Hematological changes in mice by a single and repeated administrations of trichothecenes, *J. Toxicol. Sci.,* 3, 335, 1978.
17. **Hayes, M. A., Bellamy, J. E. C., and Schiefer, H. B.,** Subacute toxicity of dietary T-2 toxin in mice: morphological and hematological effects, *Can. J. Comp. Med.,* 44, 203, 1980.
18. **Hayes, M. A. and Schiefer, H. B.,** Subacute toxicity of dietary T-2 toxin in mice: influence of protein nutrition, *Can. J. Comp. Med.,* 44, 219, 1980.
19. **Hayes, M. A. and Schiefer, H. B.,** Comparative toxicity of dietary T-2 toxin in rats and mice, *J. Appl. Toxicol.,* 2, 207, 1982.
20. **Schiefer, H. B., Nicholson, S., Kasali, O. B., Hancock, D. S., and Greenhalgh, R.,** Pathology of acute 3-acetoxydeoxynivalenol toxicity in mice, *Can. J. Comp. Med.,* 49, 315, 1985.

21. **Kasali, O. B., Schiefer, H. B., Hancock, D. S., Blakley, B. R., Tomar, R. S., and Greenhalgh, R.,** Subacute toxicity of dietary 3-acetyldeoxynivalenol in mice, *Can. J. Comp. Med.,* 49, 319, 1985.
22. **Yarom, R., Sherman, Y., More, R., Ginsburg, I., Borinski, R., and Yagen, B.,** T-2 toxin effect on bacterial infection and leukocyte functions, *Toxicol. Appl. Pharmacol.,* 75, 60, 1984.
23. **Chan, P. K.-C. and Gentry, P. A.,** LD50 values and serum biochemical changes induced by T-2 toxin in rats and rabbits, *Toxicol. Appl. Pharmacol.,* 73, 402, 1984.
24. **Schoental, R. and Gibbard, S.,** Increased excretion of urinary porphyrins by white rats given intragastrically the chemical carcinogens diethylnitrosamine, monocrotaline, T-2 toxin and ethylmethanesulphonate, *Biochem. Soc. Trans.,* 7, 127, 1979.
25. **Segal, R., Milo-Goldzweig, I., Joffe, A. Z., and Yagen, B.,** Trichothecene-induced hemolysis. I. The hemolytic activity of T-2 toxin, *Toxicol. Appl. Pharmacol.,* 70, 343, 1983.
26. **Matsuoka, Y., Kubota, K., and Ueno, Y.,** General pharmacological studies of Fusarenon-X, a trichothecene mycotoxin from *Fusarium* species, *Toxicol. Appl. Pharmacol.,* 50, 87, 1979.
27. **Saito, M. and Ohtsubo, K.,** Trichothecene toxins of Fusarium species, in *Mycotoxins,* Purchase, I. F. H., Ed., Elsevier, New York, 1974, chap. 12.
28. **Saito, M., Horiuchi, T., Ohtsubo, K., Hatanaka, Y., and Ueno, Y.,** Low tumor incidence in rats with long-term feeding of Fusarenon-X, a cytotoxic trichothecene produced by *Fusarium nivale, Jpn. J. Exp. Med.,* 50, 293, 1980.
29. **DeNicola, D. B., Rebar, A. H., Carlton, W. W., and Yagen, B.,** T-2 toxin mycotoxicosis in the guinea-pig, *Food Cosmet. Toxicol.,* 16, 601, 1978.
30. **Cosgriff, T. M., Bunner, D. P., Wannemacher, R. W., Jr., Hodgson, L. A., and Dinterman, R. E.,** The hemostatic derangement produced by T-2 toxin in guinea pigs, *Toxicol. Appl. Pharmacol.,* 76, 454, 1984.
31. **Gyongyossy-Issa, M. I. C., Khanna, V., and Khachatourians, G. G.,** Characterization of hemolysis induced by T-2 toxin, *Biochim. Biophys. Acta,* 838, 252, 1985.
32. **Gentry, P. A. and Cooper, M. L.,** Effect of Fusarium T-2 toxin on hematological and biochemical parameters in the rabbit, *Can. J. Comp. Med.,* 45, 400, 1981.
33. **Gentry, P. A.,** The effect of administration of a single dose of T-2 toxin on blood coagulation in the rabbit, *Can. J. Comp. Med.,* 46, 414, 1982.
34. **Murphy, W. K., Burgess, M. A., Valdivieso, M., Livingston, R. B., Bodey, G. P., and Freireich, E. J.,** Phase I clinical evaluation of anguidine, *Cancer Treat. Rep.,* 62, 1497, 1978.
35. **Coppock, R. W.,** Studies on the Pharmacokinetics and Toxicopathy of Diacetoxyscirpenol and Deoxynivalenol in Swine, Cattle and Dogs, Ph.D. thesis, University of Illinois, Urbana-Champaign, 1984.
36. **Sato, N., Ueno, Y., and Enomoto, M.,** Toxicological approaches to the toxic metabolites of *Fusaria.* VIII. Acute and subacute toxicities of T-2 toxin in cats, *Jpn. J. Pharmacol.,* 25, 263, 1975.
37. **Lutsky, I., Mor, N., Yagen, B., and Joffe, A. Z.,** The role of T-2 toxin in experimental alimentary toxic aleukia: a toxicity study in cats, *Toxicol Appl. Pharmacol.,* 43, 111, 1978.
38. **Weaver, G. A., Kurtz, H. J., Bates, F. Y., Chi, M. S., Mirocha, C. J., Behrens, J. C., and Robison, T. S.,** Acute and chronic toxicity of T-2 mycotoxin in swine, *Vet. Rec.,* 103, 531, 1978.
39. **Lorenzana, R. M., Beasley, V. R., Buck, W. B., and Ghent, A. W.,** Experimental T-2 toxicosis in swine. II. Effect of intravascular T-2 toxin on serum enzymes and biochemistry, blood coagulation, and hematology, *Fundam. Appl. Toxicol.,* 5, 893, 1985.
40. **Weaver, G. A., Kurtz, H. J., Mirocha, C. J., Bates, F. Y., Behrens, J. C., Robinson, T. S., and Gipp, W. F.,** Mycotoxin-induced abortions in swine, *Can. Vet. J.,* 19, 72, 1978.
41. **Weaver, G. A., Kurtz, H. J., Mirocha, C. J., Bates, F. Y., Behrens, J. C., and Robison, T. S.,** Effect of T-2 toxin on porcine reproduction, *Can. Vet. J.,* 19, 310, 1978.
42. **Patterson, D. S. P., Matthews, J. G., Shreeve, B. J., Roberts, B. A., McDonald, S. M., and Hayes, A. W.,** The failure of trichothecene mycotoxins and whole cultures of *Fusarium tricinctum* to cause experimental haemorrhagic syndromes in calves and pigs, *Vet. Rec.,* 105, 252, 1979.
43. **Weaver, G. A., Kurtz, H. J., Bates, F. Y., Mirocha, C. J., Behrens, J. C., and Hagler, W. M.,** Diacetoxyscirpenol toxicity in pigs, *Res. Vet. Sci.,* 31, 131, 1981.
44. **Friend, S. C. E., Hancock, D. S., Schiefer, H. B., and Babiuk, L. A.,** Experimental T-2 toxicosis in sheep, *Can. J. Comp. Med.,* 47, 291, 1983.
45. **Rukhlyada, V. V.,** Effect of *Fusarium sporotrichiella* T-2 toxin on sheep, *Veterinariya,* 5, 61, 1983.
46. **Weaver, G. A., Kurtz, H. J., Mirocha, C. J., Bates, F. Y., Behrens, J. C., Robison, T. S., and Swanson, S. P.,** The failure of purified T-2 mycotoxin to produce hemorrhaging in dairy cattle, *Can. Vet. J.,* 21, 210, 1980.
47. **Gentry, P. A., Ross, M. L., and Chan, P. K.-C.,** Effect of T-2 toxin on bovine hematological and serum enzyme parameters, *Vet. Hum. Toxicol.,* 26, 24, 1984.
48. **Osweiler, G. D., Hook, B. S., Mann, D. D., Buening, G. M., and Rottinghaus, G. E.,** Effects of T-2 in cattle, *Proc. Annu. Meet. U.S. Anim. Health Assoc.,* 85, 214, 1981.

49. **Buening, G. M., Mann, D. D., Hook, B., and Osweiler, G. D.,** The effect of T-2 toxin on the bovine immune system: cellular factors, *Vet. Immunol. Immunopathol.,* 3, 411, 1982.

50. **Mann, D. D., Buening, G. M., Hook, B., and Osweiler, G. D.,** Effects of T-2 mycotoxin on bovine serum proteins, *Am. J. Vet. Res.,* 44, 1757, 1983.

51. **Gentry, P. A. and Cooper, M. L.,** Effect of intravenous administration of T-2 toxin on blood coagulation in calves, *Am. J. Vet. Res.,* 44, 741, 1983.

52. **Rukmini, C., Prasad, J. S., and Rao, K.,** Effects of feeding T-2 toxin to rats and monkeys, *Food Cosmet. Toxicol.,* 18, 267, 1980.

53. **Jagadeesan, V., Rukmini, C., Vijayaraghavan, M., and Tulpule, P. G.,** Immune studies with T-2 toxin: effect of feeding and withdrawal in monkeys, *Food Chem. Toxicol.,* 20, 83, 1982.

54. **Cosgriff, T. M., Bunner, D. P., Wannemacher, R. W., Hodgson, L. A., and Dinterman, R. E.,** The hemostatic derangement produced by T-2 toxin in Cynomolgus monkeys, *Toxicol. Appl. Pharmacol.,* 82, 539, 1985.

55. **Thigpen, J. T., Vaughn, C., and Stuckey, W. J.,** Phase II trial of anguidine in patients with sarcomas unresponsive to prior chemotherapy: a southwest oncology group study, *Cancer Treat. Rep.,* 65, 881, 1981.

56. **Bukowski, R., Vaugh, C., Bottomley, R., and Chen, T.,** Phase II study of anguidine in gastrointestinal malignancies, *Cancer Treat. Rep.,* 66, 381, 1982.

57. **Adler, S. S., Lowenbraun, S., Birch, B., Jarrell, R., and Garrard, J.,** Anguidine: a broad phase II study of the Southeastern cancer study group, *Cancer Treat. Rep.,* 68, 423, 1984.

58. **Yap, H. Y., Murphy, W. K., DiStefano, A., Blumenschein, G. R., and Bodey, G. P.,** Phase II study of anguidine in advanced breast cancer, *Cancer Treat. Rep.,* 63, 789, 1979.

59. **DeSimone, P. A., Greco, F. A., and Lessner, H. F.,** Phase I evaluation of a weekly schedule of anguidine, *Cancer Treat. Rep.,* 63, 2015, 1979.

60. **Goodwin, W., Stephens, R., McCracken, J. D., and Groppe, C.,** Therapy for advanced colorectal cancer with a combination of 5-FU and anguidine: a southwest oncology group study, *Cancer Treat. Rep.,* 65, 359, 1981.

61. **Goodwin, W., Haas, C. D., Fabian, C., Bettinger, I. H., and Hoogstraten, B.,** Phase I evaluation of anguidine (diacetoxyscirpenol, NSC-141537), *Cancer,* 42, 23, 1978.

62. **Belt, R. J., Haas, C. D., Joseph, U., Goodwin, W., Moore, D., and Hoogstraten, B.,** Phase I study of anguidine administered weekly, *Cancer Treat. Rep.,* 63, 1993, 1979.

63. **Marasas, W. F. O., Bamburg, J. R., Smalley, E. B., Strong, F. M., Ragland, W. L., and Degurse, P. E.,** Toxic effects on trout, rats and mice of T-2 toxin produced by the fungus *Fusarium tricinctum* (Cd.) Snyd. et Hans., *Toxicol. Appl. Pharmacol.,* 15, 471, 1969.

64. **Woodward, B., Young, L. G., and Lun, A. K.,** Vomitoxin in diets for rainbow trout (*Salmo Gairdneri*), *Aquaculture,* 35, 93, 1983.

65. **Palyusik, M. and Kovacs, E. K.,** Effect of feed containing T_2 and F_2 toxins on laying geese, *Magyar Allatorvosok Lagja,* 30, 842, 1975.

66. **Greenway, J. A. and Puls, R.,** Fusariotoxicosis from barley in British Columbia. I. Natural occurrence and diagnosis, *Can. J. Comp. Med.,* 40, 12, 1976.

67. **Puls, R. and Greenway, J. A.,** Fusariotoxicosis from barley in British Columbia. II. Analysis and toxicity of suspected barley, *Can. J. Comp. Med.,* 40, 16, 1976.

68. **Pearson, A. W.,** Biochemical changes produced by *Fusarium* T-2 toxin in the chicken, *Res. Vet. Sci.* 24, 92, 1978.

69. **Huff, W. E., Doerr, J. A., Hamilton, P. B., and Vesonder, R. F.,** Acute toxicity of vomitoxin (deoxynivalenol) in broiler chickens, *Poult. Sci.,* 60, 1412, 1981.

70. **Doerr, J. A., Huff, W. E., Tung, H. T., Wyatt, R. D., and Hamilton, P. B.,** A survey of T-2 toxin, ochratoxin, and aflatoxin for their effects on the coagulation of blood in young broiler chickens, *Poult. Sci.,* 53, 1728, 1974.

71. **Doerr, J. A., Hamilton, P. B., and Burmeister, H. R.,** T-2 toxicosis and blood coagulation in young chickens, *Toxicol. Appl. Pharmacol.,* 60, 157, 1981.

72. **Ueno, Y., Sato, N., Ishii, K., Sakai, K., and Enomoto, M.,** Toxicological approaches to the metabolites of *Fusaria*. V. neosolaniol, T-2 toxin and butenolide, toxic metabolites of *Fusarium sporotrichioides* NRRL 3510 and *Fusarium poae* 3287, *Jpn. J. Exp. Med.,* 42, 461, 1972.

73. **Rousseaux, C. G., Nicholson, S., and Schiefer, H. B.,** Fatal placental hemorrhage in pregnant CD-1 mice following one oral dose of T-2 toxin, *Can. J. Comp. Med.,* 49, 95, 1985.

74. **Ueno, Y., Ueno, I., Tatsuno, T., Ohokubo, K., and Tsunoda, H.,** Fusarenon-X, a toxic principle of *Fusarium nivale*-culture filtrate, *Experientia,* 25, 1062, 1969.

75. **Kosuri, N. R., Smalley, E. B., and Nichols, R. E.,** Toxicologic studies of *Fusarium tricinctum* (Corda) Snyder et Hansen from moldy corn, *Am. J. Vet. Res.,* 32, 1843, 1971.

76. **Smalley, E. B., Marasas, W. F. O., Strong, F. M., Bamburg, J. R., Nichols, R. E., and Kosuri, N. R.,** Mycotoxicoses associated with moldy corn, in *Proc. 1 U.S.-Japan Conference on Toxic Micro-Organisms,* Herzberg, M., Ed., UJNR Joint Panels on Toxic Micro-Organisms and the U.S. Department of the Interior, Washington, D.C., 1970.

77. **Tremel, H., Strugala, G., Forth, W., and Fichtl, B.,** Dexamethasone decreases lethality of rats in acute poisoning with T-2 toxin, *Arch. Toxicol.,* 57, 74, 1985.
78. **Abbas, H. K., Mirocha, C. J., and Shier, W. J.,** Mycotoxins produced from fungi isolated from foodstuffs and soil: comparison of toxicity in fibroblasts and rat feeding tests, *Appl. Environ. Microbiol.,* 48, 654, 1984.
79. **Tremel, H., Szinicz, L., Fichtl, B., and Fortn, W.,** Blood coagulation disorders in rabbits following acute poisoning with T-2 toxin, in *Proc. 6th Eur. Symp. Animal, Plant and Microbial Toxins,* Meier, J., Stocker, K., Freyvogel, T. A., Eds., 1984.
80. **Lutsky, I. and Mor, N.,** Experimental alimentary toxic aleukia in cats, *Lab. Anim. Sci.,* 31, 43, 1981.
81. **Mirocha, C. J., Pathre, S. V., Schauerhamer, B., and Christensen, C. M.,** Natural occurrence of *Fusarium* toxins in feedstuff, *Appl. Environ. Microbiol.,* 32, 553, 1976.
82. **Smalley, E. B.,** T-2 toxin, *J. Am. Vet. Med. Assoc.,* 163, 1278, 1973.
83. **Elistratov, I. S., Bespalov, V. L., Kaplun, V. I., Kolyvanova, G. E., and Bordyug, V. F.,** Fusari-otoxicosis of swine and its prevention, *Veterinariya,* 5, 63, 1984.
84. **Pang, V., Haschek, W., Lambert, R., Biehl, M., Beasley, V., and Buck, W.,** unpublished data, 1985.
85. **Pang, V., Hascheck, W., Lorenzana, R., Beasley, V., and Buck, W.,** unpublished data, 1985.
86. **Young, L. G., McGirr, L., Valli, V. E., Lumsden, J. H., and Lun, A.,** Vomitoxin in corn fed to young pigs, *J. Anim. Sci.,* 57, 655, 1983.
87. **Gentry, P. A.,** unpublished data, 1986.
88. **Danko, G.,** *Stachybotrys* toxicosis of sheep, *Magyar Allatorvosok Lagja,* 31, 226, 1976.
89. **Schneider, D. J., Marasas, W. F. O., Kuys, J. C. D., Kriek, N. P. J., and van Schalkwyk, G. C.,** A field outbreak of suspected stachybotryotoxicosis in sheep, *J. South Afr. Vet. Assoc.,* 50, 73, 1979.
90. **Harrach, B., Bata, A., Bajmocy, E., and Benko, M.,** Isolation of satratoxins from the bedding straw of a sheep flock with fatal Stachybotryotoxicosis, *Appl. Environ. Microbiol.,* 45, 1419, 1983.
91. **Mortimer, P. H., Campbell, J., DiMenna, M. E., and White, E. P.,** Experimental myrotheciotoxicosis and poisoning in ruminants by Verrucarin A and Roridin A, *Res. Vet. Sci.,* 12, 508, 1971.
92. **Gentry, P. A., Socha, A., and Ross, M. L.,** Ovine platelet function and its inhibition by T-2 toxin, *Vet. Res. Commun.,* 11, 457, 1987.
93. **Hsu, I.-C., Smalley, E. B., Strong, F. M., and Ribelin, W. E.,** Identification of T-2 toxin in moldy corn associated with a lethal toxicosis in dairy cattle, *Appl. Microbiol.,* 24, 684, 1972.
94. **Hibbs, C. M., Osweiler, G. D., Buck, W. B., and Macfee, G. P.,** Bovine hemorrhagic syndrome related to T-2 mycotoxin, in *Proc. 17th Annu. Meet. Am. Assoc. Vet. Lab. Diagnosticians,* 1974, 305.
95. **Dahlgren, R. R. and Williams, D. E.,** Clinical report: hemorrhagic syndrome in feedlot cattle, *Bovine Pract.,* 7, 52, 1972.
96. **Petrie, L., Robb, J., and Stewart, A. F.,** The identification of T-2 toxin and its association with a haemorrhagic syndrome in cattle, *Vet. Rec.,* 101, 326, 1977.
97. **Danko, G.,** Stachybotryotoxicosis of cattle in Hungary, *Magyar Allatorvosok Lagja,* 27, 241, 1972.
98. **Forgacs, J.,** Stachybotryotoxicosis, in *Microbial Toxins VIII Fungal Toxins,* Kadis, S., Ciegler, A., and Ajl, S. J., Eds., Academic Press, New York, 1972, chap. 4.
99. **Grove, M. D., Yates, S. G., Tallent, W. H., Ellis, J. J., Wolff, I. A., Kosuri, N. R., and Nichols, R. E.,** Mycotoxins produced by *Fusarium tricinctum* as possible causes of cattle disease, *J. Agric. Food Chem.,* 18, 734, 1970.
100. **Kosuri, N. R., Grove, M. D., Yates, S. G., Tallent, W. H., Ellis, J. J., Wolff, I. A., and Nichols, R. E.,** Response of cattle to mycotoxins of *Fusarium tricinctum* isolated from corn and fescue, *J. Am. Vet. Med. Assoc.,* 157, 938, 1970.
101. **Pier, A. C., Cysewski, S. J., Richard, J. L., Baetz, A. L., and Mitchell, L.,** Experimental mycotoxicoses in calves with aflatoxin, ochratoxin, rubratoxin, and T-2 toxin, *Annu. Meet. U.S. Anim. Health Assoc.,* 130, 1976.
102. **Chan, P. K.-C. and Gentry, P. A.,** Inhibition of bovine platelet function by T-2 toxin, HT-2 toxin, diacetoxyscirpenol and deoxynivalenol, *Food Chem. Toxic.,* 22, 643, 1984.
103. **Gentry, P. A.,** unpublished data, 1986.
104. **Bondy, G. S. and Gentry, P. A.,** The effects of T-2 toxin alone and in combination with known platelet inhibitors on platelet function in vitro. *Proc. Can. Fed. Biol. Sci.* 29, 167, 1986.
105. **Gajdusek, D. C.,** Acute infectious hemorrhagic fevers and mycotoxicoses in the Union of Soviet Socialist Republics, *Medical Science Publication 2,* Walter Reed Army Medical Center, Washington, D.C., 1953.
106. **Lutsky, I. I. and Mor, N.,** Alimentary toxic aleukia (septic angina, endemic panmyelotoxicosis, alimentary hemorrhagic aleukia) T-2 toxin-induced intoxication of cats, *Am. J. Pathol.,* 104, 189, 1981.
107. **Haig, A. M.,** *Chemical Warfare in Southeast Asia and Afghanistan,* Spec. Rep. No. 98, U.S. Department of State, Washington, D.C., 1982.
108. **Schiefer, H. B.,** A Study of Possible Use of Chemical Warfare Agents in Southeast Asia, A Report to the Department of External Affairs, DEA, Ottawa, Canada, 1982.
109. **Marshall, E.,** Yellow rain: filling in the gaps, *Science,* 217, 31, 1982.

110. **Spyker, M. S. and Spyker, D. A.,** Yellow rain: chemical warfare in Southeast Asia and Afghanistan, *Vet. Hum. Toxicol.*, 25, 335, 1983.
111. **Mirocha, C. J., Pawlosky, R. A., Chatterjee, K., Watson, S., and Hayes, W.,** Analysis for *Fusarium* toxins in various samples implicated in biological warfare in Southeast Asia, *J. Assoc. Off. Anal. Chem.*, 66, 1485, 1983.
112. **Rosen, R. T. and Rosen, J. D.,** Presence of four *Fusarium* mycotoxins and synthetic material in "yellow rain", *Biomed. Mass Spectrom.*, 9, 443, 1982.
113. **Greenhalgh, R., Miller, J. D., Neish, G. A., and Schiefer, H. B.,** Toxigenic potential of some *Fusarium* isolates from Southeast Asia, *Appl. Environ. Microbiol.*, 50, 550, 1985.
114. **Lorenzana, R. M., Beasley, V. R., Buck, W. B., Ghent, A. W., Lundeen, G. R., and Poppenga, R. H.,** Experimental T-2 toxicosis in swine. I. Changes in cardiac output, aortic mean pressure, cate-cholamines, 6-keto-PGF$_{1\alpha}$, thromboxane B$_2$ and acid-base parameters, *Fundam. Appl. Toxicol*, 5, 879, 1985.
115. **Yarom, R., More, R., Eldor, A., and Yagen, B.,** The effect of T-2 toxin on human platelets, *Toxicol. Appl. Pharmacol.*, 73, 210, 1984.

Chapter 3

EFFECTS ON THE DIGESTIVE SYSTEM AND ENERGY METABOLISM

H. B. Schiefer and V. R. Beasley

TABLE OF CONTENTS

I. INTRODUCTION

Digestive system effects, and direct or indirect effects on appetite and/or energy metabolism, may account for the principle economic losses due to trichothecene mycotoxicoses. With regard to overt clinical manifestations of trichothecene toxicoses, the effects on the digestive tract are most obvious and, therefore, among the most commonly reported. In many instances, trichothecene-induced digestive system alterations affect animal performance, general health, and sometimes survival. Whether due to digestive system damage or dysfunction, nervous system effects on appetite, or other factors, animals given feeds containing toxic concentrations of trichothecenes tend to exhibit reduced intake. These alterations in feed intake are discussed further in the chapter "Lethal Toxicity and Nonspecific Effects". Decreased intake alone reduces energy available for growth and sustenance. An untested hypothesis is that attempts to compensate for processes impaired due to trichothecene-induced protein synthesis inhibition and/or to repair tissue damage may account for increased energy demand. Alternatively, specific trichothecene effects on energy metabolism may exist. *In vitro* assays, however, must be interpreted in view of actual toxic doses of trichothecenes in animals and the potency of trichothecenes as inhibitors of protein synthesis, as discussed in previous chapters.

II. DIGESTIVE SYSTEM EFFECTS

The digestive system effects of trichothecenes are presented on a species-affected basis. As becomes evident in this chapter, the trichothecenes may affect feed intake, digestion, maintenance of natural barriers to infection, and blood supply to the digestive system. Effects on the mucosa are of major importance because of the relative uniqueness of the lesions. Pancreatic lesions have been described for some species subjected to acute trichothecene toxicoses. Hepatic lesions, however, tend to be the exception rather than the rule.

As discussed in the chapter "Absorption, Metabolism, Distribution, and Excretion of Trichothecene Mycotoxins", cleavage of the epoxide group of trichothecene mycotoxins by microorganisms of the gastrointestinal tract clearly varies between species (and almost certainly between individuals of the same species). This process is likely to be influenced by multiple factors including the particular microorganisms present, diet, feed additives, etc. This important detoxification mechanism is likely to influence both local (digestive tract) and systemic toxic effects of trichothecenes.

Some of the effects of trichothecenes on lymphoid tissues of the digestive system are discussed in the chapter "Immunotoxicity of Trichothecene Mycotoxins", and hemorrhagic effects are discussed in the chapter "Effects on Hemostasis and Red Blood Cell Production".

A. Trout

Effects on trout given T-2 toxin have included intestinal mucosal damage (with acutely toxic doses) and increased hepatic storage of vitamin A (with chronic feeding of the toxin). A single dose of 2, 4, or 8 mg T-2 toxin per kilogram administered in the diet of trout did not cause death, but did result in shedding of the intestinal mucosa.[1,2] The mucosa was completely regenerated by 10 weeks after dosing. The administration of T-2 toxin at 15 mg/kg to adult trout (*Salmo gairdneri*) by stomach tube resulted in intestinal hemorrhage and regurgitation, but 16 weeks of exposure of 1 g fingerling rainbow trout to T-2 toxin at 1 to 15 ppm in the diet had no effect on the activities of intestinal lumen chymotrypsin or trypsin, or on nitrogen digestibility or metabolizable energy.[3]

No hepatic lesions were found in rainbow trout fed a diet containing T-2 toxin at 200 or 400 ppb for 9 to 12 months.[2] Nevertheless, the hepatic storage of vitamin A in rainbow trout fingerlings was increased in relation to the concentration of T-2 toxin added to the feed.[3] With a diet containing T-2 toxin at 16 ppm, the vitamin A concentration in the liver was almost twice that of controls. Since it had been demonstrated previously that brook trout (*Salvelinas fontinalis*) on protein-restricted diets had increased hepatic vitamin A concentrations, toxin-associated feed refusal or inhibition of protein synthesis may have produced a related effect in the rainbow trout. Gall bladder enlargement was present in fingerling trout given T-2 toxin in the feed at 15 ppm for 4 d. Overall, therefore, these results were consistent with a primary effect of starvation rather than inefficient use of nutrients.[3]

B. Gallinaceous Birds
1. Oral Lesions

Mucosal effects of the more toxic trichothecenes have been amply demonstrated by the production of oral lesions in birds fed diets containing T-2 toxin. When young chicks and hens were given T-2 toxin in the feed at 4 to 20 ppm for 3 weeks, oral lesions first appeared on the palatine areas of the oral cavity and then on the tongue, corners of the mouth, and margin of the beak.[4,5] These changes frequently appeared as circumscribed yellowish-white caseous plaques or ulcers.[4-7] They began as small necrotic foci, but in time expanded to as much as 1 cm in diameter. In birds fed T-2 toxin at 0.5 to 8.0 ppm, oral lesions were dose-related with regard to both incidence and severity.[6,8] At 8 ppm, some hens developed singular small ulcers in the gizzard.

The feeding of 1-d-old chicks with diets containing 5 ppm of either T-2 toxin or diacetoxyscirpenol (DAS) for 3 weeks caused the development of yellowish plaque-type lesions on the beak, tongue, and angle of the mouth; however, crotocin at 10 ppm in the diet did not cause any such lesions nor apparent clinical effects.[9] Similar oral lesions appeared as soon as 8 and 14 d in chicks fed T-2 toxin in the diet at 4 and 8 ppm, respectively.[6,8] In birds fed diets containing T-2 toxin at 0.4 or 0.5 ppm, oral lesions first appeared at 2 and 5 weeks, respectively.[5,6,8] In most such investigations, the oral lesions became more severe with time. In one study, however, in which birds were fed T-2 toxin at 0.5 to 8.0 ppm, the frequency of oral lesions was maximal in all groups at 14 d and declined spontaneously thereafter, regardless of the concentration of T-2 toxin continually fed.[8] Therefore, in order to avoid false negatives in differential diagnosis, oral lesions must be regarded as potentially temporary.

When a comparative study in turkey poults and Leghorn chicks was conducted over a 4-week period using feeds containing T-2 toxin at 2 and 10 ppm, the turkey poults on the high dose diet developed oral lesions by week 2, and the extent and severity of the lesions increased during the remainder of the experimental period.[10] Tongue lesions consisted of alternate layers of necrotic epithelium and bands of heterophils, suggesting degeneration and necrosis with regeneration, followed by repetition of this sequence of events. Oral lesions were not observed in poults fed the toxin at 2 ppm, however, white caseous plaques were present in the crops of poults fed 2 ppm and were prominent in the high-dose poults. In contrast, no lesions were noted at any time point when young chickens were fed the same rations. These studies demonstrated wide variation in susceptibility to T-2 toxin-induced oral lesions, both within and between species.

2. GI and Hepatic Effects

In oral LD_{50} studies with day-old broiler chicks, several group A trichothecenes (T-2 toxin, HT-2 toxin, DAS, deacetyl-HT-2 toxin, and T-2 tetraol) caused diarrhea within 4 to 10 h after dosing, regardless of which toxin was administered.[11] Chickens given oral doses of T-2 toxin in an LD_{50} study did not vomit, but developed mucus-laden diarrhea.[11] Survivors voided large amounts of blue-colored excreta for 2 to 3 d, but had no clinical signs thereafter. Hens given lethal doses developed a covering of chalk-like material, possibly uric acid crystals, over much of the abdominal viscera. Dying birds also had enlarged gall bladders and blue contents of the gizzard. In a few of the high-dose birds, necrosis of the mucosa of the gizzard and thickening, sloughing, and necrosis of the mucosal epithelium of the crop were noted at 10 and 30 d after T-2 toxin administration. No lesions were found in the livers.

In addition to the severe reduction in egg production observed in a flock of hens fed a diet containing T-2 toxin at 3.5 ppm and HT-2 toxin at 0.7 ppm, a blue-green discoloration of the droppings was noted in some birds. Despite these effects, the mortality rate was no greater than before the feeding of the contaminated feed, and no lesions were found on necropsy.[12]

To assess whether estrogens affected sensitivity to T-2 toxin, 6-week-old male chickens were dosed with T-2 toxin intramuscularly (i.m.) at approximately 0.75 mg/kg with or without concurrent i.m. injection of estradiol-17-β-dipropionate at 4.25 mg/kg.[13] When killed at 96 h, both of the T-2 dosed groups had increased liver:body weight ratios. The toxin-associated change was attributable to increased liver weights, rather than an alteration of body weight; there was no increase in total DNA in liver and the toxin had not produced hyperplasia.

In a comparative investigation of the effects of trichothecenes on 7-week-old broiler chicks, single doses of either T-2 toxin (at 2.0 or 2.5 mg/kg) or DAS (at 2.7 mg/kg) were given by crop gavage.[14] Birds were periodically killed from 1 to 168 h postdosing. With either toxin, birds necropsied during the first 24 h had clear-fluid contents in the small intestine and distended gall bladders. Histologic changes in the liver were more severe in those chicks given T-2 toxin and, from 1 to 24 h, were comprised of disseminated foci of coagulation, or infrequently as widely disseminated foci of either coagulation or fibrinoid necrosis with hemorrhage. The extent of fibrinoid necrosis of vessels was deemed insufficient to explain the foci of parenchymal necrosis occurring primarily in the portal region and sometimes involving the entire portal triad. Bile ductiles were usually intact, but a few were necrotic. Whether concentration of T-2 toxin or its metabolites in the portal region had resulted in this localization of hepatocellular and vascular injury was not determined. Bile duct hyperplasia also occurred in chickens given either T-2 toxin or DAS. T-2 toxin induced diffuse reddening and a greater degree of necrosis of the gall bladder mucosa than DAS. Necrosis and ulceration of the gall bladder mucosa at 24 h were followed by cholecystitis at 72 h.

In the first 24 h, DAS caused hyperemia and both toxins caused mild necrosis of the proventriculus.[14] DAS caused red cecal contents, while T-2 toxin was associated with focal or diffuse reddening of the small intestinal mucosa. By 6 h, either toxin had caused necrosis of the tips of the duodenal villi and by 12 h necrosis had become more extensive, affecting the crypt epithelium of both the small and large intestine. Mitotic figures were reduced in both of these areas at 18 and 24 h.

3. Pancreatic Effects

In the study by Pearson[13] described under the section "Gastrointestinal and Hepatic Effects", the pancreas:body weight ratio was decreased in the T-2/nonestrogen treated birds. Further, pancreatic lipase of young chickens was moderately decreased by T-2 toxin at 8 ppm or higher concentrations.[15] T-2 toxin at 8 and 16 ppm also had a slightly depressing effect on the activities of pancreatic trypsin, amylase, and RNA-ase. Thus, at greater than 8 ppm, the effects of T-2 toxin on digestive function included a moderate depression of pancreatic enzymes and induction of steatorrhea. It would be of interest to determine whether the reductions in these enzyme activities were a direct result of inhibition of protein synthesis and whether absorptive capacity of the intestine was altered.

4. Effects on Intestinal and Hepatic Enzymes and Uric Acid

In the survivors of an oral intubation LD_{50} study of T-2 toxin in laying hens, serum activities of alanine aminotransferase and lactate dehydrogenase were not altered at 10 d postdosing;[11] however, alkaline phosphatase activity was decreased. Similarly, in response to the feeding of T-2 toxin to broiler chicks, alkaline phosphatase activity was decreased, and in birds given diets with 4.0 ppm T-2 toxin, the activities were less than 1/3 of control values.[5]

In contrast, feeding T-2 toxin to laying hens at up to 8 ppm in the ration for 8 weeks resulted in increases in serum alkaline phosphatase and lactate dehydrogenase as well as in uric acid.[6] At the highest feeding level there were decreases in alanine aminotransferase. Liver and gizzard weights were unaffected.

The results with regard to lactate dehydrogenase were quite different in a subsequent study, whereas the uric acid results were similar. Although serum lactate dehydrogenase was decreased by feeding broiler chicks T-2 toxin at 2 or 4 ppm for 9 weeks, serum uric acid was increased by toxin concentrations as low as 0.2 ppm.[5] There was no evidence of kidney damage on histologic examination and no evidence of dehydration. The increased serum uric acid, therefore, may have been due to poor utilization of dietary amino acids for protein synthesis rather than decreased renal function.

In both the estrogen and the nonestrogen-treated chickens mentioned previously,[13] T-2 toxin was associated with modest increases in activities of aspartate aminotransferase, alanine aminotransferase, and lactate dehydrogenase, but there were very notable decreases in alkaline and acid phosphatase activities. Furthermore, the estradiol-induced increase in acid phosphatase was prevented by T-2 toxin. Since T-2 toxin had no significant effect on gamma glutamyl transpeptidase, it was suggested that at these doses it had not seriously harmed the pancreas or biliary tract of the chickens.

Some of the differences between the various studies in chickens evaluating the effects of T-2 toxin on aspartate transaminase and lactate dehydrogenase may be related to differences in route of administration and the subsequent effects on feed intake.[13] However, most reports of T-2 toxin administration to chickens in which alkaline phosphatase has been measured have revealed reductions in activity. In the fowl, the intestinal isoenzyme makes a major contribution to the total activity in the plasma and the amount produced is diminished by restriction of feed intake or starvation. T-2 may have an additional effect by harming intestinal mucosal cells which produce this enzyme. The reduction occurs even when the toxin is injected i.m.[15] The fall in acid phosphatase following T-2 toxin dosing may also be due to an effect on the intestinal mucosa, but the proportion of serum activity originating from various organs has not been determined.

5. Malabsorption

In order to produce lipid malabsorption in young chickens, it was necessary to feed concentrations of T-2 toxin greater than 8 ppm for the first 3 weeks after hatching.[15] Even then, the lipid malabsorption was mild. Although it was associated with a mild reduction in pancreatic lipase and steatorrhea, it was not accompanied by hypocarotenoidemia; however, hypocarotenoidemia, which may result in reduced consumer acceptance of chicken carcasses and eggs, did follow the consumption of feed containing either aflatoxin or ochratoxin. Aflatoxin was a potent producer of both malabsorption and steatorrhea, while ochratoxin did not increase fecal lipids. Thus, there was a lack of correlation between hypocarotenoidemia and steatorrhea with either T-2 toxin or ochratoxin ingestion. This suggested separate processes for lipid and carotenoid absorption which was contrary to generally accepted scientific doctrine. Total serum lipid concentrations were slightly depressed by feed containing ochratoxin, and greatly reduced by aflatoxin, but unaffected by T-2 toxin despite the steatorrhea. Although aflatoxin depressed the concentrations of bile salts in bile, neither ochratoxin nor T-2 at up to 16 ppm had any such effect.[15] Total bile flow and absorptive capacity of the intestine were not measured.

C. Ducks and Geese

An outbreak of T-2 toxicosis occurred when geese were fed barley naturally contaminated with 25 ppm T-2 toxin.[17] There was extreme necrosis of the esophagus, and the mucosa of the gizzard turned from gray to black, and became thickened, "shredded", and necrotic. The fact that geese have no crop may have increased the duration of contact of the ingesta with the esophageal mucosa. Severe necrosis of the proventriculus and intense enteritis were seen and histologic examination revealed necrosis and sloughing of the keratinized epithelium of the esophagus.

When a goose was dosed with 30 g of the barley on days 1, 2, 3, 4, 7, 8, and 9, polydipsia, greenish droppings, and a temperature of 106.8°F (41.6°C) developed on the 3rd day.[18] After death on day 10, the entire digestive tract from the epiglottis to the gizzard contained barley. The esophagus and proventriculus were distended, and necrosis of the mucosa began in the upper esophagus and extended into the gizzard.

Geese, fed for 10 d on a diet inoculated with *Fusarium tricinctum* and containing 3 ppm T-2 toxin, refused part of the feed and gradually lost weight.[19] After feeding a ration containing T-2 toxin at 1.5 ppm for another 25 to 60 weeks, necrotic and diphtheroid lesions of the oral and pharyngeal mucosae developed and the birds did not resume normal feed consumption after withdrawal of the toxic ration. Some of the geese also developed hemorrhagic enteritis.

Vomiting in 10-d-old ducklings occurred within 5 to 10 min of administration of fusarenon-X, regardless of the route of administration. The minimum effective subcutaneous (s.c.) dose to induce emesis with T-2, HT-2, and neosolaniol was 0.1 mg/kg body weight and the respective doses for other trichothecenes were 0.2 for DAS, 0.4 for diacetylnivalenol, 1.0 for nivalenol, and 13.5 for deoxynivalenol (DON).[20] Shortly after vomiting the ducks actively drank water. The cycle of vomiting and drinking was frequently repeated for 20 to 30 min. Degeneration and necrosis were present in mucosal cells of both the gizzard and the glandular stomach.

Young mallard ducks (*Anas platyrynchos*) fed diets containing T-2 toxin at 20 or 30 ppm had reduced weight gain and delayed development of adult plumage. The ducks developed caseonecrotic plaques throughout the alimentary tract, and some developed severe, ulcerative, proliferative esophagitis and proventriculitis; however, significant alterations were not detected in either the concentration of plasma and serum protein, and cholesterol, or in the activities of glutamate pyruvate transaminase, glutamate oxaloacetate transaminase, and alkaline phosphatase.[21]

D. Pigeons

Pigeons vomited within 35 min after administration of T-2 toxin.[22] The ED_{50} for emesis were 0.72 and 0.15 mg/kg when given by the oral and intravenous (i.v.) routes, respectively. As the ED_{90} corresponded to the LD_{25}, doses exist at which vomiting would be detected as the predominant clinical effect. This observation was developed into a bioassay for trichothecenes using either ducklings or pigeons.[23] Vomiting may occur 53 to 10 min after s.c. administration of doses from 0.1 mg/kg (with T-2 toxin or HT-2 toxin), to 0.2 mg/kg (with DAS), 0.4 mg/kg (with trichothecin), 1.0 mg/kg (with nivalenol), and 13.5 mg/kg (with DON).

E. Rodents and Rabbits

Investigations of trichothecene-related digestive system effects in rodents and rabbits are comprised primarily of studies of changes related to pathology and motility. These are discussed on an organ basis to allow for comparison between toxins and dosage regimens.

1. Oral Mucosa, Esophagus, and Stomach

To compare effects of ATA isolates of *Fusarium poae* and *F. sporotrichioides* strains, the organisms were cultured and extracts administered to mice and rats in graded, single, or multiple doses by topical, s.c., intraperitoneal (i.p.), intragastric, or p.o. administration.[24] Extracts of both organisms caused similar effects in mice and rats. The p.o. administration to baby rats of a drop of either extract caused death within 2 to 3 d, apparently as a result of swelling of the tongue and inability to suckle. Fusarial extracts administered by stomach tube to weanling rats caused ulceration, hyperkeratosis, and desquamation of the mucosa of the esophagus and the squamous part of the gastric mucosa. Smaller doses of extract were well tolerated by rats, even when administered daily or weekly. With subsequently increased doses, however, the rats died within a few days and acute upper gastrointestinal lesions were found to be superimposed on chronic ones.[24] In both the esophagus and the squamous part of the stomach, foci of ulceration and edema of the muscular wall were adjacent to areas of mucosal epithelial hyperplasia. Animals killed after low doses of extract had no gross lesions, but histologic examination revealed invagination and pocked formation in the esophageal mucosa and a thickened, hyperplastic layer of basal cells in the squamous portion of the stomach.

When rats were intragastrically administered 3 to 8 doses of T-2 toxin at 0.2 to 4.0 mg/ kg at approximately monthly intervals, 2/3 of the animals died.[25] These rats usually developed a hunched posture, diarrhea, and bleeding from the body orifices. The stomachs were distended with soft, often blood-stained contents. There were petechial hemorrhages and erosions in the stomach as well as microscopically evident glandular atrophy with "cellular" infiltrates and submucosal edema. The stomach contents were blood stained. Rats surviving weeks or months after the last of three to eight treatments with T-2 toxin consistently had hyperkeratosis and hyperplasia of the epithelium of the esophagus and of the squamous portion of the stomach. In the glandular portion of the stomach and in the duodenum "atypical" glandular elements were frequently present and there were foci of calcification of the muscularis, "infiltration" of crypts, and thickening of walls of the arteries.

Mice fed diets containing T-2 toxin at either 10 or 20 ppm for 3 weeks and longer developed perioral dermatitis.[26] The squamous portion of the stomach became hyperkeratotic and hyperplastic, with an associated increase in stomach weight. No differences in the severity of gastric hyperkeratosis were seen in mice given T-2 toxin in their diets at 20 ppm as a function of variation in protein content of 8 to 16% protein.[27] Gastric mucosal hyperplasia was also reported in mice fed a diet containing T-2 toxin at 15 ppm for 52 weeks.[28]

Intragastric administration of T-2 toxin to guinea pigs (doses listed below) induced gastric mucosal hyperemia, hemorrhage, and necrosis.[29] Similar gastric mucosal necrosis was observed in the guinea pigs of an i.p. LD_{50} study using fusarenon-X.[20] The gastric glandular cells of rats were more markedly damaged than those of mice when both were used in LD_{50} studies of fusarenon-X, using 5 different doses from 2.4 to 5.0 mg/kg.[20]

2. Intestine, Cecum, and Pancreas

Diarrhea occurred in rats given T-2 toxin and DAS orally at up to 8 mg/kg.[30] In these rats, hemorrhage into intestinal lumens also occurred and focal areas of necrosis were present in the liver. Similar effects have been observed in rats treated with T-2 toxin topically.[31]

In the duodenum of rats that died after one of a series of intermittent 0.2 to 4.0 mg/kg intragastric doses of T-2 toxin, there were hemorrhages and erosions and a mild degree of mucosal loss.[25] The small intestine was often full of blood. Rats that died shortly after treatment had interlobular edema of the pancreas. Those surviving weeks or months after the last treatment had frequent partial or total occlusion in the pancreas. Other pancreatic lesions included arteritis, proliferation of the islets, hyperplasia of the ducts, and benign and malignant tumors of both endo- and exocrine cells. Moreover, feeding mice a diet containing fusarenon-X at 10 ppm for 4 weeks was associated with pancreatic atrophy.[32]

Single intragastric doses of T-2 toxin (in DMSO/ethanol 1:1) given to male guinea pigs at 1.85 to 5.0 mg/kg caused dramatic lesions, including hyperemia, hemorrhage, and necrosis in the mucosa of the cecum, distension of the cecum with watery fluid, edema of intestinal lymphoid tissues, and adrenal hemorrhage.[29] In the small intestine and to a lesser extent in the large intestine, there were focal areas of villar necrosis with pseudomembrane formation and casts within crypts. At 4.66 to 3.43 mg/kg, deaths took place within 6 to 12 h and at 1.85 mg/kg animals continued to die until 36 h.

Histologic examination of tissues from guinea pigs given fusarenon-X in an i.p. LD_{50} study revealed necrosis of the mucosal epithelium of the small and large intestine.[20] In LD_{50} studies using mice, fusarenon-X caused changes in the crypt epithelium of the duodenum and jejunum which included atypical mitoses, pyknoses of nuclei, and nuclear swelling or fragmentation.[20] Some mice appeared to have died from intestinal bleeding caused by ulceration of the mucosa.

During LD_{50} studies of fusarenon-X using mice and rats, it was noted that diarrhea was more prevalent in animals with longer survival times of 3 to 4 d than in those which died more acutely.[20] Matsuoka and Kubota[33] found that in 90% of rats treated 24 h earlier with fusarenon-X at 1 mg/kg i.p., the small intestine was hyperemic and filled with yellow mucus, but intestinal hemorrhage was rare. Histologic examination revealed marked shortening of the intestinal villi. Not surprisingly, the i.p. injection was followed by a rapid decrease in intake of both water and food. The diarrhea became violent from the 36th to the 48th hour and then subsided to the point of resolution by the 4th day.

3. Antimitotic Effects of Trichothecenes

In mice given fusarenon-X at 3 mg/kg i.p. (a dose near an LD_{50}), inhibition of mitosis of the small intestinal mucosal cells started later but persisted longer than similar effects on lymphoid tissues apart from the thymus.[34] It must be noted, however, that these comparisons were made over a period of only 4 h. A similar mitotic inhibition was observed in the pancreas from 1 to 3 h with mitotic recovery beginning by the 4th hour.

A detailed sequential study (1 to 96 h) following intragastric administration of 2.5 mg of T-2 toxin to young male white Swiss mice revealed that mitotic activity in intestinal crypts ceased within 2 h.[35] By 3 to 4 h, numerous round bodies had appeared in the cytoplasm of intestinal crypt cells. Many such bodies were evident by 12 h, and often they formed into plugs of necrotic debris at the base of the crypts. Regenerative activity was evident by 9 h and this increased until the crypt epithelium had become hyperplastic between 24 and 48 h. After 48 h, the crypts were distorted in shape and the villi were shortened. This pattern of lesion development could be expected to be associated with malabsorption syndromes. Similar lesions were observed in mice given various trichothecenes topically; the lesions differed in extent and severity, depending on the trichothecenes employed.[36]

4. Other Pathophysiologic Events

Several investigators have attempted to characterize intestinal effects apart from clinical signs, mitotic inhibition, or descriptions of necrosis. For example, when rats were given fusarenon-X i.p. at 1 mg/kg and Evans Blue dye i.v. 23 h later, the increased amount of dye in the intestinal lumen indicated increased permeability and loss of plasma protein into the lumen.[33] There was, however, neither Evans Blue leakage into the peritoneal cavity nor significant increase in hemoglobin in the intestinal lumen. These findings indicate a partial reduction in vascular functional integrity in the gut mucosa of trichothecene dosed animals.

D-Xylose is absorbed from the intestine by both passive and active (energy requiring) mechanisms.[37] Intestine taken from rats 24 h after being treated with fusarenon-X at 1 mg/kg was characterized by increased rapidity of D-xylose absorption *in vitro*, an indication of increased intestinal mucosal permeability. A separate group of rats given the toxin i.p. at 1 mg/kg developed lesions including marked shortening of intestinal villi and "an infiltration of erythrocytes into the lamina propria", which may explain, in part, the observed changes in permeability. Fusarenon-X-induced diarrhea in mice could not, however, be associated with altered intestinal digestion of starch, intestinal absorption of glucose, or a secondary osmotic attraction of water into the gut.[38] These findings seem to contradict the report of Suneja et al.,[39] who dosed young rats orally with T-2 toxin for 4 d at 1.5 mg/kg/ d. After removal of intestinal loops, they observed a 73% reduction in glucose absorption and a 67% drop in tryptophan absorption. They also noted marked reductions in intestinal brush border sucrase whereas reductions in brush border lactase and Na^+-K^+-ATPase were comparatively mild. Intestinal lysosomal enzymes (acid phosphatase and acid ribonuclease) were higher in T-2 dosed animals, but the increases were not statistically significant. Whether the observed reductions in enzyme activities were due to reduced synthesis, inhibition or preformed enzymes (far less likely) or mucosal damage was not determined.

When rat jejunum or ileum was perfused *in vitro* using Tyrode's solution containing T-2 toxin at 1 to 100 μmol/l (0.0046 to 0.46 ppm), there were no changes in the absorption of glucose, water, sodium, or potassium.[40] In a companion study, rats were pretreated with T-2 toxin either orally (at 0.5, 1.0, or 1.5 mg/kg) or i.v. (at 0.25, 0.5, or 0.75 mg/kg) and the jejunal or ileal segments were removed 12 h later and perfused for a 2-h observation period without further addition of toxin. Unlike the previous study, whether pretreated orally or i.v., dose-dependent reductions (as high as 60%) were observed in glucose absorption by the jejunum. Absorption of water and sodium was impaired after the oral but not the i.v. pretreatment. In the ileum, orally administered T-2 toxin caused no change in absorption of glucose, water, or sodium, but after i.v. administration at the 0.25 mg/kg dose, elevated rates of absorption of glucose, water, and sodium were observed. No effects were noted at the 0.5 mg/kg i.v. dose, but at 0.75 mg/kg sodium absorption was impaired. Potassium absorption was increased in the jejunum from i.v. pretreated rats. The results seem to suggest that systemic effects of the toxin on the animal (including shock) may secondarily (or indirectly) influence intestinal capacity for absorption since perfusion of isolated intestine with toxin had little effect in itself. It is important to recognize that the intestinal trichothecene exposure of the dosed animals was almost certainly substantially higher than that used with the toxin perfused during *in vitro* exposures. Therefore, despite the absence of effects in the *in vitro* system, the differences between effects observed after oral administration and those after i.v. dosing suggest that both systemic and local toxic effects are likely to be of importance.

Injection of male mice with fusarenon-X at 15 mg/kg i.p. caused hemoptysis (expectoration of blood) and diarrhea with expansion and hyperemia of the intestine.[41] Similarly, fusarenon-

X at 3 mg/kg i.p. or i.v. caused hyperemia of the intestine but the incidence of intestinal dilation was lower, and 0.7 mg/kg i.p. caused no visceral changes. When 10^{-5} M (approximately 3.5 ppm) fusarenon-X was applied to the isolated gastric fundus of the rat or to the ileum of the guinea pig, neither relaxation nor contraction was observed. In addition, none of the following responses to agonists were affected: ileum to acetylcholine, nicotine or histamine, and gastric fundus to serotonin. Similarly, the spontaneous movement of isolated rabbit duodenum was not changed by fusarenon-X addition to the organ bath even after 60 min of incubation at 50 ppm.

In spite of the above evidence suggesting absence of a local effect, but in agreement with the "expansion of the intestine" mentioned above, the i.v. injection of guinea pigs with fusarenon-X at 1 mg/kg caused partial inhibition of intestinal peristalsis 20 to 30 min after the injection and complete inhibition after 40 min. The inhibition lasted over 2 h, but it could be antagonized by pilocarpine, indicating retention of smooth muscle contractibility. With administration of fusarenon-X at 0.2 mg/kg, suppression of peristalsis still occurred, but it lasted less than 2 h, and at 0.1 mg/kg peristalsis was unaffected. In contrast, fusarenon-X administered to mice at 1 mg/kg i.p. did not affect intestinal propulsion of charcoal 30 min later, and from 6 to 12 h after administration, propulsion was increased by up to 25%.[41] The influence of charcoal as an adsorbent of trichothecenes, however, may have compromised the usual effects on the gut. The work of Kosuri et al.[30] also provided results different from most of the fusarenon-X reports. They found that the frequency of peristaltic waves in isolated rat colon segments doubled after exposure to extracts of *F. tricinctum*, although the useful life of segments decreased as the toxin concentration was increased.

In view of the usual absence of direct effects on motility and the failure to influence the effects of agonists, it is possible that the increased propulsion of intestinal contents develops as a result of increased fluid content and volume of the intestinal contents. Considering that trichothecenes induce inhibition of small intestinal mucosal epithelial cell growth, followed by karyorrhexis and necrosis,[35,42] it is indeed plausible that trichothecene-associated damage and desquamation of intestinal epithelium may cause loss of fluid and electrolytes into the intestinal lumen with the resultant enhancement of intestinal propulsion. This may be analogous to the effect of cholera toxin, which instead acts by stimulating adenylate cyclase, resulting in increases in cyclic AMP (cAMP) in the intestinal mucosal cells, but nevertheless causes a similar increase in the fluidity of intestinal contents and diarrhea.[41] The more recently documented stimulation of "prostaglandin" synthesis by cholera toxin[43] may be similar to the increase in prostaglandin concentrations in T-2 toxin-dosed animals.[44,45] In an effort to lessen cholera toxic effects, indomethacin treatment was evaluated and found to reduce cAMP concentrations and fluid loss into the gut. Thus, evaluation of inhibitors of prostaglandin synthesis with respect to trichothecene effects on the gut may also be of value.

5. Liver

In spite of some of the effects in poultry mentioned earlier, the trichothecene mycotoxins are not generally known for their effects on the liver. It is therefore not surprising that neither large (LD_{50} to LD_{70}) doses of *F. tricinctum* extracts, which killed most mice and rats within 3 d, nor small repeated sublethal doses, caused specific lesions in the liver.[24] Similarly, when mice were given i.p. injections of *F. tricinctum* crude extracts at 1/2 LD_{50} on day 0 followed by 1/4 LD_{50} on day 1, histologic lesions were not observed in the liver when the animals were killed on days 3 through 33.[46] Furthermore, liver weights of mice were not affected by 7 daily i.p. injections of either T-2 toxin or DAS at up to 2.0 mg/kg/24 h.[47,48] Similarly, rats fed 5 to 15 ppm T-2 toxin in complete diets for weeks to months developed minimal or, most often, no hepatic lesions.[2,49]

Additional evidence for the absence of significant hepatic dysfunction in trichothecene exposed rodents was provided by the finding that, at 12 h after rats were given either T-2 toxin at 2 mg/kg i.p. or lyophilized *F. tricinctum* cultures at 100 mg/kg orally, sulfobrom-ophthalein (BSP) retention was only slightly increased with values of 12% for controls and 15% for treated rats.[30]

In contrast to these negative findings, pathologic alterations were described only in the liver when mice were fed naturally contaminated barley containing approximately 25 ppm T-2 toxin free choice for 77 d.[18] Lesions included centrilobular necrosis, nuclear degeneration, fatty degeneration of hepatocytes, and increased extramedullary hematopoiesis. In view of the possibility of other toxins being present, however, an absolute cause and effect relationship was not established. Another exception to the general absence of hepatic lesions in trichothecene dosed rodents was the finding in mice treated twice weekly with fusarenon-X at 3 to 5 mg/kg i.p. of amyloid deposition in the arterial walls of portal regions, as well as in the sinusoidal walls of the liver.[28]

As mentioned with regard to metabolism, the liver is an important site of trichothecene detoxification. It is, therefore, noteworthy that mice exposed to T-2 toxin at 20 ppm in the diet developed increased liver weights, especially after the 5th week.[26] Similarly, during a 4-week trial, liver:body weight ratios of mice fed T-2 toxin at 20 ppm in 12 or 16% protein diets increased when compared to control mice fed diets containing similar protein levels. At 8% protein, however, no increase in this ratio had occurred by the 28th day.[27] These findings are compatible with an induction of mixed function oxidase enzymes in the liver as a result of prolonged trichothecene mycotoxin exposure, which is dependent upon adequate protein intake.

6. Hepatic and Intestinal Enzymes

After a single i.v. injection of T-2 toxin at 0.5 mg/kg, serum alkaline phosphatase activity of rabbits was decreased by 2 d and thereafter remained depressed for at least 9 d.[50] Oral T-2 toxin given to rabbits at 2 mg/kg for 4 d caused similar decreases on days 5 to 10 but not before or after this interval. These reductions in alkaline phosphatase are, of course, similar to those described for chickens above. Although the i.v. dose administered to rabbits produced a transient increase in serum alanine aminotransferase activity, oral administration had no effect and toxin administration by either route failed to cause changes in total serum protein or albumin.

In view of the formation and elimination of T-2 metabolites by the liver, Gentry and Cooper[50] suggested that the observed decrease in alkaline phosphatase may be due to a reduction in hepatic enzyme production, especially in the biliary tree. It would appear that reduction in alkaline phosphatase is a fairly consistent effect of repeated T-2 toxin administration in several species. Additional effects on alkaline phosphatase are discussed in subsequent portions of this chapter.

F. Ruminants

Evaluations of effects of trichothecenes on ruminants have involved parenteral injections of T-2 toxin, oral administration of fungal extracts and purified toxins via gelatin capsules, and very limited feeding studies. The results described must be interpreted in light of the route of administration and the presence of a single purified toxin vs. multiple metabolic intermediates. As a rule, exposures via feedstuffs have not involved the more toxic trichothecenes.

1. Forestomachs, Abomasum, and Intestine

The administration of T-2 toxin at 0.44 mg/kg by esophageal intubation to a parturient Holstein cow for 16 d was associated with localized mucosal ulceration in the anterior ventral rumen.[51] The duodenum of the cow appeared normal but the jejunal mucosa was moderately to severely congested. The small intestinal congestion became severe near the ileocecocolic junction. The jejunal and ileal contents were very fluid. On histologic examination there was congestion of the rumen and abomasum and submucosal edema of the reticulum. Moderate congestion of the duodenal mucosa and severe congestion of the tips of the mucosal villi and the lamina propria of the jejunum and ileum were seen. The cecum and colon were edematous in the submucosal muscular and serosal layers. Comparison of samples from days 1, 8, and 16 revealed no notable alterations in blood urea nitrogen, alanine or aspartate aminotransferases, total protein, or lactate dehydrogenase.

When T-2 toxin was administered in gelatin capsules daily for 30 d to 30-d-old Jersey calves, the minimum dosage which caused clearly discernible clinical signs was 0.32 mg/kg/d and signs first developed at 9 d.[52] These consisted of bloody feces, anorexia, dehydration, and rough hair coat. The voiding of semisolid feces, potentially attributable to T-2 toxin, occurred on day 24 in one calf at 0.08 mg/kg/d, and on day 12 at 0.16 mg/kg/d in another. A Jersey calf given T-2 toxin orally in gelatin capsules at 0.64 mg/kg/d voided soft stools after 1 d and subsequently developed bloody feces, inappetence, and loss of over 25% of its body weight, a rough hair coat, and a hunched-up posture.[52] Death occurred on day 20. The two calves given 0.16 and 0.32 mg/kg/d were killed at 30 d. At necropsy, there were abomasal ulcers in the calf given the lowest dose, and ruminal ulcers and abomasitis in the calves at the two higher doses. Mild enteritis was present in the calves given the lower and intermediate doses. Histologic changes in the calves at the two higher doses included focal suppurative rumenitis and abomasitis. Calves given T-2 toxin at 0.6 mg/kg/d in gelatin capsules for 6 weeks developed intermittent soft tan or dark semifluid feces.[53] Calves dosed at 0.3 mg/kg/d, however, were unaffected.

In two calves given T-2 toxin i.v. at 0.6 mg/kg (one of which was killed at 5.5 h and the other at 25 h postdosing), the colon contents were fluid and, in one, the jejunal contents contained mucus.[54] Histologically evident GI lesions in these calves were limited to lymphoid necrosis.

In a calf given T-2 toxin i.v. at 1.2 mg/kg and killed 24 h later, the entire mucosal surface of the abomasum was dark red,[54] The duodenal mucosa near the abomasum was also red and the jejunal mucosa was both red and thickened. The ruminal contents of this calf were drier than normal, whereas the contents of the remainder of the digestive tract were of increased fluidity. Apart from lymphoid necrosis, however, no notable lesions were histologically observed in the forestomachs, abomasum, duodenum, or jejunum of this calf. By contrast, in the ileum, crypts were dilated and contained necrotic debris, and in some areas extensive hemorrhage was present.

A second calf, given the toxin at 1.2 mg/kg, passed normal feces prior to and initially after dosing; however, at 2.5 h, an increased amount of mucus was present in the feces, and by 3 h, diarrhea with mucus and blood clots was present.[54] Thereafter, the calf developed persistent watery diarrhea which rapidly became bloody. Shortly after the onset of diarrhea, the calf displayed apparent attempts to vomit, as evidenced by repeated abdominal contractions with the head lowered, the neck extended, and the tongue protruding from the mouth. The calf subsequently became recumbent and developed severe bloat and shock and died 10.5 h postdosing. Digestive tract lesions were marked in this calf. Diffuse redness was present in the ruminal and abomasal mucosae and hemorrhage was present in the pyloric mucosa. Marked edema was present in the mesentery adjacent to the duodenum and liver and there were multiple ecchymotic hemorrhages in the duodenal mucosa. In the jejunum, ecchymotic hemorrhages were present and the mucosa became progressively more purple aborally. In the ileum, multiple petechial and ecchymotic hemorrhages were scattered over the mucosa. The cecal serosa was purple and there were multiple ecchymotic hemorrhages and fibrin strands on the mucosal surface. The mucosa of the spiral colon was red, and in the large colon multiple ecchymotic hemorrhages were scattered over the mucosa with numerous adherent clots. The jejunal, ileal, spiral colon, and cecal contents resembled watery blood. This calf apparently developed an acute coagulopathy as evidenced by the concurrent development of pleural and microscopically evident brain hemorrhages.

In a calf given T-2 toxin orally at a dose of 2.4 mg/kg via a gelatin capsule and killed 24 h later, there were no notable gross lesions observed in the forestomachs, abomasum, duodenum, cecum, or colon.[54] In the jejunum, however, the mucosa was increasingly congested aborally such that severe redness was present near the ileum; and the ileum was a similar red color. The only notable degenerative changes in lymphoid tissues of this calf occurred in Peyer's patches which were moderately shrunken and contained increased numbers of mononuclear cells. Other than ballooned epithelial cells in the stratum spinosum of the ruminal mucosa, no other gastroentreric lesions were encountered in the tissues of this calf.

Lambs given T-2 toxin over a 3-week period, at 0.3 or 0.6 mg/kg/d in a propylene glycol vehicle via gelatin capsules, developed prolonged diarrhea and a focal rumenitis with parakeratosis and polymorphonuclear cell infiltration.[55] Diarrhea was more severe in lambs given the higher amount of T-2 toxin. The study, however, was compromised by concurrent coccidiosis and perioral lesions of contagious ecthyma, but the authors felt that these were not substantially affected by T-2 toxin administration. There was also no effect on the liver:body weight ratios and no GI or other hemorrhages were observed.

2. Liver

Serum aspartate and alanine aminotransferases and lactate dehydrogenase activities were not notably affected by oral administration of T-2 toxin to calves at 0.6 mg/kg/d.[53] Although alkaline phosphatase was decreased at this dosage, controls, pair-fed to reflect the intake of the 0.6 mg/kg group, had almost identical activities. The suggestion that the reduction in alkaline phosphatase was related to decreased consumption of feed is in agreement with one offered in relation to the reduction of alkaline phosphatase in T-2 dosed chickens and may partially explain this largely consistent finding (*Editor's Note*: see the section "Rodents and Rabbits" for an alternate theory). Liver:body weight ratios in the 0.6 mg/kg group were not significantly different from controls or pair-fed controls.

When a 300-kg heifer was given daily injections of 0.24, 0.06, and especially 0.12 mg/kg T-2 toxin over 60 d, the animal developed elevated aspartate aminotransferase activity (150 increased to 640 IU), an increase in uric acid concentration (0.9 increased to 8.4 mg/100 ml), and a reduction in alkaline phosphatase activity (80 decreased to 20 IU).[56] At necropsy, severe GI hemorrhage and hepatic fatty degeneration were present. Similarly, when a 300-kg heifer was given T-2 toxin at 0.12 mg/kg T-2 toxin and butenolide (another *Fusarium* metabolite) at 1.8 mg/kg for 5 d followed by 0.06 mg T-2 per kilogram and 0.9 mg butenolide per kilogram for 2 d, there were increases in aspartate aminotransferase activity (124 to 450 IU) and reductions in alkaline phosphatase activity (43 to 20 IU).

3. Effects of Macrocyclic Trichothecenes on Sheep

In a study to evaluate the toxic effects of macrocyclic trichothecenes, sheep were orally dosed with cultures of a cytotoxic strain of *Myrothecium roridum* or *M. verrucaria*.[57] At sublethal to lethal acute doses, sheep developed anorexia, ruminal tympany, and diarrhea. The lips and nostrils were frequently stained with regurgitated ingesta. Sheep that died had watery or mucoid GI contents, especially when death was less immediate. Ruminal ulcerations occurred together with hemorrhage. The ruminal papillae and superficial ridges in the reticular mucosa were congested and there was necrosis of the epithelium of the omasal folds. More deeply in the omasal folds and in the abomasum, there were variable degrees of submucosal hemorrhage. Severe hemorrhages sometimes occurred in the abomasum. In the small intestine, lesions were localized, less frequent, and included areas of inflammation, edema, and occasional submucosal hemorrhage. Lesions of the spiral colon, large intestine, and cecum were often extensive and sometimes included submucosal hemorrhage and ulceration. The livers were enlarged and mottled and the gall bladders were occasionally edematous and ulcerated.

With subacute toxicosis, dosed animals developed many of the above lesions plus extensive areas of caseous necrosis in the mucosa of the forestomachs. However, after 30 daily doses of as much as 1/2 of the dose which killed 3 of 4 sheep within 10 d, sheep developed only thickening of the abomasal mucosa.

Similarly, after "stomach tube" administration of lethal doses of partially purified crude verrucarin A, sheep became anorexic and developed diarrhea.[57] Portions of the ruminal mucosa were congested, and there was a severe, hemorrhagic abomasitis as well as mild enteritis with fluid intestinal contents.

After oral administration of purified verrucarin A at 4 mg/kg, an affected lamb developed hepatic hemorrhage, mucosal erosions, and hemorrhages in the small intestine.[57] At 2 mg/kg, there were no macroscopic liver lesions, but hemorrhagic erosions of the abomasal mucosa were noted. Similarly, after a lethal oral dose of purified roridin A at 4 mg/kg, the liver of the treated lamb was icteric and the lobular pattern increased. There was a very severe hemorrhagic gastroenteritis with marked edema and severe erosions of the mucosa of the abomasum. The small intestinal lumen contained firm casts of clotted blood and epithelial debris, which were removable in long cords. At 2 mg/kg, liver injury was not pronounced, but the abomasal mucosa was hemorrhagic and lined with green-black, caseous necrotic material. In addition, the small and large intestines were both hemorrhagic and eroded.

Apparent ovine stachybotryotoxicosis has also been documented in South Africa.[58] The animals experienced intermittent hemorrhagic diarrhea; the causative lesions were confirmed on necropsy. Subsequently, the causative organism was identified as *Stachybotrys chartarum*, and the field observations were experimentally reproduced.[59] Hemorrhagic enteritis was the predominant feature in both bovine and ovine stachybotryotoxicosis in Hungary.[60]

4. Effects of Macrocyclic Trichothecenes on Calves

In calves that died within 30 h of an oral dose of either *Myrothecium verrucaria* or *M. roridum* cultures, the livers were pale and enlarged.[57] The small intestine had areas of inflammation and severe submucosal hemorrhage. Milder lesions were present in the abomasum and large intestine. When death occurred after a more prolonged illness, there were no obvious changes in the liver. However, the mucosae of the forestomachs were markedly degenerated and the intestine contained increased fluid but little ingesta.

G. Swine

1. T-2 Toxin

When a group of swine were fed barley naturally contaminated with approximately 25 ppm of T-2 toxin "in a mixture with oats", clinical signs included first, vomiting, and later, diarrhea, feed refusal, and polydipsia. When turned out to pasture, the pigs ate inordinate amounts of grass.[17]

Sows fed T-2 toxin at 12 ppm in a complete ration for a prolonged time displayed multiple pinpoint-sized anterior esophageal mucosal erosions, a tenacious fibrin-like coating on the duodenal mucosa, and moderate congestion of the ileal mucosa which became progressively more severe aborally.[61] The spiral colon and gallbladder mucosa were congested and the major bile ducts were severely edematous. Activities of alkaline phosphatase and alanine and aspartate aminotransferases remained within normal limits.

Similarly, administration of T-2 toxin in the diet of growing swine at concentrations up to 8 ppm for 8 weeks (which is equivalent to a daily dose on the order of 0.35 mg/kg/d) did not cause serum lactate dehydrogenase, aspartate aminotransferase, alanine aminotransferase, alkaline phosphatase, or total protein to fall outside normal limits.[61] No hepatic or pancreatic lesions were detected in these swine nor in swine given single i.v. injections of T-2 toxin in an LD_{50} study and necropsied after death or from 1 to 12 d after dosing. Gross examination of swine that died due to single i.v. administration of T-2 toxin revealed stomachs filled with ration and an intestinal tract virtually devoid of ingesta or fecal material. Similar results, the presence of feed in the stomach, and more fluid/less voluminous contents of the remainder of the digestive tract were also observed at death or at 24 h postdosing in swine given T-2 toxin i.v. at 0.6 or 1.2 mg/kg.[54]

An intravascular dose of 0.15 mg T-2 toxin per kilogram did not cause vomiting;[62] however, the oral administration of T-2 toxin at 0.2 mg/kg reportedly caused "almost immediate" emesis in pigs.[63] Similarly, the administration of T-2 toxin intravascularly at 0.3, 0.6, 1.2, or 4.8 mg/kg or orally at 2.4 mg/kg was rapidly followed by salivation, bruxism (grinding of the teeth), and vomiting.[44,54] After T-2 toxin administration by the intravascular and oral routes, vomiting began within 8 to 30 and 30 to 60 min, respectively. Emesis persisted for approximately 1, 1.5, 2.5, and 7 h, after intravascular doses of 0.3, 0.6, and 1.2 mg/kg and the oral dose of 2.4 mg/kg, respectively. In the intravascularly dosed swine, tenesmus was sometimes severe (even at the 0.3 mg/kg dose) and was occasionally associated with watery diarrhea or flatulence. Diarrhea appeared as early as 2 h postdosing. Both intravascularly and intragastrically dosed swine sometimes assumed an "arched-up" stance with the hind legs positioned well forward, possibly indicating abdominal pain.

Redness of the gastric fundus, often with erosion, is the most consistent gross lesion in swine given high (1.2 mg/kg and greater) doses of T-2 toxin. At doses of 1.2, 4.8, or 5.4 mg/kg, multiple erosions have been observed with areas of hemorrhage, and a thick covering with mucus.[64] When compared to the 4.8 or 5.4 mg/kg doses, the lesions were less prominent at the 1.2 mg/kg dose and they were only occasionally observed at the 0.6 mg/kg dose. Histologic changes in the stomach of animals dosed at 1.2 to 5.4 mg/kg were described as a severe necrohemorrhagic gastritis. Fibrin thrombi were commonly observed in the capillaries and venules of the lamina propria associated with the necrosis. Severe epithelial cell necrosis in the gastric crypts occurred within or adjacent to the injured areas; however, individual parietal cell necrosis was observed in the absence of generalized necrosis. Similar gastric lesions have been observed in pigs dosed with T-2 toxin by inhalation.[65] It is widely known that swine are prone to similar gastric lesions in conjunction with other conditions causing circulatory shock, such as acute bacterial septicemias.

Gastric lesions in rats given endotoxin could be minimized by the concurrent administration of naloxone or proglumine,[66] suggesting the possible involvement of endorphins or gastrin, respectively. Based on a hemorrhagic shock model, it has been suggested that gastric ulceration in shock may be due to a reduction in the clearance of back-diffusing hydrogen ions, probably as a result of hypoperfusion.[67]

In swine that died after an oral dose at 2.4 mg/kg, the T-2 toxin induced gastric lesions were no worse, and in some instances were milder than those in animals given an intravascular dose at 1.2 mg/kg.[54] These findings and the presence of fibrin thrombi suggested the probable involvement of a vascularly mediated reaction, rather than a strictly cytotoxic (local gastric epithelial) effect. This was confirmed when it was found that the blood supply to the stomach of pigs dosed with T-2 toxin was severely compromised.[68] The rate of reduction in blood flow to the stomach was considerably greater than the rapid drop in cardiac output which occurred in the same pig. A the present time, however, the significance of the elaboration of thromboxane and/or catecholamines (vasoconstrictors known to be produced in T-2-dosed pigs[44]) in the development of gastric lesions is uncertain. Potentially adverse effects on gastric blood flow secondary to a direct toxic effect on the mucosal cells must also be considered. It is presently suggested, however, that the principal adverse effects on the stomach of T-2 dosed swine are due to impairment of blood supply, perhaps coupled with a degree of mechanical trauma associated with emesis. In a preliminary study in pigs dosed intravascularly with T-2 toxin, there was no increase in plasma histamine or serotonin concentrations.[44] This is of importance since histamine is known to stimulate gastric acid secretion.

A singular intravascular dose of 4.8 mg T-2 toxin per kilogram caused an increase in the serum activity of alkaline phosphatase while aspartate aminotransferase activity was increased by either 0.6 or 4.8 mg/kg.[69]

Pancreatic lesions induced by sublethal (0.6 mg/kg) i.v. doses of T-2 toxin have been characterized at the light microscopic and ultrastructural levels.[70] Severe pancreatic edema occasionally developed in T-2-dosed pigs. Microscopic changes were much more consistent. These included multifocal acinar degeneration and necrosis. Lesions found on electron microscopic examination included irregular dilation and coalescence of rough endoplasmic reticulum and zymogen granules which were sometimes irregular, "smudgy", or electron-lucent. In necrotic cells, the degenerate nucleus was displaced to the margin of the cell membrane by large cytoplasmic vacuoles. These lesions have also been observed in swine dosed with the toxin by inhalation (see the chapter "Inhalation Toxicity of the Trichothecene Mycotoxin T-2 Toxin"). Pancreatic damage is of particular interest for two reasons: it illustrates another instance in which blood flow to a target organ is severely impaired and it probably results in the elaboration of the myocardial depressant factor which follows pancreatic ischemia in shock states caused by other agents. The significance of these findings is discussed further in the chapter "Circulatory System Effects of Trichothecenes". The significance of pancreatic dysfunction, if any, at lower doses is less certain. The reader is reminded that the pancreatic lesions reported above for rats exposed to trichothecenes were observed after a series of acutely toxic parenteral doses.

2. Diacetoxyscirpenol

When given DAS i.v. in an LD_{50} study in which the doses ranged from 0.3 to 0.5 mg/kg, pigs started to vomit repeatedly beginning 20 min postinjection and continuing for 3 h.[71] The animals had increased frequency of defecation leading to watery diarrhea. The LD_{50} derived was 0.376 ± 0.043 mg/kg. Of the 15 pigs, 7 died within 24 h. At necropsy, stomachs were generally filled with feed. Although five out of seven that died reportedly had "no gross or microscopic DAS attributable lesions", two had severe GI lesions. These included severe congestion of the jejunum, the spiral colon, and especially the ileum, filling of the cecum with blood, and severe cecal mucosal hemorrhage. On the small intestinal mucosa, there was an overlying, yellow, fibrin-like coating. Microscopic lesions included hemorrhages in the lamina propria of the small intestine and severe submucosal edema. Many small intestinal mucosal cells were necrotic and there were multiple erosions with catarrhal exudation. Considerable hemorrhage and mucosal necrosis in the colon was present as well. In one animal, all sections of affected small and large intestines showed the presence of multiple fibrin thrombi in vessels and severe edema of the submucosa.

When given i.v. to swine at 0.5 to 1.0 mg/kg, DAS caused severe hemorrhagic, necrotizing, erosive gastritis limited to the glandular stomach.[72] The upper 1/2 to 2/3 of the gastric mucosa was necrotic and numerous thrombi were observed in the deep mucosal veins. Parietal cells in the gastric crypts were necrotic and sometimes sloughed. One pig that died 4 h after dosing also had necrosis of the fundic surface epithelium. The squamous epithelium, however, did not appear to be affected. Enteric lesions included a lack of mitotic activity in crypts. Necrosis of crypt enterocytes was noted and some of the cells contained eosinophilic intracytoplasmic inclusions. In severe cases, some crypts were packed with debris. Brunner's and Paneth cells, however, were spared. Congestion and hemorrhage were more prominent in areas overlying the Peyer's patches. As expected, these lymphoid structures were severely damaged by the toxicosis. Thrombi were present in the deep mucosal veins of the cecum. The predominant cells in the lamina propria of the control pigs were lymphocytes and plasma cells, but in these DAS-treated pigs (as in T-2 dosed pigs[54,64]), these areas contained debris and a few eosinophils.

In the study of DAS in pigs just mentioned,[72] pancreatic lesions were also observed, including extensive areas of necrosis affecting both acinar and islet cells with occasional saponification of the peripancreatic fat. These lesions, therefore, represent more severe and extensive damage than that mentioned previously for T-2 toxin. Like T-2 toxin, however, the acinar cells were still more sensitive than the islet cells. Alanine aminotransferase was mildly elevated in the DAS-dosed pigs.

3. Deoxynivalenol

The i.p. "emetic dose" of deoxynivalenol (DON) in young pigs was 0.1 mg/kg or lower, and the minimal oral emetic dose of DON in swine was 0.1 to 0.2 mg/kg.[73] Although DON has been called vomitoxin, in a survey of the effects of DON contaminated feed on swine, vomition was not a prevalent sign.[74] Clearly, reductions in feed intake occur much more readily than vomiting. It is, therefore, desirable to use only the term deoxynivalenol rather than the confusing use of both terms.

In swine given DON i.v. at 0.5 mg/kg, clinical signs included vomiting (which commenced at 6 to 7 min postdosing), as well as diarrhea, muscular weakness, tremors, and coma.[75] Emesis or retching persisted for up to 4 h. Diarrhea was observed at 1.5 h. Marked tenesmus, partial rectal prolapse, and mucoid diarrhea was first observed at 2 h and persisted through hour 10. Formed feces were present in the colon at necropsy 24 h postdosing, indicating a transient intestinal effect. Microscopic lesions were few, but included mild lymphoid necrosis of B-cell areas of the mesenteric lymph nodes and necrosis of the pancreatic acinar and islet cells.

In swine fed diets containing DON, a different gastric lesion has been observed as compared to the one associated with acutely toxic doses of T-2 toxin or DAS. The lesions were more like those described above for laboratory animals chronically fed diets containing T-2 toxin. Stomach weights of the swine (as a percentage of body weight) increased with elevations in DON content.[76] At higher concentrations (maximum: 5 ppm) in the diet, there was thickening and keratinization of the esophageal portion of the stomach. Longitudinal folds of the mucosa of the esophagus were also observed. In a prior study in which pigs were fed a diet reportedly containing 43 ppm of DON for 21 d, "no lesions attributable to DON" were reported.[77] A dietary concentration of 20 ppm caused vomiting.

H. Cats

Cats have been orally dosed for 13 to 34 d with T-2 toxin at 0.06 to 0.1 mg/kg/d as either pure compound or in a crude extract.[78] The animals developed multiple hemorrhagic erosions in the gastric mucosa and along the length of the intestinal tract. The superficial gastric mucosa was markedly necrotic. The small intestinal villi were frequently desquamated and the crypts of Lieberkuhn were consistently dilated and often filled with necrotic cells. Extensive necrosis in the mucosa of the small and large intestine of T-2 dosed cats had been previously reported.[79]

When an adult cat and a 1-week-old kitten died after single respective s.c. doses of fusarenon-X at 5.0 and 1.0 mg/kg, both had marked necrosis of "intrasinusoidal cells" of the liver.[20] Each cat exhibited marked vomiting within 30 min of the lethal s.c. injection of fusarenon-X.

I. Dogs

Fusarenon-X at 0.3 mg/kg i.v. caused vomiting in dogs which began 5 to 15 min postdosing and occurred repeatedly at intervals of 30 to 40 min for 1 to 3 h.[41] Increased frequency of fecal evacuation and urination occurred for the first 3 h; however, at a lower dose of 0.1 mg/kg, only 1 of 4 dogs vomited. The emetic effect of i.v. fusarenon-X at 0.3 mg/kg could be antagonized by injection of metaclopramide hydrochloride at 0.5 mg/kg, or chlorpromazine hydrochloride at 1.0 mg/kg at 1 h before toxin administration. The effectiveness of the latter drug suggests a possible stimulatory effect of fusarenon-X on the chemoreceptor trigger zone and secondarily the emetic center in the medulla oblongata. In a study of deoxynivalenol using 6-month-old dogs, the minimum effective s.c. dosages causing emesis and diarrhea were 0.1 and 0.2 mg/kg.[80]

When DAS was administered (apparently by the i.v. route) to beagle dogs in 5 single daily doses of 2.5 or 5.0 mg/m²/d, which corresponds to approximately 0.12 and 0.23 mg/kg/d, respectively, toxic signs included emesis, ptyalism, and diarrhea. There were also elevations of serum alkaline phosphatase, and alanine and aspartate aminotransferases.[81] In lethal regimens of 5 mg/m²/d, the same toxic effects occurred and necropsy revealed moderate congestion, with lymphoid infiltration, of the mucosa of the stomach. The only hepatic lesion described was congestion.

In dogs i.v. dosed with DAS at 0.5 mg/kg, clinical signs included panting, excessive salivation, emesis, defecation, apparent abdominal distress, diarrhea, and cyanosis.[82] At 8 h postdosing, when the animals were killed, the bone marrow was "void of cellular elements".

J. Nonhuman Primates

Adult Rhesus monkeys given T-2 toxin orally at 1 mg/kg/d vomited and some of the animals developed diarrhea. The toxic effects were more pronounced in males than in females.[83] When African Green monkeys were administered T-2 toxin by gastric intubation in doses varying from 0.25 to 10 mg/kg 3 times per week, animals given the high dosages died acutely with hemorrhagic diarrhea, and there were characteristic necrotic lesions in the intestine.[59]

K. Humans
1. Alimentary Toxic Aleukia (ATA)

In the early states of human ATA, changes occurred primarily in the mouth and GI tract.[84] Shortly after consuming toxic grains, individuals complained of burning sensations similar to a scalding of the mouth, tongue, throat, palate, esophagus, and stomach. In some people, the tongue felt stiff and swollen and the oral mucosa became hyperemic. Diarrhea, nausea, and vomition developed within a few days and, although accompanied by perspiration, there was generally no elevation of the body temperature. In severe cases of the first stage of ATA, however, fever sometimes exceeded 102°F (38.9°C) and was accompanied by acute esophagitis, esophageal pain, and sialorrhea, or gastroenteritis and abdominal pain.

In the third stage of ATA, multiple hemorrhages in the oral cavity and necrotic lesions of 5 to 7 mm in diameter occurred. A severe gangrenous pharyngitis was often accompanied by additional necrotic lesions extending to the soft palate, gingiva, cheeks, larynx, and vocal cords. These lesions, which were usually contaminated with an array of opportunistic bacteria, were accompanied by associated pain on swallowing.

Soft palate injuries sometimes caused regurgitation of food from the nose, while esophageal and epiglottal lesions were accompanied by laryngeal edema and laryngitis. Of deaths in persons during the third stage of ATA, approximately 30% were attributed to stenosis of the glottis! Although there was hemosiderosis and reticulosis in the liver, no marked hepatic degeneration occurred and serum bilirubin concentration were unaffected.

2. Anticancer Trials with Diacetoxyscirpenol

When DAS was administered in clinical studies as an anticancer drug at greater than 3 mg/m^2 i.v. for 5 d in repeated courses of treatment, toxic signs included moderate to severe nausea and vomiting.[81] Other immediate effects included diarrhea and stomatitis. Similarly, in breast cancer patients being given DAS at 5.0 mg/m^2 for 5 d once every 3 weeks, 87% of courses were associated with nausea and vomition.[85]

In human cancer patients being given 4-h infusions of DAS, GI manifestations were still among the dose-limiting factors.[86] Nausea, vomiting, and occasionally diarrhea occurred at doses over 4.0 mg/m^2 for patients with liver dysfunction, and at doses above 6.0 mg/m^2 for patients without hepatic dysfunction. GI toxicity was decreased somewhat when the dose, previously given in 4-h infusions, was instead administered over 8 h.

Of 27 cancer patients given DAS at 4.5 mg/m^2/d in 4-h infusions daily in 5-d courses, repeated every 21 d, and in which the dose was increased or decreased depending on toxicity, 13 had nausea and emesis.[87] Similarly, in other clinical anticancer trials, weekly administration of DAS at 1.5 mg/m^2 by i.v. infusion over 3 h caused only minimal nausea and vomiting, but at doses greater than 3.0 mg/m^2 these signs consistently occurred.[88] Diarrhea was infrequent, occurring only at 7.5 mg/m^2. When given DAS in regimens at 3.0 to 4.5 mg/kg/d × 5, 49% of human patients with GI or pancreatic malignancies experienced moderate to severe nausea and emesis. Two persons died from drug-related causes, one from sepsis and the other from hypotension.[89]

3. Carcinogenesis in Man

Cancer of the esophagus of man has been described in South Africa and northern China, and in both areas workers have suggested that *Fusarium* toxins might be involved, namely deoxynivalenol, zearalenone, moniliformin[90,91] and, more recently, the mutagenic metabolite fusarin C.[92] This remains an area of intense scientific interest.

4. Conclusions — Human Effects

The toxic effects observed in repeatedly treated cancer patients as well as the benefit of changing to several-hour-long infusions indicate that *in vivo* processes of distribution and detoxification limits some of the toxic effects of DAS. With naturally occurring ATA and the probable frequent oral ingestion of trichothecenes, both local and systemic effects were more severe. Unlike the anti-cancer trials with DAS, many of the digestive system effects observed in victims of ATA were highly suggestive of two primary effects of trichothecenes: local cytotoxicity and immunosuppression. In addition, dose-response differences, the mix of toxins present, nutritional imbalances, and other varying stresses undoubtedly affected these persons.

III. EFFECTS ON ENERGY METABOLISM

The lag period seen between the administration of trichothecene mycotoxins and severe clinical manifestations was suspected as being due to either production of a reactive metabolite, or to a direct effect of altered energy utilization on "some other enzyme process".[16] Several aspects of defective lipid and carbohydrate utilization have been experimentally produced by trichothecene mycotoxins. One can readily speculate that interference with energy metabolism may be a secondary manifestation of circulatory shock in *acute* toxicosis, and may result from enzyme depletion after interference with protein and/or DNA synthesis in either *acute or chronic* toxicosis. For the present, however, evidence demonstrating specific linkages between enzyme depletion and energy metabolism is limited.

A. Cholesterol

Synthesis of cholesterol in the liver is suppressed by dietary cholesterol and by fasting, whereas high fat diets accelerate this process.[93] Diminished food intake subsequent to trichothecene administration would, therefore, be expected to reduce serum cholesterol concentrations. This is in agreement with the modest reductions in serum cholesterol concentrations in broiler chicks fed T-2 toxin at as high as 4 ppm in the diet.[5] Moreover, the treatment of 6-week-old male chickens with single doses of T-2 toxin at 0.75 mg/kg i.m., concurrently with or without estradiol-17 β-dipropionate at 4.25 mg/kg i.m., revealed that T-2 toxin delayed the estradiol-induced increase in plasma triglyceride concentrations, and both delayed and lessened the estradiol-induced increase in plasma cholesterol concentrations.[13] When neither group was given estradiol, however, mean plasma cholesterol concentrations were only slightly less in T-2 treated chickens as compared with the solvent-treated controls. Similarly, serum cholesterol was not significantly affected by feeding chickens a ration containing T-2 toxin at up to 8 ppm for 8 weeks.[6] In contrast, when 4-week-old male broiler chicks were intubated with a single dose of T-2 toxin at 2.5 mg/kg, serum cholesterol was modestly increased at 4 and 12 h postadministration.[94]

After either 3 intragastric doses of a lyophilized *F. tricinctum* culture at 75 mg/kg/d or 2 i.p. doses of T-2 toxin at 2 mg/kg/d, rats exhibited a 33% increase in both serum cholesterol and serum total lipids;[30] however, the feeding of T-2 toxin at up to 8 ppm in swine rations for 8 weeks did not affect serum cholesterol sufficiently to result in abnormal concentrations.[95] Similarly, sows chronically fed 12 ppm T-2 toxin had normal serum cholesterol concentrations.[61]

Administration of T-2 toxin at 0.44 mg/kg/d to a Holstein cow for 16 d caused no change in serum cholesterol concentrations.[51] In addition, when this cow's calf was dosed beginning on the 4th postparturient day and continuing at daily or periodic intervals for a total of 16 doses, cholesterol was unaltered.

In consideration of these studies, the overall effects of *Fusarium* cultures and T-2 toxin on cholesterol concentrations appear to be slight and, therefore, the significance of these alterations is questionable.

B. Lipids and Fat-Soluble Vitamins

Unlike the trichothecene-associated increase in blood lipids described by Kosuri,[30] trichothecene mycotoxins have also been associated with reductions in blood lipids, as well as reductions in blood glucose concentrations. For example, when T-2 toxin was added at 20 ppm to diets of 30-week-old laying hens for 3 weeks, feed intake and plasma glucose and lipid concentrations declined.[4] The plasma lipids declined by 60% by 3 weeks; however, liver lipid concentrations and pancreas sizes were not altered.

In chicks fed a diet containing T-2 toxin at up to 15 ppm, there were dose-related decreases in plasma vitamin E concentrations of as much as 65%.[8] This was not explainable by lipid malabsorption as steatorrhea did not occur and total fecal lipids were not significantly affected. Furthermore, in chicks fed T-2 toxin at up to 5 ppm, there was no impairment of absorption of vitamin D_3.

Despite the evidence suggesting adequate lipid absorption, micelle-promoting compounds, when added to T-2 amended diets, alleviated the T-2 toxin-associated depressions of growth, feed efficiency, plasma vitamin E activity, and reduced liver and pancreas relative weights. Considering the minimal effects on lipid digestion and absorption, the effect on vitamin E transport may have been caused by T-2 induced reduction in the plasma lipoproteins required for vitamin E transport.[8] The micelle promoters apparently improved vitamin E absorption to overcome this limitation. These observations would also be compatible with an increase in vitamin E utilization (perhaps a result of lipid peroxidation) and agree with the finding of a preventive benefit of vitamin E administration as discussed in the chapter "Treatment and Prophylaxis for Trichothecene Mycotoxicosis".

When DON was fed to laying hens at up to 0.7 mg/kg of diet, a 15% increase in liver lipid and a 50% elevation of liver triglyceride were observed.[76]

C. Carbohydrates

In rats given 3 daily oral doses of lyophilized *Fusarium tricinctum* at 75 mg/kg or 2 daily
i.p. doses of T-2 toxin at 2 mg/kg, the mean serum glucose concentration was 61 mg/100
ml; the mean control concentration was 85 mg/100 ml.[30] Moreover, in glucose tolerance
tests using mice treated i.p. with fusarenon-X at 3 mg/kg, the normal initial increase in the
blood glucose concentration vs. time profile (at 15 min after oral administration of glucose)
was decreased by 60% and thereafter the curve remained rather flat.[34] This could have been
caused by either glucose malabsorption or accelerated glucose degradation, but was not
attributable to glycosuria. In view of the adverse effects of T-2 toxin on glucose absorption
mentioned previously,[39] glucose malabsorption is probable. Evidence for the accelerated
glucose utilization is also likely as suggested by the finding that the liver glycogen stores,
of mice injected i.v. with tritiated DAS, were markedly decreased by the second hour
postinjection and completely depleted by 6 h. Similarly, male mice, injected i.p. with a
sublethal dose of fusarenon-X at approximately 3 mg/kg and killed 1 to 4 h thereafter,
rapidly developed modest reductions in blood glucose followed by depletion of liver glycogen.[34] Liver glycogen was markedly decreased at 2 h postinjection and had almost disappeared at 3 h. In addition, the disappearance of liver glycogen did not result in a simultaneous
increase in serum glucose concentrations. It seems, therefore, that both glucose malabsorption
and accelerated glycolysis may combine to reduce liver glycogen. The accelerated disappearance of glucose and glycogen is probably not due, however, to an immediate, direct
effect on glycolysis since verrucarin A had no significant effect on aerobic or anaerobic
glycolysis in cells or tissues.[16] Similarly, in the liver of the pigs given a single, acutely toxic
i.v. dose of DAS, glycogen depletion was observed and this was correlated with antemortem
hypoglycemia observed in some of the pigs.[72] In pigs given DON i.v. at 0.5 mg/kg, as with
DAS, in spite of pancreatic damage, hypoglycemia was noted. With this dose of DON, the
hypoglycemia was moderate and transient, with values returning to normal by 24 h. Glycogen
synthesis may also be decreased due to depletion of amylophosphorylase activity as documented in the tissues of rats dosed with T-2 toxin at 3 mg/kg.[30]

In view of the increase in plasma cortisol concentrations observed in T-2 toxin-dosed
swine,[96] it seems probable that the physiologic effects of glucocorticoids are somehow
disrupted or overwhelmed during acute trichothecene toxicosis. In the absence of these
toxins, glucocorticoids alter carbohydrate and lipid metabolism, glucose is spared with a
tendency to induce hyperglycemia, there is release of free fatty acids into the blood, and
hepatic glycogen is increased. Glucocorticoids are also highly active in the induction of
enzymes involved in hepatic gluconeogenesis, which are required to convert carbon skeletons
of amino acids into glucose.[93]

Considering that fact that the protein synthesis inhibitor, cycloheximide, blocks gluconeogenesis by inhibition of the *de novo* synthesis of indispensible enzymes, it would be
worthwhile to determine whether this occurs during trichothecene toxicosis.

It was determined by autoradiography that ^{14}C-labeled d-glucose markedly accumulated
in and then very slowly disappeared from the brains of mice recovering from a sublethal
dose of fusarenon-X.[16] This phenomenon also occurs in rats recovering from radiation injury.

Effects on energy metabolism associated with the circulatory disturbances, tissue hypoxia,
and metabolic acidosis that occur during acute trichothecene toxicosis are also probable.

D. Oxidative Phosphorylation and Glucose Utilization

When the growth of *Saccharomyces* yeast cells on various carbohydrate sources were
compared, T-2 toxin caused varying degrees of growth inhibition.[97] From least to most
inhibited were yeast growing on glucose, galactose, maltose, sucrose, raffinose, and glycerol.
The authors suggested that an effect on mitochondrial enzymes may have been responsible
for these observations. In a subsequent study, it was suggested that the ability of T-2 toxin

to inhibit the growth of *S. cerevisiae* growing on glycerol and the lesser ability to affect the yeast when growing on glucose were indicative of inhibition of mitochondrial electron transport.[98] In the same study, increased resistance of yeast cells to mutagenesis induced by ethidium bromide and reduced pigment production by a mutated strain were taken as further proof of a T-2 toxin-associated reduction of cellular "energy levels".

T-2 toxin had no effect on oxidative phosphorylation in rat liver mitochondria,[16] and histochemical evaluations of tissues of rats dosed with T-2 toxin at 3 mg/kg revealed no inhibition of NADH oxidation or cytochrome oxidase activity.[30] Furthermore, the rates of oxygen consumption of kidney and brain tissues maintained on glucose, lactate, succinate, or butyrate substrates were not significantly affected after treatment of rats with T-2 toxin at 2 mg/kg.[30]

In contrast, oxygen consumption in liver tissue from these rats measured with glucose as a substrate was decreased by 46% and was decreased by 21 to 32% with the other substrates. Similarly, oxygen consumption by the gastrocnemius muscle from treated rats was decreased by approximately 35% with glucose, lactate, or butyrate as substrates. This suggested a decrease in the metabolic rate or a defect in oxygen utilization by these tissues. The failure to use glucose may imply decreased glucose uptake and, since liver and muscle were affected while brain and kidney were not, it is possible that an insulin deficiency or a reduction in insulin effect may have occurred.

Pace[99] suggested that T-2 toxin may inhibit mitochondrial oxygen consumption in either adenosine diphosphate coupled or dinitrophenol uncoupled systems. The toxin was tested *in vitro* at concentrations of from 0.05 to 2.2 mM which are equivalent to 23.1 to 1018 ppm. The highest concentration caused an approximately 40% reduction in oxygen consumption when the substrate succinate, pyruvate and malate, or glutamate was added simultaneously with the toxin. Preincubation with the high concentration of T-2 toxin prior to adding substrate could increase this effect. Also, T-2 could prevent the dinitrophenol-associated increase in oxygen uptake. The significance of these effects *in vivo*, however, is questionable in view of the high concentration of toxin requried to elicit an effect. These observations are in close agreement with those of Schiller and Yagen[100] who also reported a T-2 toxin-induced increase in hepatic mitochondrial latent ATPase. Of greater significance, perhaps, was the observed 45% reduction in pyruvate + malate-associated oxygen consumption of liver mitochondria from rats dosed 10 h previously with T-2 toxin s.c. at an LD$_{50}$ dose.[94] The actual biochemical mechanism for this trichothecene action is uncertain.

The P/O ratio is defined as the number of molecules of inorganic phosphate used to phosphorylate ADP per atom of oxygen consumed.[93] After oral administration to rats of T-2 toxin at 4.1 mg/kg or lyophilized *F. tricinctum* at 160 mg/kg, oxidative phosphorylation (P/O) ratios of liver mitochondria were not changed; however, oxygen consumed increased by approximately 30%.[30] These findings, overall, suggest intact function of F$_1$ ATPase and oxidative phosphorylation in T-2 intoxicated animals.

When the effects of fusarenon-X on the ciliated protozoan, *Tetrahymena pyriformis*, were investigated in a medium containing glucose, peptone, and yeast extract, 15 and 44% reductions of oxygen consumption were observed at mycotoxin concentrations of 1 and 5 ppm, respectively.[101] Nevertheless, a maximal 46% decrease in oxygen consumption occurred at 10 and 50 ppm of fusarenon-X. Thus, as in rat tissues, a significant inhibition of oxygen consumption occurred when glucose was the principal energy source even though insulin would not be involved in *Tetrahymena*.

Areas that have apparently not yet been investigated are effects of trichothecenes on either the citric acid cycle or the hexosemonophosphate shunt. In view of the diminished efficacy of glucose utilization in the presence of apparently increased oxygen consumption, study of these pathways could be worthwhile.

E. Phosphate Uptake and Phosphocreatine

The effects of fusarenon-X on lipid synthesis in *Tetrahymena pyriformis* were assessed by measurement of the incorporation of ^{14}C-acetate into neutral lipids and phospholipids and ^{32}P-phosphate into the latter.[101] Fusarenon-X at 50 ppm inhibited acetate incorporation into tetrahymanol, a pentacyclic triterpenoid alcohol, by about 1/2, but stimulated its incorporation into triglycerides 10-fold. The increased triglyceride synthesis was presumed to be caused by a 50% decrease in ^{14}C-acetate incorporation into phospholipids and an almost complete inhibition of ^{32}P-phosphate incorporation. The phosphate incorporation was apparently decreased as a result of fusarenon-X-induced inhibition of cellular ^{32}P-phosphate uptake. The inhibition of phosphate entry into the cells was rapid, as a considerable degree of inhibition was observed even when ^{32}P-phosphate was added simultaneously with fusarenon-X. Whether phosphate entry into mammalian or avian cells is affected by trichothecenes apparently has not been investigated.

Creatine phosphate is of paramount importance in muscle and nerve cells as a large store of high energy for the phosphorylation of ADP to form the 1/5 as abundant, slightly lower energy ATP.[93] If creatine phosphate were depleted as a result of defective phosphorus uptake and/or creatinuria, this could be a significant factor in the toxicity of trichothecenes. Creatine kinase, also called ATP creatine-phosphotransferase or creatine phosphokinase, catalyzes the reaction ADP + phosphocreatine $\rightarrow$ ATP + creatine in which both creatine and ADP are bound to the active site and after which they leave in either sequence. Creatine kinase is present in the sarcoplasm, and at normal sarcoplasmal pH of about 6, the creatine kinase equilibrium lies very much in favor of the formation of ATP. This fact explains why ATP concentrations of muscle do not decline during a single contraction as the terminal phosphate lost from ATP is instantly replenished from phosphocreatine. In view of the fact that the rephosphorylation of creatine phosphate is an energetically unfavored reaction, a functional enzyme and high ATP concentration are necessary for normal function. If creatine kinase were inhibited or somehow depleted by trichothecenes, one would expect creatine to be lost in the urine as the only known pathway of formation of creatine phosphate is by reversal of the same reaction which phosphorylates ATP.[93]

Rats treated with verrucarin A or J developed creatinuria.[102] The creatinuria was far greater than that attributable to starvation but it could be prevented by large doses of vitamin E. Elevations of inorganic phosphorus concentrations are found in the serum of swine given acutely toxic doses of T-2 toxin.[69] Both creatinura in rats and increased inorganic phosphorus in swine may indicate failure of phosphate entry into cells as seen in *Tetrahymena* or increased ATP degradation due to stress with decreased production of creatine phosphate. In acute toxicosis it is possible that hypoxia in skeletal muscle as a result of circulatory shock may be involved. Another hypothesis is that the creatinuria and/or hyperphosphatemia are a result of severe ATP depletion, perhaps due to depletion of creatine kinase from protein synthesis inhibition with a secondary reduction in the amount of creatine being converted into creatine phosphate. This deserves investigation.

The Sanger reagent 2,4-dinitrofluorobenzene has been used to completely inhibit creatine kinase. In muscles poisoned in this manner, ATP quickly declines on stimulation, but phosphocreatine remains unchanged. Epoxides of many compounds react enzymatically or nonenzymatically with sulfhydryl groups of amino acids and proteins. Creatine kinase, alcohol dehydrogenase, and lactate dehydrogenase all possess thiol (sulfhydryl) groups in their catalytic centers.[103] Significant reaction with the epoxy groups of trichothecenes and resulting inhibition of creatine kinase is, however, unlikely in trichothecene mycotoxicosis. Although creatine kinase was inhibited by trichothecenes *in vitro*, the EC_{50} for this inhibition were 7×10^{-4} *M* and 28×10^{-4} *M* for verrucarins A and J, respectively.[102] These concentrations correspond to unrealistically high concentrations of 3500 and 13,000 ppm.

In agreement with Guarino et al.,[102] Ueno and Matsumoto[103] found that T-2 toxin, neosolaniol, and fusarenon-X did not inactivate creatine kinase or two other sulfhydryl-containing enzymes when added in the presence of their substrates at 10 mM (400 to 500 ppm). Inactivation occurred, however, when the toxins, at the same 10 mM concentration, were preincubated with creatine kinase before the addition of the substrate. Also, the inhibitory effect of the fusarenon-X on one of the other enzymes tested, alcohol dehydrogenase, could be prevented by the addition of glutathione or dithiothreitol. Alcohol dehydrogenase has 36 thiol residues, of which 4 react with sulfhydryl reagents. Gel filtration of this enzyme and incubation with labeled toxin identified a complex with a molar ratio of approximately four trichothecene molecules to one alcohol dehydrogenase molecule. These findings are compatible with the hypothesis that trichothecenes can bind to these reactive sulfhydryl residues. The actual significance of effects on sulfhydryl groups of enzymes, however, clearly remains to be demonstrated because of the extremely high toxin concentrations tested.

It may be noted that liver and kidney do not rely heavily on creatine phosphate, and they are among the more resistant tissues to trichothecenes despite their disproportionately high exposure in the body. Phosphocreatinine is not used by invertebrates. Instead, phosphoarginine is the storage reservoir of phosphate-bond energy of muscles in invertebrates and this compound operates under the influence of arginine kinase. Whether the differences between these compounds are of importance in the susceptibility of invertebrates to trichothecenes may be worthy of consideration.

F. Interplay between Energy Balance, Metabolic Rates, and Susceptibility to Trichothecenes

Metabolic rates of rats fasted for 2 d and then dosed with crude T-2 toxin at 100 mg/kg declined rapidly, and the animals died within 48 h;[104] however, in nonfasted rats dosed with T-2 toxin, metabolic rates declined for 1 to 2 d and then returned to normal by the 3rd day. None of the nonfasted animals died. Therefore, fasting clearly increases susceptibility to T-2 toxin and increases the associated depression of metabolic rate. Similarly, in persons or poor diets, ATA was more often of severe or lethal consequences.

IV. SUMMARY AND CONCLUSIONS

In a range of species, reduced feed intake seems to be one of the most sensitive indicators of dietary exposure to trichothecenes. At higher doses or with repeated exposure, this may be followed by actual feed refusal, emesis in capable species, and possibly the development of perioral, oral, pharyngeal, esophageal or gastroenteric lesions or a combination of these. Perioral and oral lesions have been most thoroughly documented in birds, swine, and horses. Humans with ATA sometimes suffered from severe necrotic stomatitis, pharyngitis, and even suffocation. It seems logical to assume that immunosuppression probably interacts with cytotoxic and possibly vascularly mediated mucosal damage.

Clearly the trichothecene mycotoxins affect the digestive tract by virtue of both local cytotoxic effects and, at least at acutely toxic doses, by altering its blood supply. Lesions include damage to and partial loss of the mucous membrane, which may involve not only crypt necrosis, but also loss of the tips of microvilli. Fluid loss into the gut appears to be a result of a loss of vascular functional integrity and damage to the mucosal epithelium. Perhaps as a result of actual mucosal loss or inhibition of enzyme synthesis, absorption of glucose, amino acids, and sodium are reduced and activities of Na^+-K^+-ATPase and especially sucrase may decline. Fluid loss into the gut (and not a direct trichothecene stimulation of peristalsis) seems to be the primary mechanism for diarrhea. Whether autonomic nervous system stimulation is involved (as discussed in the chapter "Effects of Trichothecene Mycotoxins on the Nervous System") is less certain, but the intestine probably retains responsiveness to neural stimulation unless its motility is inhibited by shock-associated hypoxia. Either hypo- or hyperglycemia may occur. The former seems to be more common and is likely to be related to both reduced absorption and increased utilization; the latter may potentially be a response to secretion of glucocorticoids and to reduced utilization.

Gastric lesions in animals experiencing trichothecene-induced shock appear to be mediated by reduced blood flow and, perhaps, a secondary decrease in clearance of hydrogen ions from the mucosa. Chronic hypertrophic changes in the squamous portion of the stomach may be a response to local cytotoxicity.

The liver appears to be spared from the adverse effects of highly toxic doses of trichothecenes, at least in part, by virtue of increased blood flow, despite overall vascular collapse in many other sites. In some studies, however, damage to bile ducts and gall bladder can occur, probably due to disproportionately high exposure to toxic metabolites.

Alkaline phosphatase activity may be elevated acutely, perhaps as a result of circulatory collapse and ischemia of the gut. More important is the characteristic reduction in alkaline phosphatase in response to repeated exposure to trichothecenes. This is likely to be a manifestation of the combined processes of elimination of trichothecene metabolites in the bile with local protein synthesis inhibition and reduced intake of food.

Reductions in blood flow to the pancreas have been observed after exposure to comparatively high doses of trichothecenes and seem to be associated with pancreatic necrosis.

Hemorrhagic enteropathies have been associated with trichothecene exposures of livestock in the field, but have been somewhat difficult to reproduce in the laboratory, occurring only after comparatively high doses with the more toxic trichothecenes. These are likely to be a combined result of trichothecene-induced vascular and mucosal damage and reduced activities of clotting proteins.

Cholesterol synthesis and concentrations do not appear to change in a consistent manner as a result of trichothecene exposure. Concentrations of plasma lipids may be expected to decline, possibly due to a reduction in lipoprotein synthesis and possibly due to increased utilization of lipids as glucose availability declines. Plasma vitamin E activity is also reduced. Micelle-promoting agents, however, were able to alleviate T-2 toxin-associated reductions in vitamin E, as well as liver and pancreas weights.

A reduction in glucose utilization by tissues requiring insulin (muscle and liver) and not tissues that do not require insulin (brain and kidney) suggested that defective insulin production or secretion might be involved. Whether creatine kinase is directly involved (by reduced synthesis or inhibition), trichothecene toxicosis is likely to deplete ATP, to reduce stores of creatine phosphate, and to cause creatinuria. Finally, preexistent energy depletion increases susceptibility to trichothecene toxicosis.

REFERENCES

1. **Marasas, W. F. O., Smalley, E. B., Degurse, P. E., Bamburg, J. R., and Nichols, R. E.,** Acute toxicity to rainbow trout (*Salmo gairdneri*) of a metabolite produced by the fungus *Fusarium tricinctum*, *Nature*, 214, 817, 1967.
2. **Marasas, W. F. O., Bamburg, J. R., Smalley, E. B., Strong, F. M., Ragland, W. L., and Degurse, P. E.,** Toxic effects on trout, rats, and mice of T-2 toxin produced by the fungus *Fusarium tricinctum* (Cd.) Snyd. et. Hans., *Toxicol. Appl. Pharmacol.*, 15, 471, 1969.
3. **Poston, H. A., Coffin, J. L., and Combs, G. F.,** Biological effects of dietary T-2 toxin on rainbow trout, *Salmo gairdneri*, *Aquat. Toxicol.*, 2, 79, 1982.
4. **Wyatt, R. D., Doerr, J. A., Hamilton, P. B., and Burmeister, H. R.,** Egg production, shell thickness, and other physiological parameters of laying hens affected by T-2 toxin, *Appl. Microbiol.*, 29, 641, 1975.
5. **Chi, M. S., Mirocha, C. J., Kurtz, H. J., Weaver, G., Bates, F., and Shimoda, W.,** Subacute toxicity of T-2 toxin in broiler chicks, *Poult. Sci.*, 56, 306, 1977.

6. **Chi, M. S., Mirocha, C. J., Kurtz, H. J., Weaver, G., Bates, F., and Shimoda, W.,** Effects of T-2 toxin on reproductive performance and health of laying hens, *Poult. Sci.,* 56, 628, 1977.

7. **Speers, G. M., Mirocha, C. J., Christensen, C. M., and Behrens, J. C.,** Effects on laying hens of feeding corn invaded by two species of *Fusarium* and pure T-2 toxin, *Poult. Sci.,* 56, 98, 1977.

8. **Coffin, J. L. and Combs, G. F.,** Impaired vitamin E status of chicks fed T-2 toxin, *Poult. Sci.,* 60, 385, 1981.

9. **Chi, M. S. and Mirocha, C. J.,** Necrotic oral lesions in chickens fed diacetoxyscirpenol, T-2 toxin and crotocin, *Poult. Sci.,* 57, 807, 1978.

10. **Richard, J. L., Cysewski, S. J., Pier, A. C., and Booth, G. D.,** Comparison of effects of dietary T-2 toxin on growth, immunogenic organs, antibody formation, and pathologic changes in turkeys and chickens, *Am. J. Vet. Res.,* 39, 1674, 1978.

11. **Chi, M. S., Mirocha, C. J., Kurtz, H. J., Weaver, G., Bates, F., Shimoda, W., and Burmeister, H. R.,** Acute toxicity of T-2 toxin in broiler chicks and laying hens, *Poult. Sci.,* 56, 103, 1977.

12. **Shlosberg, A., Weisman, Y., Handji, V., Yagen, B., and Shore, L.,** A severe reduction in egg laying in a flock of hens associated with trichothecene mycotoxins in the feed, *Vet. Hum. Toxicol.,* 26, 384, 1984.

13. **Pearson, A. W.,** Biochemical changes produced by *Fusarium* T-2 toxin in the chicken, *Res. Vet. Sci.,* 24, 92, 1978.

14. **Hoerr, F. J., Carlton, W. W., and Yagen, B.,** Mycotoxicosis caused by a single dose of T-2 toxin or diacetoxyscirpenol in broiler chickens, *Vet. Pathol.,* 18, 652, 1981.

15. **Osborne, D. J., Huff, W. E., Hamilton, P. B., and Burmeister, H. R.,** Comparison of ochratoxin, aflatoxin, and T-2 toxin for their effects on selected parameters related to digestion and evidence for specific metabolism of carotenoids in chickens, *Poult. Sci.,* 61, 1646, 1982.

16. **Bamburg, J. R. and Strong, F. M.,** 12,13-Epoxytrichothecenes, in *Microbial Toxins,* Vol. 7, Kadis, S., Ciegler, A., and Ajl, S. J., Eds., Academic Press, New York, 1971, 207.

17. **Greenway, J. A. and Puls, R.,** Fusariotoxicosis from barley in British Columbia. I. National occurrence and diagnosis, *Can. J. Comp. Med.,* 40, 12, 1976.

18. **Puls, R. and Greenway, J. A.,** Fusariotoxicosis from barley in British Columbia. II. Analysis and toxicity of suspected barley, *Can. J. Comp. Med.,* 40, 16, 1976.

19. **Palyusik, M. and Koplik-Kovacs, E.,** Effect on laying geese of feeds containing the fusariotoxins T-2 and F-2, *Acta Vet. Acad. Sci. Hung.,* 25, 363, 1975.

20. **Ueno, Y., Yeno, I., Iitoi, Y., Tsunoda, H., Enomoto, M., and Ohtsubo, K.,** Toxicological approaches to the metabolites of *Fusaria.* III. Acute toxicity of fusarenon-X, *Jpn. J. Exp. Med.,* 41, 521, 1971.

21. **Hayes, M. A. and Wobeser, G. A.,** Subacute toxic effects of dietary T-2 toxin in young mallard ducks, *Can. J. Comp. Med.,* 47, 180, 1983.

22. **Ellison, R. A. and Kotsonis, F. N.,** T-2 toxin as an emetic factor in moldy corn, *Appl. Microbiol.,* 26, 540, 1973.

23. **Black, R. M.,** The Detection and Analysis of Trichothecene Mycotoxins, A Review, Tech. Note No. 553, Chemical Defence Establishment, Salisbury, U.K., 1983.

24. **Schoental, R. and Joffe, A. Z.,** Lesions induced in rodents by extracts from cultures of *Fusarium poae* and *F. sporotrichioides, J. Pathol.,* 112, 37, 1974.

25. **Schoental, R., Joffe, A. Z., and Yagen, B.,** Cardiovascular lesions and various tumors found in rats given T-2 toxin, a trichothecene metabolite of *Fusarium, Cancer Res.,* 39, 2179, 1979.

26. **Hayes, M. A., Bellamy, J. E. C., and Schiefer, H. B.,** Subacute toxicity of dietary T-2 toxin in mice: morphological and hematological effects, *Can. J. Comp. Med.,* 44, 203, 1980.

27. **Hayes, M. A. and Schiefer, H. B.,** Subacute toxicity of dietary T-2 toxin in mice: influence of protein nutrition, *Can. J. Comp. Med.,* 44, 219, 1980.

28. **Ohtsubo, K.,** Pathology of trichothecene toxicosis, *Proc. Jpn. Assoc. Mycotoxicol.,* 13, 19, 1981.

29. **DeNicola, D. B., Rebar, A. H., Carlton, W. W., and Yagen, B.,** T-2 toxin mycotoxicosis in the guinea-pig, *Food Cosmet. Toxicol.,* 16, 601, 1978.

30. **Kosuri, N. R., Smalley, E. B., and Nichols, R. E.,** Toxicologic studies of *Fusarium tricinctum* (Corda) Snyder et Hansen from moldy corn, *Am. J. Vet. Res.,* 32, 1843, 1850, 1971.

31. **Schiefer, H. B., Hancock, D. S., and Bhatti, A. R.,** Systemic effects of topically applied trichothecenes. II. Studies with T-2 toxin in rats, *J. Vet. Med.,* A33, 384, 1986.

32. **Ueno, Y. and Ueno, I.,** Toxicology and biochemistry of mycotoxins, in *Toxicology, Biochemistry and Pathology of Mycotoxins,* Uraguchi, K. and Yamazaki, M., Eds., Kodansha, Tokyo and Halstad Press, New York, 1978, 107.

33. **Matsuoka, Y. and Kubota, K.,** Studies on mechanisms of diarrhea induced by fusarenon-X, a trichothecene mycotoxin from *Fusarium* species, *Toxicol. Appl. Pharmacol.,* 57, 293, 1981.

34. **Shimizu, T., Nakano, N., Matsui, T., and Aibara, K.,** Hypoglycemia in mice administered with fusarenon-X, *Jpn, J. Med. Sci. Biol.,* 32, 189, 1979.

35. **Hayes, M. A.,** Morphological and Toxicological Studies on Experimental T-2 Mycotoxicosis, Ph.D. thesis, University of Saskatchewan, Saskatoon, Canada, 1979.

36. **Schiefer, H. B. and Hancock, D. S.,** Systemic effects of topically applied trichothecenes. I. Comparative study of various trichothecenes in mice, *J. Vet. Med.,* A33, 373, 1986.
37. **Sherding, R. G.,** Diseases of the small bowel, in: *Textbook of Veterinary Internal Medicine Diseases of the Dog and Cat,* Ettinger, S. J., Ed., 1983, 1294.
38. **Matsuoka, Y. and Kubota, K.,** Studies of mechanisms of diarrhea induced by fusarenon-X, a trichothecene mycotoxin from *Fusarium* species; the effects of fusarenon-X and various cathartics on the digestion and the absorption in the mouse intestine, *Yakagakn Zasshi,* 105, 77, 1985.
39. **Suneja, S. K., Ram, G. C., and Wagle, D. S.,** Effects of T-2 toxin on glucose and tryptophan uptake and intestinal mucosal enzymes, *Toxicon,* 22, 39, 1984.
40. **Riess, G., Strugala, G. J., Fichtl, B., and Forth, W.,** Effects of T-2 toxin on the intestinal absorption of glucose, water, and electrolytes in vitro, in Proceedings of 6th European *Symposium on Animal, Plant and Microbial Toxins,* Meler, J., Stocker, K., and Freyrogel, T. A., Eds., S. Karger, Basel, 1984, 117.
41. **Matsuoka, Y., Kubota, K., and Ueno, Y.,** General pharmacological studies of fusarenon-X, a trichothecene mycotoxin from *Fusarium* species, *Toxicol. Appl. Pharmacol.,* 50, 87, 1979.
42. **Saito, H., Enomoto, M., and Tatsuno, T.,** Radiomimetic biological properties of the new scirpene metabolites of *Fusarium nivale, Gann,* 60, 599, 1969.
43. **Duebbert, I. E. and Peterson, J. W.,** Enterotoxin-induced fluid accumulation during experimental salmonellosis and cholera: involvement of prostaglandin synthesis by intestinal cells, *Toxicon,* 23, 157, 1985.
44. **Lorenzana, R. M., Beasley, V. R., Buck, W. B., Ghent, A. W., Lundeen, G. R., and Poppenga, R. H.,** Experimental T-2 toxicosis in swine. I. Changes in cardiac output, aortic mean pressure, catecholamines, 6-keto-PGF 1 alpha, thromboxaneB$_2$, and acid-base parameters, *Fundam. Appl. Toxicol.,* 5, 879-892, 1985.
45. **Feuerstein, G., Goldstein, D. S., Ramwell, P. W., Zerbe, R. L., Lux, W. E., Jr., Faden, A. I., and Bayorh, M. A.,** Cardiorespiratory, sympathetic and biochemical responses to T-2 toxin in the guinea pig and rat, *J. Pharmacol. Exp. Ther.* 232, 786, 1985.
46. **Lafarge-Frayssinet, C., Lespinats, G., Lafont, P., Louisillier, F., Mousset, S., Rosenstein, Y., and Frayssinet, C.,** Immunosuppressive effects of *Fusarium* extracts and trichothecenes: blastogenic response of murine splenic and thymic cells to mitogens (40439), *Proc. Soc. Exp. Biol. Med.,* 160, 302, 1979.
47. **Rosenstein, Y., Lafarge-Frayssinet, C., Lespinats, G., Loisillier, F., Lafont, P., and Frayssinet, C.,** Immunosuppressive activity of *Fusarium* toxins. Effects on antibody synthesis and skin grafts of crude extracts, T-2 toxin, and diacetoxyscirpenol, *Immunology,* 36, 111, 1979.
48. **Rosenstein, Y., Kretschmer, R. R., and Lafarge-Frayssinet, C.,** Effect of *Fusarium* toxins, T-2 toxin, and diacetoxyscirpenol on murine T-independent immune responses, *Immunology,* 44, 555, 1981.
49. **Bamburg, J. R., Marasas, W. F., Riggs, N. V., Smalley, E. B., and Strong, F. M.,** Toxic spiroepoxy compounds from *Fusaria* and other hyphomycetes, *Biotechnol. Bioeng.,* 10, 445-455, 1968.
50. **Gentry, P. A. and Cooper, M. L.,** Effects of *Fusarium* T-2 toxin on hematological and biochemical parameters of the rabbit, *Can. J. Comp. Med.,* 45, 400, 1981.
51. **Weaver, G. A., Kurtz, H. J., Mirocha, C. J., Bates, F. Y., Behrens, J. C., Robison, T. S., and Swanson, S. P.,** The failure of purified T-2 mycotoxin to produce hemorrhaging in dairy cattle, *Can. Vet. J.,* 21, 210, 1980.
52. **Pier, A. C., Cysewski, S. J., Richard, J. L., Baetz, A. L., and Mitchell, L.,** Experimental mycotoxicoses in calves with aflatoxin, ochratoxin, rubratoxin, and T-2 toxin, *Proc. U.S. Anim. Health Assoc.,* 130, 1976.
53. **Osweiler, G. D., Hook, B. S., Mann, D. D., Buening, G. M., and Rottinghaus, G. E.,** Effects of T-2 toxin in cattle, *Proc. U.S. Anim. Health Assoc.,* 214, 1981.
54. **Beasley, V. R.,** The Toxicokinetics and Toxicodynamics of T-2 Toxin in Swine and Cattle, Ph.D. thesis, University of Illinois, Chicago, 1983.
55. **Friend, S. C. E., Hancock, D. S., Schiefer, H. B., and Babiuk, L. A.,** Experimental T-2 toxicosis in sheep, *Can. J. Comp. Med.,* 47, 291, 1983.
56. **Kosuri, N. R., Grove, M. D., Yates, S. G., Tallent, W. H., Ellis, J. J., Wolff, I. A., and Nichols, R. E.,** Response of cattle to mycotoxins of *Fusarium tricinctum* isolated from corn and fescue, *J. Am. Vet. Med. Assoc.,* 157, 938, 1970.
57. **Mortimer, P. H., Campbell, J., DeMenna, M. E., and White, E. P.,** Experimental myrotheciotoxicosis and poisoning in ruminants by verrucarin A and roridin A, *Res. Vet. Sci.,* 12, 508, 1971.
58. **Schneider, D. J., Marasas, W. F. O., Dale Kuys, J. C., Kriek, N. P. J., and Van Schalkwyk, G. C.,** A field outbreak of suspected stachybotryotoxicosis in sheep, *J. S. Afr. Vet. Assoc.,* 50, 73, 1979.
59. **Kriek, N. P. J. and Marasas, W. F. O.,** Trichothecene research in South Africa, *in Trichothecenes—Chemical, Biological and Toxicological Aspects,* Ueno, Y., Eds., Kodansha, Tokyo and Elsevier, Amsterdam, 1983, 273.
60. **Szathmary, C. I.,** Toxicoses and natural occurrence in Hungary, *in Trichothecenes - Chemical, Biological and Toxicological Aspects,* Ueno, Y., Ed., Kodansha, Tokyo and Elsevier, Amsterdam, 1983, 229.

61. **Weaver, G. A., Kurtz, H. J., Mirocha, C. J., Bates, F. Y., Behrens, J. C., and Robison, T. S.,** Effect of T-2 toxin on porcine reproduction, *Can. Vet. J.,* 19, 310, 1978.

62. **Corley, R. A., Swanson, S. P., Gullo, G. J., Johnson, L., Beasley, V. R., and Buck, W. B.,** Disposition of T-2 toxin, a trichothecene mycotoxin, in intravascularly dosed swine, *J. Agric. Food Chem.,* 34, 868, 1986.

63. **Patterson, D. S. P., Matthews, J. G., Shreeve, B. J., Roberts, B. A., McDonald, S. M., and Hayes, A. W.,** The failure of trichothecene mycotoxins and whole cultures of *Fusarium tricinctum* to cause experimental haemorrhagic syndromes in calves and pigs, *Vet. Rec.,* 105, 252, 1979.

64. **Pang, V. F.,** T-2 Mycotoxicosis in Swine Following Topical Application, Intravascular Administration and Inhalation Exposure, Ph.D. thesis, University of Illinois, Chicago, 1986.

65. **Pang, V. F., Lambert, R. J., Felsberg, P. J., Beasley, V. R., Buck, W. B., and Haschek, W. M.,** Experimental T-2 toxicosis in swine following a single inhalation exposure: clinical signs, pathology, and effects on systemic and local pulmonary immunity, *Toxicol. Pathol.,* in press.

66. **Parmer, N. S.,** Gastric mucosal damage induced by endotoxin shock and its prevention by naloxone and anti-ulcer drugs in rats, *Toxicon,* 24, 611, 1986.

67. **Kivilaakso, E., Fromm, D., and Silen, W.,** Relationship between ulceration and intraruminal pH of gastric mucosa during hemorrhagic shock, *Surgery,* 84, 70, 1978.

68. **Beasley, V. R., Lundeen, G. R., Poppenga, R. H., and Buck, W. B.,** Distribution of blood flow to the gastrointestinal tract of swine during T-2 toxin induced shock, *Fundam. Appl. Toxicol.,* 1987.

69. **Lorenzana, R. M., Beasley, V. R., Buck, W. B., and Ghent, A. W.,** Experimental T-2 toxicosis in swine. II. Effect of intravascular T-2 toxin on serum enzymes and biochemistry, blood coagulation and hematology, *Fundam. Appl. Toxicol.,* 5, 893, 1985.

70. **Pang, V. F., Adams, J. H., Beasley, V. R., Buck, W. B., and Haschek, W. M.,** Myocardial and pancreatic lesions induced by T-2 toxin, a trichothecene mycotoxin in swine, *Vet. Pathol.,* 23, 13, 1986.

71. **Weaver, G. A., Kurtz, H. J., Mirocha, C. J., Bates, F. Y., and Behrens, J. C.,** Acute toxicity of the mycotoxin diacetoxyscirpenol in swine, *Can. Vet. J.,* 19, 267, 1978.

72. **Coppock, R. W., Gelberg, H. B., Hoffman, W. E., and Buck, W. B.,** The acute toxicopathy of intravenous diacetoxyscirpenol (anguidine) administration in swine, *Fundam. Appl. Toxicol.,* 5, 1034, 1985.

73. **Forsyth, D. M., Yoshizawa, T., Morooka, N., and Tuite, J.,** Emetic and refusal activity of deoxynivalenol to swine, *Appl. Environ. Microbiol.,* 34, 547, 1977.

74. **Beasley, V. R., Swanson, S. P., Reynolds, R. D., Coppock, R. W., Corley, R. A., Cote, L. M., and Buck, W. B.,** Current status of toxicokinetics and residue detection of trichothecene mycotoxins in swine, cattle, and feedstuffs, *Proc. U.S. Anim. Health Assoc.,* 82, 245, 1982.

75. **Coppock, R. W., Swanson, S. P., Gelberg, H. B., Koritz, G. D., Hoffman, W. E., Buck, W. B., and Vesonder, R. F.,** Preliminary study of the pharmacokinetics and toxicopathy of deoxynivalenol (vomitoxin) in swine, *Am. J. Vet. Res.,* 46, 169, 1985.

76. **Trenholm, H. L., Hamilton, R. M. G., Friend, D. W., Thompson, B. K., and Hartin, K. E.,** Feeding trials with vomitoxin (deoxynivalenol)-contaminated wheat: effects on swine, poultry and dairy cattle, *J. Am. Vet. Med. Assoc.,* 185, 527, 1984.

77. **Young, L. G., McGirr, L., Valli, V. E., Lumsden, J. H., and Lun, A.,** Vomitoxin in corn fed to young pigs, *J. Anim. Sci.,* 57, 655, 1983.

78. **Lutsky, I., Mor, N., Yagen, B., and Joffe, A. Z.,** The role of T-2 toxin in experimental alimentary toxic aleukia: a toxicity study in cats, *Toxicol. Appl. Pharmacol.,* 43, 111, 1978.

79. **Sato, N., Ueno, Y., and Enomoto, M.,** Toxicological approaches to the toxic metabolites of *Fusaria.* VIII. Acute and subacute toxicities of T-2 toxin in cats, *Jpn. J. Pharmacol.,* 25, 263, 1975.

80. **Yoshizawa, T. and Morooka, N.,** Studies on the toxic substances in the infected cereals III. Acute toxicities of new trichothecene mycotoxins: Deoxynivalenol and its monoacetate, *J. Food Hyg. Soc. Jpn.,* 15, 261, 1974.

81. **Murphy, W. K., Burgess, M. A., Valdivieso, M., Livingston, R. B., Bodey, G. P., and Freireich, E. J.,** Phase I clinical evaluation of anguidine, *Cancer Treat. Rep.,* 62, 1497, 1978.

82. **Coppock, R. W.,** Studies on the Pharmacokinetics and Toxicopathy of Diacetoxyscirpenol and Deoxynivalenol in Swine, Cattle, and Dogs, Ph.D. thesis, University of Illinois, Chicago, 1984.

83. **Rukmini, C., Prasad, J. S., and Rao, K.,** Effects of feeding T-2 toxin to rats and monkeys, *Food Cosmet. Toxicol.,* 18, 267, 1980.

84. **Joffe, A. Z.,** *Fusarium Species: Their Biology and Taxonomy,* John Wiley & Sons, New York, 1986, 225.

85. **Yap, H. Y., Murphy, W. K., DiStefano, A., Blemenschein, G. R., and Bodey, G. P.,** Phase II study of anguidine in advanced breast cancer, *Cancer Treat. Rep.,* 63, 789, 1979.

86. **Belt, R. J., Haas, C. D., Joseph, U., Goodwin, W., Moore, D., and Hoogstraten, B.,** Phase I study of anguidine administered weekly, *Cancer Treat. Rep.,* 63, 1993, 1979.

87. **Thigpen, T., Vaughn, C., and Stuckey, W. J.,** Phase II trial of anguidine in patients with sarcomas unresponsive to prior chemotherapy: a Southwest oncology group study, *Cancer Treat. Rep.,* 65, 9, 1981.

88. **DeSimone, P. A., Greco, F. A., and Lessner, H. F.,** Phase I evaluation of a weekly schedule of anguine, *Cancer Treat. Rep.,* 63, 2015, 1979.
89. **Bukowski, R., Vaughn, C., Bottomley, R., and Chen, T.,** Phase II study of anguidine in gastrointestinal malignancies: a southwest oncology group study, *Cancer Treat. Rep.,* 66, 381, 1982.
90. **Marasas, W. F. O., van Rensburg, S. J., and Mirocha, C. J.,** Incidence of *Fusarium* species and the mycotoxins, deoxynivalenol and zearalenone, in corn produced in esophageal cancer areas in Transkei, *J. Agric. Food Chem.,* 27, 1108, 1979.
91. **Thiel, P. J., Meyer, C. J., and Marasas, W. F. O.,** Natural occurrence of moniliformin together with deoxynivalenol and zearalenone in Transkeian corn, *J. Agric. Food Chem.,* 30, 308, 1982.
92. **Gelderblom, W. C. A., Thiel, P. G., Marasas, W. F. O., and van der Merwe, K. J.,** Natural occurrence of fusarin C, a mutagen produced by *Fusarium moniliforme,* in corn, *J. Agric. Food. Chem.,* 32, 1064, 1984.
93. **Lehninger, A. L.,** *Biochemistry, the Molecular Basis of Cell Structure and Function,* 2nd ed., Worth Publishers, New York, 1977.
94. **Chi, M. S., El-Halawani, M. E., Waibel, P. E., and Mirocha, C. J.,** Effects of T-2 toxin on brain catecholamines and selected blood components in growing chickens, *Poult. Sci.,* 60, 137-141, 1981.
95. **Weaver, G. A., Kurtz, H. J., Bates, F. Y., Chi, M. S., Mirocha, C. J., Behrens, J. C., and Robison, T. S.,** Acute and chronic toxicity of T-2 mycotoxin in swine, *Vet. Rec.,* 103, 531, 1978.
96. **Rafai, P. and Tuboly, S.,** Effect of T-2 toxin on adrenocorticol function and immune response in growing pigs, *Zentralbl. Vet. Med. B,* 29, 558, 1982.
97. **Schappert, K. T. and Khachatourians, G. G.,** Effects of fusariotoxin T-2 on *Saccharomyces cerevisiae* and *Saccharomyces carlsbergensis, Appl. Environ. Microbiol.,* 45, 862, 1983.
98. **Schappert, K. T. and Khachatourians, G. G.,** Effects of T-2 toxin on induction of petite mutants and mitochondrial functions in *Saccharomyces cerevisiae, Curr. Genet.,* 10, 671, 1986.
99. **Pace, J. G.,** Effects of T-2 mycotoxin on rat liver mitochondrial electron transport system, *Toxicon,* 21, 675, 1983.
100. **Schiller, C. M. and Yagen, B.,** Inhibition of mitochondrial respiration by trichothecene toxins from *Fusarium sporotrichioides., Fed. Proc.,* 40, 1579, 1981.
101. **Chiba, J., Nakano, N., Morooka, N., Nakazawa, S., and Watanabe, Y.,** Inhibitory effects of fusarenon-X, a sesquiterpene mycotoxin, on lipid synthesis and phosphate uptake in *Tetrahymena pyriformis. Jpn. J. Med. Sci. Biol.,* 25, 291, 1972.
102. **Guarino, A. M., Mendillo, A. B., and DeFeo, J. J.,** Toxic and inflammatory properties of two antibiotics: muconomycin A and B. *Biotechnol. Bioeng.,* 10, 457, 1968.
103. **Ueno, Y. and Matsumoto, H.,** Inactivation of some thiol-enzymes by trichothecene mycotoxins from *Fusarium* species, *Chem. Pharm. Bull.,* 23, 2439, 1975.
104. **Smalley, E. B., Marasas, W. F. O., Strong, F. M., Bamburg, J. R., Nichols, R. E., and Kosuri, N. R.,** Mycotoxicoses Associated with Moldy Corn. Proc. 1st U.S.-Japan Conf. on Toxic Micro-Organisms, 1983, 163.

Chapter 4

EFFECTS ON THE CIRCULATORY SYSTEM*

James K. Bubien, Gregg Lundeen, Charles Templeton, and W. T. Woods, Jr.

TABLE OF CONTENTS

* This work was supported in part by USAMRDC, DAMD 17-86-C-6075, and DAMD 17-83-C-2179.

I. INTRODUCTION

This chapter describes the cardiovascular toxicity of trichothecene mycotoxins in mammals and is organized according to the species in which the trichothecene toxicoses (either accidental or experimental) have been observed. *In vivo* effects and *in vitro* experiments (if any) are described and interpreted. A common observation in most species after sufficient exposure to trichothecene has been initial tachycardia followed by bradycardia and hypotension. In cases of severe toxicosis, a shock-like syndrome has often been described. The available experimental evidence indicates that the effects of trichothecenes on the cardiovascular system are both direct and indirect (mediated through reflex mechanisms, hormones, shock, other tissues damaged, etc.). In laboratory tests, initial tachycardia and increased arterial blood pressure were prevented by either sympathetic blockers or brain stem ablation, indicating that these effects were centrally reflexively mediated. At very high degrees of exposure, trichothecene-induced hypotension, bradycardias and/or tachycardias, and arrhythmias have been demonstrated *in vivo*. These effects could not be reversed by drugs and were not present after brain stem ablation. Therefore, these cardiovascular effects resulted, at least in part, from trichothecene-induced central nervous system dysfunction. Alternate hypotheses, that trichothecenes interfere with myocyte transmembrane ion fluxes and that trichothecenes inhibit protein synthesis, are discussed in the context of observed cardiovascular effects.

II. HUMANS

One of the first diseases associated with trichothecene mycotoxicosis in humans was alimentary toxic aleukia (ATA), outbreaks of which followed ingestion of moldy cereal grains or their products.[21] *Fusarium poae* and *F. sporotrichoides* isolated from samples of infected grain were shown to produce trichothecenes, particularly T-2 toxin.[23] A common cardiovascular effect in patients with ATA is tachycardia.[15]

When phase I and II human clinical trials were undertaken to evaluate the trichothecene diacetoxyscirpenol (DAS, anguidine) as a cancer chemotherapeutic agent,[4,11,35,64] a consistent effect was hypotension. The hypotension was dependent upon dose and frequency of administration and was associated with dizziness and light-headedness. In some of the studies, patients developed hypotension requiring fluid therapy, and in one patient, infusion of 7.5 mg/m^2 (approximately 0.21 mg/kg) resulted in life-threatening hypotension (60/40 mmHg; systolic/diastolic). Of two treatment-related deaths reported, one was attributed to myelosuppression and sepsis and the other to hypotension.[7]

HT-2 (a reduced metabolite of T-2 toxin) has been identified in myocardial tissue from an alleged "yellow rain" victim.[33] Some of the signs and symptoms of the victim included tachycardia, dyspnea, cyanosis, angina, syncope, fatigue, and dizziness. Thin sections of myocardium taken 31 d after the alleged exposure showed acute interstitial hemorrhage, intramural hemorrhage of medium-sized coronary arteries, acute myocarditis, and hyperacute ischemic myocardial lesions. The detection of the toxin metabolites and, perhaps, the acute character of the myocardial lesion are suggestive of much more recent exposure.

III. NONHUMAN PRIMATES

Cynomolgus monkeys were given T-2 toxin intramuscularly (0.33, 0.65, or 2.00 mg/kg).[19] Cardiovascular parameters were evaluated noninvasively using electrocardiography, echocardiography, and assessment of cuff blood pressure. Blood gases and respiratory rates were also followed. All animals given 0.33 mg/kg survived. The monkeys dosed at 0.65 or 2.00 mg/kg died within 12 to 27 h and 11 to 12 h, respectively. Hemodynamic alterations were characterized by reductions in arterial pressure, peripheral resistance, cardiac output, and stroke volume. Indices of cardiac output suggested a direct negative inotropic effect on the heart. A slight tachycardia was observed. These observations are consistent with shock. Arterial oxygen tension decreased, and arterial carbon dioxide tension increased. There were no attempts at respiratory compensation. Rhesus monkeys given T-2 toxin (1 mg/kg/d) orally developed apathy and weakness of the lower limbs.[44]

IV. HORSES AND CATTLE

Trichothecene toxicosis in horses has been associated with contamination of feed and bedding by the saprophytic fungus *Stachybotrys atra*.[14] Macrocyclic trichothecenes have been produced from isolates of *S. atra* by Harrach et al.[18] Stachybotryotoxicosis has been classified into typical and atypical forms. Typical stachybotryotoxicosis is subdivided into three stages. Stage I consists of stomatitis and usually occurs when the animals are chronically exposed to low levels of moldy feed.[14] Signs of the second stage of intoxication include thrombocytopenia, leukopenia, agranulocytosis, and increased clotting time. Necrosis of the oral mucosa can also be observed.[14] The third stage of intoxication is characterized by arrhythmias, new areas of necrosis of the oral mucosa, fever, depression, a weak pulse, and usually death.[13]

The atypical ("shocking") form of stachybotryotoxicosis is associated with the consumption of large quantities of mold-infected fodder. It occurs within 10 to 12 h after feeding and is almost always fatal. Central nervous system effects are often characteristic of the atypical form. Horses have reduced reflexes, blindness, and lethargy interrupted by fits of hyperexcitability. Initially cardiac activity accelerates but becomes severely depressed with time.[14] Weak pulse, cyanosis, dyspnea, increased body temperature, and mucosal hemorrhaging suggest either direct or reflex-induced cardiovascular dysfunction with atypical stachybotryotoxicosis.

Horses in several districts of Hokkaido, Japan, died when moldy bean hulls were used as fodder and bedding.[59] Signs of intoxication included convulsions, cyclic movement, impaired respiration, and bradycardia. T-2 toxin and neosolaniol were isolated from the moldy bean hulls.

Calves given daily oral doses of toxic strains of *Myrothecium* died within 4 to 8 d. The only clinical manifestations of intoxication were increased salivation and respiration.[34] T-2 toxin given orally (0.6 mg/kg/d for 6 weeks) caused no change in the ratio of heart to body weight.[36] Intravenously injected (0.6 or 1.2 mg/kg) and orally administered (2.4 or 3.6 mg/kg) T-2 toxin caused cold mucous membranes and ears in calves, indicating reduced blood circulation.[2]

Recently, T-2 toxin was shown to increase vascular resistance in an *in vitro* bovine ear perfusion system. Concentrations from 1×10^{-5} *M* to 1×10^{-2} *M* (equivalent to 4.6 to 4625 ppm) produced a dose-dependent increase in perfusion pressure and also a decreased vascular response to histamine and norepinephrine compared to toxin-free control preparations.[63]

V. SWINE

Intravascular infusion of T-2 toxin (0.6 or 4.8 mg/kg) (via the pulmonary artery) produced a syndrome similar to cardiovascular shock since early declines in both cardiac output (CO) and mean arterial pressure (MAP) were observed.[27] In animals given 0.6 mg/kg T-2 toxin, CO and MAP stabilized by 4 h postdosing. By 24 h, CO had returned to predosing levels, while MAP remained below control values (23 to 25% reduction). In those pigs given 4.8 mg/kg T-2 toxin, both variables (CO and MAP) continued to decline until death. Both groups of animals dosed with T-2 toxin exhibited significant increases in heart rate. This increase, however, was not evident until 2 h after toxin administration. Similarly, pulmonary vascular resistance was increased in response to T-2 toxin infusion.

In this same study, the authors evaluated changes in plasma catecholamine concentrations (i.e., epinephrine and norepinephrine) in response to T-2 toxin. In those animals dosed with T-2 toxin at 4.8 mg/kg, tremendous oscillations and overall elevations in both epinephrine and norepinephrine were noted. Although concentrations of both norepinephrine and epinephrine were elevated in the low dose group (0.6 mg/kg T-2 toxin), these increases were somewhat attenuated as compared to the high dose. The infusion of either dose of T-2 toxin did not affect plasma concentrations of dopamine. Similarly, plasma histamine and serotonin concentrations remained unchanged.

The prostanoid, thromboxane (TX) A_2 arises from platelets and acts as a vasoconstrictor and platelet adhesion activator, and its production is reflected by the presence of increased concentrations of its stable hydrolysis product, TXB_2. In contrast, prostacyclin is a prostaglandin compound produced by vessel walls that is vasodilatory and which reduces platelet adhesion. Its production is indicated by the presence of increased amounts of 6-keto-$PGF_{1\alpha}$.

Plasma concentrations of TXB_2 and 6-keto-$PGF_{1\infty}$ increased following T-2 toxin administration. TBX_2 characteristically increased before elevations in 6-keto-$PGF_{1\alpha}$ were noted.

Arterial (aortic) oxygen tension (PaO_2) remained functionally adequate in both groups of animals given T-2 toxin. Arterial carbon dioxide tension ($PaCO_2$), however, decreased in response to the toxin. Similarly, arterial pH was significantly reduced in both T-2 toxin-dosed groups. This decline in pH was accompanied by a 15-fold increase in plasma lactic acid concentrations. Overall, therefore, the animals experienced a metabolic acidosis and attempts toward respiratory compensation were inadequate to prevent severe reductions in blood pH.

Hemodynamic and organ blood flow changes induced by T-2 toxin were also studied in swine.[28] Animals were injected with T-2 toxin (0.6 or 2.4 mg/kg) or 70% ethanol via the pulmonary artery. CO (cardiac output) and organ blood flow was determined using the radioactive microsphere technique. In pigs given 0.6 mg/kg T-2 toxin, CO decreased as compared to values of respective control (70% ethanol) animals at 3 and 4.5 h postdosing, but had returned toward control by 6 h. Mean arterial pressure (MAP) in the 0.6 mg/kg group followed a similar trend. In the high dose group (2.4 mg/kg T-2 toxin), decreases in CO and MAP did not occur until 3 h postdosing. Thereafter, these values continued to decline until termination of the experiment of 6 h postdosing. As in the study by Lorenzana et al.,[27] heart rates were increased in both T-2 treated groups in response to the hypotension and reduced cardiac output. Similarly, a metabolic acidosis, characterized by a significant decrease in arterial pH and $PaCO_2$, was observed. The administration of T-2 toxin did not alter PaO_2 or body temperature.

Brain blood flow was decreased in response to the 2.4 mg/kg dose of T-2 toxin. In those pigs given 0.6 mg/kg T-2 toxin, brain blood flow showed marked fluctuations and as a result was significantly decreased at 1.5 and 4.5 postdosing. Because of the greater reduction in total CO, however, the percentage of CO received by the brain was significantly increased, which suggests locally mediated vasodilation to preserve blood flow.

Administration of T-2 toxin caused a reduction in cerebral blood flow at all postdosing time points except at 3 h in the low dose group. These decreases are most likely explained by reductions in perfusion pressure; however, these changes in cerebral blood flow were not as rapid as the decline in MAP, again indicating a compensatory attempt to preserve blood flow to the cerebrums. The decline in cerebral blood flow may contribute to cerebral hypoxia and explain, in part, the neurologic deficits described in the chapter "Effects of Trichothecene Mycotoxins on the Nervous System".

Cerebellar blood flow was decreased only in those animals given 2.4 mg/kg T-2 toxin.

Again, these reductions were not as extreme as the fall in arterial pressure. Since the main function of the cerebellum is to maintain equilibrium and coordination, these reductions could be partially responsible for the ataxia and incoordination associated with T-2 toxicosis.

Brain stem blood flow was altered in a fashion similar to that described for cerebellar blood flow. The respiratory center is located in areas of the brain stem. In those animals given T-2 toxin at 2.4 mg/kg, the resultant decrease in brain stem blood flow could have impaired centrally mediated respiratory function. This could, perhaps, contribute to the inability of animals to successfully compensate for metabolic acidosis.

Blood flow to the myocardium behaved in a fashion similar to that described for the brain. Myocardial blood flow declined, but the fraction of CO perfusing the heart increased. Left ventricular (LV) blood flow decreased from control values only at 4.5 h postdosing in those pigs given 0.6 mg/kg T-2 toxin. In the high dose group (2.4 mg/kg T-2 toxin), LV blood flow was decreased at 3, 4.5, and 6 h postdosing. These reductions were not as severe as the decline in arterial pressure. This seems to indicate the presence of functional autoregulation and a degree of coronary vasodilation in an effort to maintain myocardial blood flow.

Blood flows to the interventricular septum behaved similar to that observed for LV blood flow. Right ventricular blood flow was not affected by T-2 toxin administration despite the significant changes in MAP. This may be due to a combination of intact autoregulation in response to the lower pressure and the lower tension normally developed in the right ventricle during systole.

At 2.4 mg/kg T-2 toxin, adrenal blood flow was significantly increased. Although a similar trend appeared to occur in those animals given 0.6 mg/kg, the increase was not statistically significant. The authors have speculated that this increase in blood flow may be due to enhanced adrenal activity and oxygen consumption as catecholamine production increased in response to the hypotension and decreased cardiac output. In addition, glucocorticoid (i.e., cortisol) release has been documented in pigs given T-2 toxin.[41] It appears that the glucocorticoids may be involved in maintaining the integrity of vascular receptors to endogenous catecholamines.[16] In view of the dilatory effects of epinephrine on the adrenal vasculature (i.e., via β-receptor mediated action), it is likely that the glucocorticoids contribute to the increase in adrenal blood flow by augmenting the reduction in adrenal vascular resistance.

Renal blood flow decreased in a dose-dependent manner which paralleled the reduction in MAP. Since the decrease in absolute blood flow paralleled the drop in CO, the percentage of cardiac output received by the kidneys remained unchanged.

Pancreatic and splenic blood flows were the most severely compromised of the organs/tissues studied. In both organs, absolute blood flow was decreased up to 90% of respective control values.

Hepatic arterial blood flow increased in both groups of animals given T-2 toxin. As a result, the percentage of cardiac output going to this organ was substantially increased.

Animals given 0.6 mg/kg T-2 toxin i.v. and killed 24 and 48 h later had multifocal edema of the myocardium, myofiber hyalinization, vacuolation, and formation of contraction bands with areas of nuclear pyknosis.[38] Myocardial lesions were largely confined to the subendocardium. The lesions were similar to those induced by catecholamines.[43] All animals injected with T-2 toxin had multifocal acinar degeneration and necrosis of the pancreas, with irregular dilatations of the endoplasmic reticulum. These results and the ischemia reported by Lundeen et al.[28] suggest that the necrosis was a probable result of inadequate pancreatic blood flow and that a myocardial depressant factor (MDF) was probably released from damaged pancreatic tissue. The combination of myocardial damage and MDF would probably cause at least additive functional myocardial depression during acute trichothecene intoxication. The nature and concentrations of metabolites of T-2 toxin detected in myo-

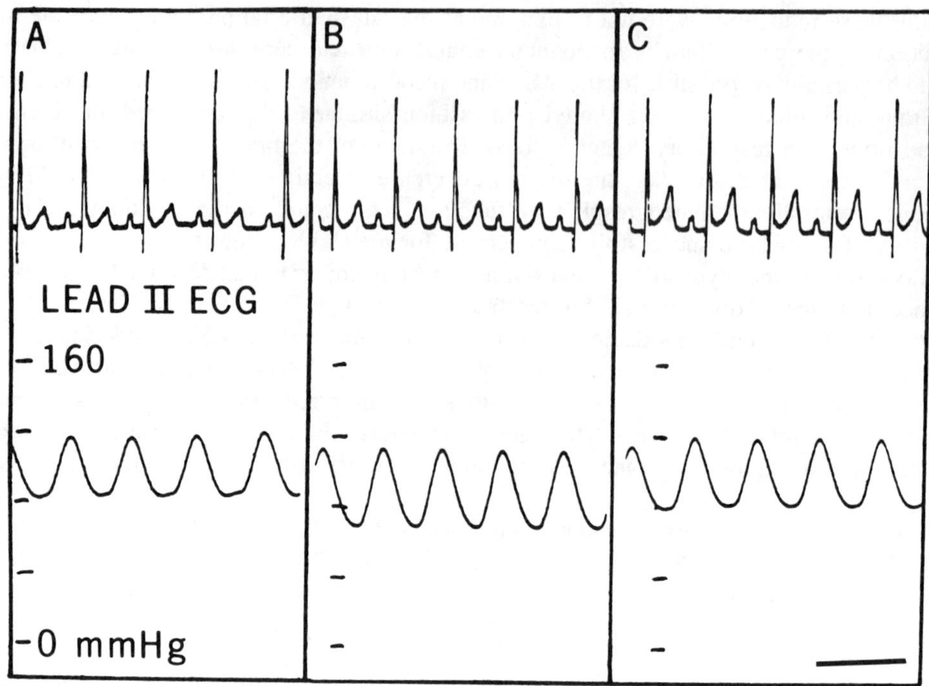

FIGURE 1.   These panels show a lead II ECG (upper) and arterial pressure (lower) in an anesthetized animal before i.v. T-2 (1.5 mg/kg panel A), 2 h after T-2 (panel B), and 1 h later following injection of propranolol (5 mg) (panel C). Note that only part of the T-2-induced tachycardia (150 to 176 beats per minute) was blocked by propranolol (165 beats per minute). The time-dependent increase in T-wave amplitude suggested hyperkalemia, but P-waves remained prominent, suggesting that K^+ concentration was normal horizontal calibration bar is 1.0 s. (Reprinted with permission from Bubien, J. K. and Woods, W. T., Jr., Direct and reflex cardiovascular effects of trichothecene mycotoxins, *Toxicon,* 25,325-331, © 1987, Pergamon Press, Ltd.)

cardium of pigs given T-2 toxin are discussed in the chapter "Absorption, Distribution, Metabolism, and Exertion of Trichothecene Mycotoxins".

VI. DOGS

Intravenous injection of T-2 toxin or roridin-A (2 mg/kg) into pentobarbital-anesthetized (30 mg/kg) dogs produced decreased systolic pressure within 30 min and atrioventricular block within 60 min.[6] Tachycardia was observed in all animals tested within 45 ± 15 min after injection with toxin. To separate direct toxin effects from reflex effects, some animals were pretreated with either propranolol (5 mg/kg i.v.) or atropine (5 mg/kg). The toxin-induced tachycardia was reduced by 50% in the propranolol-pretreated animals. Cardiovascular responses in animals pretreated with atropine sulfate, however, were not different. These results suggest that trichothecenes induce both direct (only 50% of the toxin-induced tachycardia was blocked by propranolol) and reflex cardiac effects mediated by the sympathetic nervous system. Parasympathetic nerves did not appear to contribute to the cardiovascular effects observed during trichothecene toxicosis because animals pretreated with atropine sulfate had responses to both T-2 toxin and roridin-A that were identical to those in animals that were not pretreated. The decrease in mean arterial pressure and increase in heart rate are shown in Figure 1.

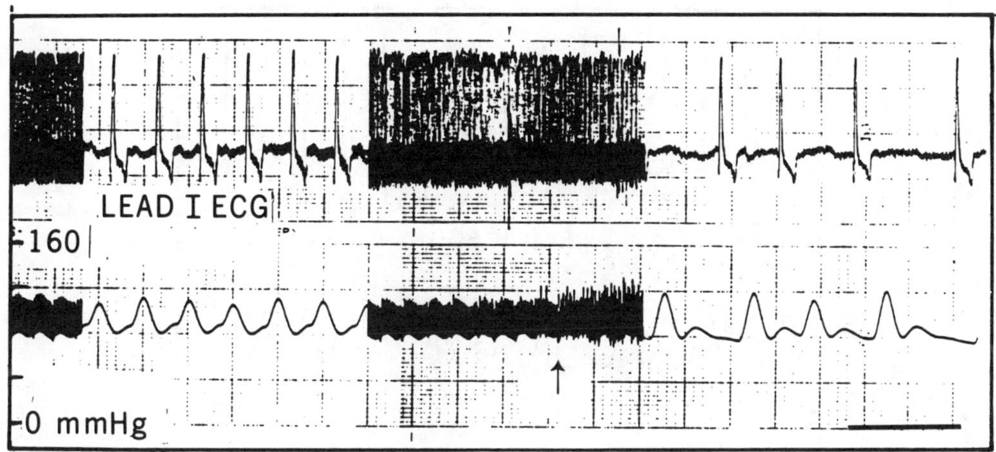

FIGURE 2. This continuous record shows the transition from normal impulse conduction to second-degree atrioventricular block observed 1 h after i.v. roridin-A (2.0 mg/kg). The lead I ECG (upper trace) and arterial pressure (lower trace) show the irregular rate associated with this arrhythmia which began at the arrow. Horizontal calibration bars are 1.0 s (fast speed) and 1.0 min (slow speed). (Reprinted with permission from Bubien, J. K. and Woods, W. T., Jr., Direct and reflex cardiovascular effects of trichothecene mycotoxins, *Toxicon*, 25,325-331, © 1987, Pergamon Press, Ltd.)

Intravenous injection of roridin-A (2 mg/kg) did not reduce the mean arterial pressure up to 6 h after it was injected; however, in all animals tested, roridin-A induced atrioventricular block within 60 min after it was administered. Subsequent infusion of sympathetic and parasympathetic blocking drugs had no effect on the arrhythmias, which persisted until death or irreversible deterioration. These results suggest that roridin-A directly depresses atrioventricular conduction in the canine heart. Figure 2 shows the onset of atrioventricular block after the injection of roridin-A into an anesthetized dog. Figure 3 shows the prolonged and irregular P-R intervals characteristic of atrioventricular block.

In addition to the evidence of direct myocardial effects *in vivo*, direct electrophysiologic effects of trichothecene toxins have been observed in *in vitro* canine cardiac preparations.[6] Spontaneous firing of isolated canine right atrial muscle perfused through the sinus node artery became depressed when trichothecenes were added to the perfusate. The firing rate slowed by 11 and 21%, respectively, when a high concentration of T-2 toxin (30 mg/1) or roridin-A (30 mg/1) was added. *In vitro* preparations were isolated from exogenous sympathetic or humeral inputs. Therefore, the toxin effects observed *in vitro* were direct effects. Dimethylsulfoxide (DMSO) was the vehicle for toxins. In separate tests, the concentration of DMSO used to dissolve the toxins (1.2% by vol) increased the rate of spontaneous beating by 9%. The vehicle, therefore, may have antagonized the toxin-induced bradycardia.

Additional *in vitro* studies of the cardiac effects of trichothecenes were performed using single cells from the sinus node region impaled with conventional microelectrodes for measurement of action potentials. Analysis of the action potentials is summarized in Table 1. T-2 toxin (30 mg/1) did not produce any significant changes in sinus node cell action potentials. Roridin-A (30 mg/1) reduced the slope of phase 4 by 51% and increased (negatively) the maximum diastolic potential by 10%. These action potential changes demonstrate that sinus node cells perfused with high concentrations of roridin-A have altered transmembrane ion fluxes. These results suggest that roridin-A directly depresses cells of the cardiac conduction system. This direct effect is a possible explanation for the atrioventricular block observed *in vivo*. Figure 4 shows action potential recorded from the sinus node prior to and after perfusion with DMSO, T-2, and roridin-A.

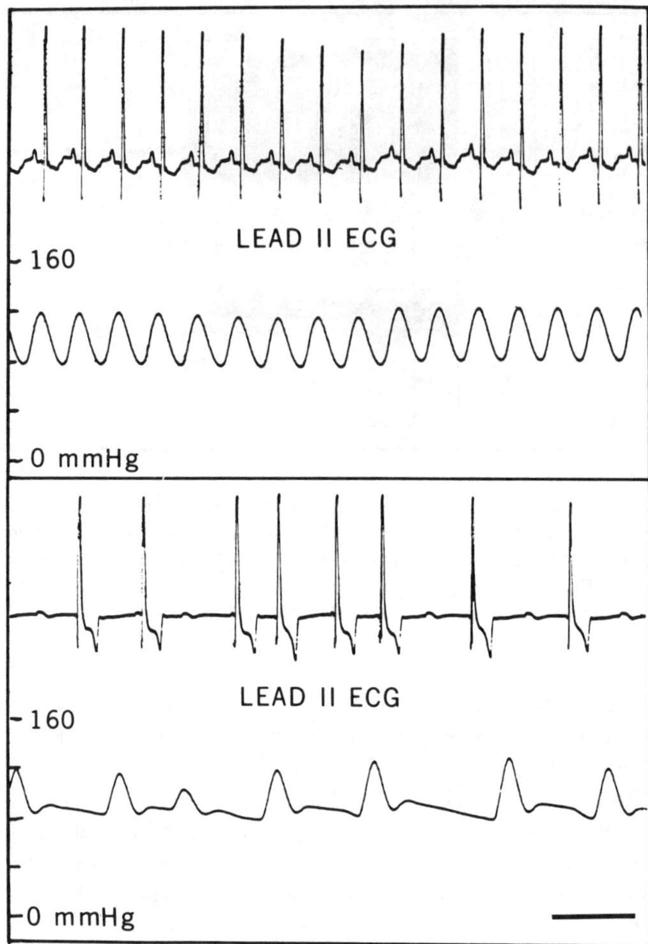

FIGURE 3.   These two records (from the same experiment as Figure 2) show that roridin-A prolonged the PR interval (80 to 320 ms) and increased the T wave amplitude. Upper panel was before and lower panel was 2 h after roridin-A was injected. Horizontal calibration bar is 1.0 s. (Reprinted with permission from Bubien, J. K. and Woods, W. T., Jr., Direct and reflex cardiovascular effects of trichothecene mycotoxins, *Toxicon,* 25,325-331, © 1987, Pergamon Press, Ltd.)

Table 2 summarizes the analysis of action potentials recorded in working canine atrial myocytes. T-2 toxin (30 mg/1) did not alter any action potential parameters. Roridin-A (30 mg/1) shortened the action potential duration by 20%, but DMSO also shortened the action potential duration by 22%. Therefore, the roridin-A had no significant effect on working atrial myocyte action potential durations.

Trichothecenes have also been tested for direct electrophysiologic effects in isolated canine ventricular tissue.[5] Isolated canine false tendons were exposed to T-2 toxin, T-2 tetraol, and scirpentriol, to examine the effects of each trichothecene on action potentials of cells from the 3 ventricular tissue types (conducting tissue, papillary muscle tissue, and ventricular septal tissue) contained in each preparation. For each cell type, 8 action potential parameters (amplitude, overshoot, maximum rate of rise of the upstroke, maximum diastolic potential, action potential duration at 20, 50, and 80% repolarization, and conduction velocity) were measured before and during trichothecene suffusion. The false tendons were stimulated through bipolar silver electrodes at a rate of 120 beats per minute. Control action potential

Table 1
EFFECTS OF ARTERIALLY PERFUSED TRICHOTHECENE MYCOTOXINS (30 MG/L) ON CANINE SINUS NODE CELL ACTION POTENTIALS

		Cycle length (ms)	V_{max} (v/s)	Overshoot (mV)	MDP (mV)	Amplitude (mV)	ADP 50 (mV)	Phase 4 slope (v/s)
Control	(n = 9)	689 ± 20	15 ± 6	6 ± 5	−54 ± 7	60 ± 9	173 ± 10	0.047 ± 0.01
DMSO	(n = 8)	631[a] ± 45	19 ± 9	−2[a] ± 6	−54 ± 8	54 ± 8	160 ± 18	0.029[a] ± 0.01
Control	(n = 8)	510 ± 21	12 ± 1	6 ± 11	−59 ± 7	65 ± 7	125 ± 19	0.047 ± 0.01
Roridin-A	(n = 10)	651[a] ± 70	12 ± 1	3 ± 7	−65[a] ± 5	68 ± 10	149 ± 44	0.024[a] ± 0.01
Control	(n = 5)	724 ± 50	20 ± 2	−0.2 ± 1	−59 ± 9	52 ± 12	133 ± 13	0.017 ± 0.00
T-2	(n = 6)	814[a] ± 16	20 ± 1	−8.0 ± 11	−63 ± 8	55 ± 8	136 ± 18	0.011 ± 0.00

[a] Significantly different from concurrent control (p <0.05). MDP = maximum diastolic potential; V_{max} = maximum upstroke velocity; ADP 50 = time to 50% repolarization.

Reprinted with permission from Bubien, J. K. and W. T. Woods, Jr., *Toxicon*, 25, 325, 1987, Pergamon Press, Ltd.

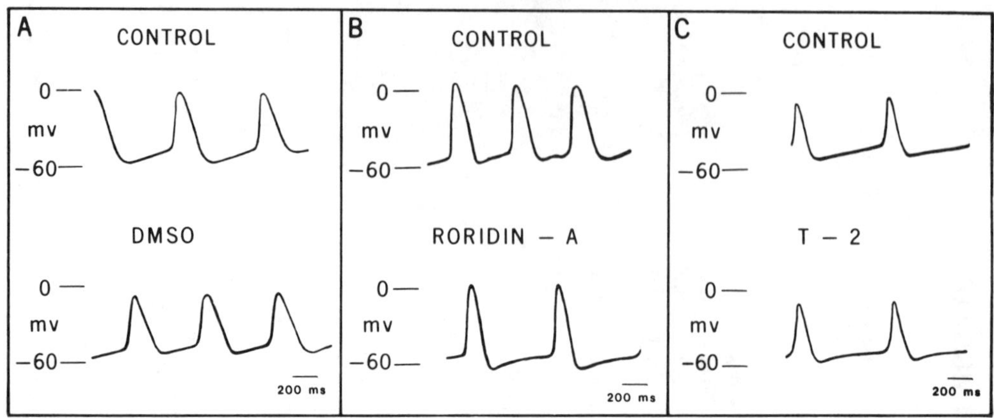

FIGURE 4.   (A) Action potentials from canine sinus node cells before and during perfusion with DMSO, 1.3% show the reduced cycle length. These action potentials served as controls. (B) Action potentials recorded from canine sinus node cells before and during perfusion with roridin-A (30 mg/l). Roridin-A perfusion hyperpolarized diastolic potentials of sinus node cells by 6 mV and reduced the slope of phase 4 depolarization by 49%. Roridin-A perfusion increased the cycle length by 37% (allowing for DMSO) corresponding to a decrease in heart rate from 118 to 74 beats per minute. (C) Action potentials recorded in canine sinus node cells before and during perfusion with T-2 toxin (30 mg/l) illustrate the 10% increase in the cycle length. The direct effect of T-2 was a 19% reduction in heart rate (allowing for a 9% DMSO-induced increase). (Reprinted wtih permission from Bubien, J. K. and Woods, W. T., Jr., Direct and reflex cardiovascular effects of trichothecene mycotoxins, *Toxicon*, 25,325-331, © 1987, Pergamon Press, Ltd.)

Table 2
EFFECTS OF ARTERIALLY PERFUSED TRICHOTHECENE MYCOTOXINS (30 MG/L) ON CANINE WORKING ATRIAL MYOCYTE ACTION POTENTIALS

		Cycle length (ms)	V_{max} (V/s)	Overshoot (mV)	MDP (mV)	Amplitude (mV)	ADP 50 (mV)
Control	(n = 10)	657 ± 17	116 ± 30	13.3 ± 5	−83 ± 4	97 ± 7	155 ± 7
DMSO	(n = 9)	676[a] ± 9	103 ± 23	13.2 ± 6	−82 ± 8	95 ± 9	120[a] ± 5
Control	(n = 9)	552 ± 57	87 ± 35	19 ± 5	−80 ± 8	98 ± 8	127 ± 20
Roridin-A	(n = 15)	639[a] ± 54	112 ± 36	21 ± 6	−80 ± 4	101 ± 6	101[a] ± 14
Washout	(n = 11)	471[a] ± 13	89 ± 36	19 ± 6	−79 ± 6	98 ± 7	98[a] ± 28
Control	(n = 8)	693 ± 5	120 ± 21	30 ± 4	−74 ± 8	104 ± 11	137 ± 6
T-2	(n = 8)	801[a] ± 14	127 ± 35	19 ± 6	−79 ± 10	97 ± 11	140 ± 15
Washout	(n = 8)	795 ± 13	139 ± 31	27 ± 6	−75 ± 6	101 ± 6	136 ± 10

[a]   Significantly different from concurrent control (p <0.05). MDP = maximum diastolic potential; V_{max} = maximum upstroke velocity; ADP 50 = time to 50% repolarization.

Reprinted with permission from Bubien, J. K. and W. T. Woods, Jr., *Toxicon*, 25,325-331, ©1987, Pergamon Press, Ltd.

measurements for each tissue type are summarized in Table 3. T-2 toxin (1 mg/1), when suffused for 60 min in false tendon cells, reduced the amplitude by 15%, the maximum diastolic potential by 11%, the overshoot by 22%, and the duration by 32% (Figure 5). The only apparent action potential changes in false tendon cells induced by scirpentriol (1 mg/1) was a 31% reduction in the action potential durations. T-2 tetraol did not induce any action potential changes in false tendon cells action potentials.

T-2 toxin (1 mg/1) reduced the amplitude of papillary muscle cells by 13%, the maximum diastolic potential by 11%, the overshoot by 22%, the maximum upstroke velocity by 24%,

Table 3
CONTROL VALUES FROM CANINE CARDIAC ACTION POTENTIALS BEFORE SUFFUSION WITH TRICHOTHECENES

Tissue type	Resting transmembrane potential (mV)	Maximal upstroke velocity (V/s)	Amplitude (mV)	Overshoot (mV)	Action potential duration (ms)		Conduction velocity (mm/s)
					APD_{20}	APD_{80}	
False tendon n = 13	−88 ± 8	258 ± 45	119 ± 9	31 ± 6	41 ± 9	208 ± 34	954 ± 325
Papillary muscle n = 15	−76 ± 10	151 ± 39	98 ± 9	23 ± 3	105 ± 33	230 ± 56	193 ± 45
Septal muscle n = 17	−77 ± 8	127 ± 36	98 ± 10	21 ± 4	107 ± 24	246 ± 26	178 ± 126

Note: Each entry in this table is the mean ± 1 standard deviation.

Reprinted with permission from Bubien, J. K. and W. T. Woods, Jr., Differential effects of trichothecenes on the canine cardia action potential, *Toxicon*, 25:325-331, ©1987, Pergamon Press, Ltd.

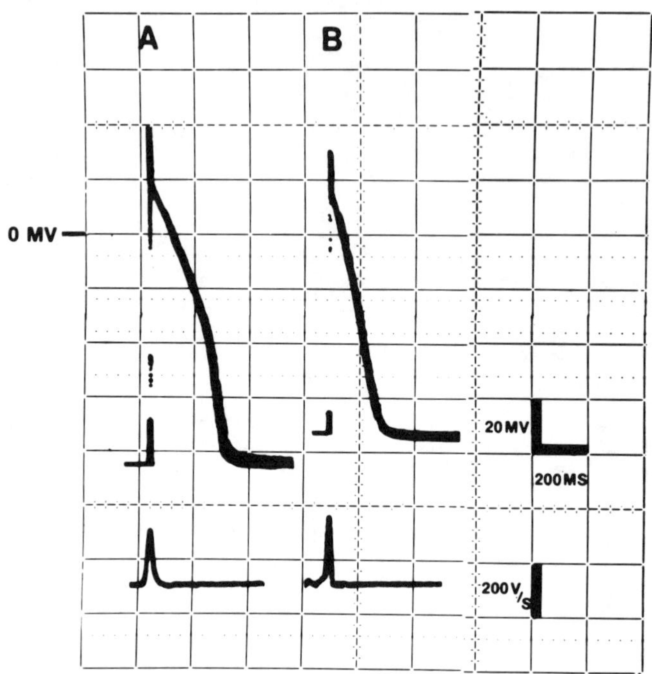

FIGURE 5.   Action potentials (AP) recorded from a canine false tendon stimulated at 2 Hz. (A) Control AP recorded immediately prior to suffusion with T-2 toxin. (B) AP from the same false tendon at 60-min suffusion with T-2 toxin (1.0 mg/1). This action potential shows the reduced MDP, OSH, and APD typically observed after suffusion with T-2 toxin. (Reprinted with permission from Bubien, J. K. and Woods, W. T., Jr., Direct and reflex cardiovascular effects of trichothecene mycotoxins, *Toxicon*, 25,325-331, © 1987, Pergamon Press, Ltd.)

and the action potential duration by 19%. T-2 tetraol and scirpentriol (1 mg/1) did not induce any significant action potential changes in papillary muscle cells.

Action potentials from interventricular septal wall cells were unaltererd by suffusion with either T-2 toxin or scirpentriol (1 mg/1 for 60 min). T-2 tetraol (1 mg/1) reduced the maximum diastolic potential by 9% and shortened the action potential duration by 42%.

Three separate papillary muscle preparations were suffused with physiological solutions containing adenosine triphosphate (ATP) (1100 mg/1). Subsequent suffusion with T-2 toxin did not produce any changes in papillary muscle cell action potentials. In papillary muscle preparations where T-2 toxin (1 mg/1) was suffused prior to the addition of ATP, action potential durations were reduced 16%. The subsequent addition of ATP reversed the T-2-induced action potential duration shortening. Figure 6 shows the effect of T-2 toxin on papillary muscle cell action potential durations and the reversal of the effect by ATP.

Trichothecene-induced action potential changes in ventricular tissue were similar to changes observed after metabolite inhibition (induced by hypoxia or dinitrophenol).[46] The effects of metabolic inhibition are reversed by the addition of high energy phosphates to the suffusates.[3,9,31] ATP reversed the effects induced by T-2 toxin in papillary muscle cells. Therefore, trichothecenes may induce an energy deficit in the cells of the ventricular myocardium.

The reduced action potential durations are consistent with a reduction in slow inward (calcium channel) conductance (which is energy dependent) as postulated by Schneider and Sperelakis.[46] Calcium channels in heart cells open more frequently at increasingly positive

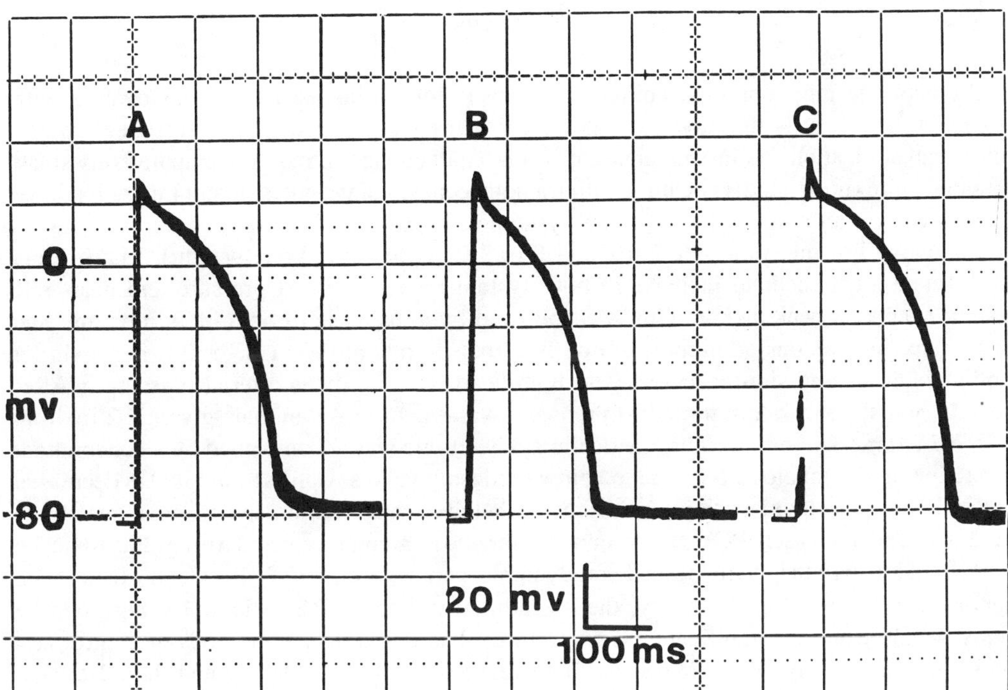

FIGURE 6.   Action potentials recorded from papillary muscle cells. (A) Action potential recorded from papillary muscle cell prior to exposure to trichothecene mycotoxins (control). The APD_{50} was 190 ms. (B) Action potential recorded from the same tissue after 60 min suffusion with 1 mg/l T-2 toxin. The APD_{50} was 160 ms. (C) Action potential recorded from the same tissue after 180 min suffusion with T-2 toxin and 60 min suffusion with ATP 2 mM/l added. The APD_{50} was 210 ms.

membrane potentials above 0 mV.[42] Therefore, the trichothecene-induced reduction in overshoot potentials is also consistent with a reduction in calcium channel conductance; however, it is unlikely that trichothecenes are calcium channel blockers (like dihydropyridines) because trichothecene-induced action potential changes are readily reversed by ATP, whereas the effects of direct calcium channel blockers are not. The maximum diastolic potential of false tendon cells was depolarized by T-2 toxin by 9 ± 6 mV. The magnitude of this effect is similar to depolarizations observed in cardiac cells when the electrogenic Na^+-K^+ pump is poisoned with ouabain.[52] This pump hydrolyzes ATP to produce the ion exchanges. Therefore, trichothecenes could reduce the ATP available for the electrogenic pump resulting in the observed depolarizations. Additional information on the interactions between trichothecenes and ATP concentrations is provided in the chapters "Effects on the Digestive system and Energy Metabolism" and "Therapy and Prophylaxis for Trichothecene Mycotoxicosis".

The postulated mechanisms of action of trichothecenes in cardiac cells may be explained by the fact that these toxins inhibit protein synthesis.[32] Generalized inhibition of protein synthesis could affect cell membrane processes. The action potential effects of trichothecenes may be relevant to the overall pathogenicity of these compounds because the concentration used in these studies was approximately equal to the LD_{50} for dogs, rats, and rabbit (1 mg/ kg).[53] The observations do not support the hypothesis that simple trichothecenes induce arrhythmias by direct effects on cardiac cell membranes, although the macrocyclic trichothecene roridin-A does seem to affect cells of the cardiac conduction system directly. The observations support the hypothesis that trichothecenes in some way reduce energy metabolism in cardiac cells.

VII. RATS

Perhaps the most common animal model used for cardiovascular studies dealing with toxins is the rat. It is the model of choice for many studies since it has sufficient size to allow catheterization and instrumentation, yet is small enough to require comparatively small amounts of toxin. In studies dealing with trichothecenes, many routes of administration have been used, yet all seem to have similar systemic effects.

Following i.v. injection of T-2 toxin (1.0 or 3.0 mg toxin/kg body weight), Matsuoka et al.[30] found an immediate increase in both systemic arterial blood pressure and heart rate which reached a peak at 1 h. This was followed by a decrease in both blood pressure and heart rate. Intravenous administration of T-2 toxin in rats at 0.5, 1.0, or 2.0 mg toxin/kg body weight caused similar increases in both heart rate and mean arterial pressure.[12] After several hours, heart rate returned to predosing values. In those animals given T-2 toxin at 1.0 and 2.0 mg/kg body weight, the decline in heart rate was accompanied by a concomitant reduction in arterial blood pressure to below predosing values. Cardiac output also decreased following toxin administration. As discussed below, hyperoxemia, hypocapnia, metabolic acidosis, and increased PCV were reported for those animals given 1.0 mg T-2 toxin/kg body weight. Similar changes in hemodynamic parameters of T-2 dosed rats have been reported by Parker.[39] In this study, the i.v. administration of T-2 toxin at 1.0 mg toxin/kg body weight caused a significant reduction in cardiac output to 21 and 58% of control at 4 and 8 h, respectively. Heart rate increased over the first 4 h postdosing and then declined. Mean arterial pressure exhibited a triphasic response which consisted of a decrease through 4 h postdosing, an increase at 6 h, and severe hypotension at 8 to 18 h. The ECG showed elongation of P-R and Q-T intervals, indicating possible conduction problems in the myocardium.

Siren and Feuerstein[49] and Feuerstein et al.[12] reported stable heart rates and blood pressures in pithed rats after i.v. injection of T-2 toxin (1 mg/kg body weight); however, in conscious intact rats given the same dose of T-2 toxin, both of these parameters become elevated as described above. These observations suggest neurogenically induced hemodynamic alterations (dysautonomia). Decreased heart rate and blood pressure appear to be two factors in the trichothecene induced shock-like syndrome in rats. Whether they are direct effects of trichothecene toxicosis or neurogenically mediated remains to be elucidated.

Increases in blood pressure, heart rate, and respiratory rate were observed following oral administration of freeze-dried cultures of *F. tricinctum* at 300 mg/kg body weight.[51] In this study, heart rates were increased 4 to 8 h after dosing but declined below normal by 10 h. Heart rates continued to decline after this point until death. These same investigators, using crude T-2 toxin administered i.v. at 1.0 mg/kg body weight, observed similar changes in heart rate as found with the orally dosed animals. In this case, however, the sequence of events followed a much quicker time course (i.e., the initial changes occurred within 1 h rather than 4 h). Kosuri et al.[25] reported similar findings following oral administration of lyophilized fungal cultures of *F. tricinctum* (300 mg/kg body weight). In addition, these same investigators used the Evans Blue dye technique to show T-2 toxin-induced vascular effects. Increased local vascular permeability was observed following an intradermal dose of 0.1 mg of T-2 toxin in rats. A similar effect on the GI vasculature was reported in rats following i.p. administration of the trichothecene fusarenon-X.[57,58]

Wilson et al.[62] intermittently administered T-2 toxin p.o. to rats over a period of 12 months with observations for a total of 17 months. Doses administered caused acute toxic effects and many of the rats died shortly after dosing. Vascular damage followed by healing resulted in thickened retinas, perivascular fibrosis, and calcification of blood vessels. These changes were ultimately associated with significant elevations in systemic arterial blood pressures when compared to rats fed normal diets.

In rats dosed i.v. at 1.0 or 2.0 mg T-2 toxin/kg body weight, $PaCO_2$ and pH declined following toxin administration, while PaO_2 showed a significant increase.[12] Parker[39] described blood gas changes similar to those described by Feuerstein et al.[12] The extent of increase in PaO_2, however, was less than that of Feuerstein's study. As discussed in the summary chapter, however, there is reason for concern with regard to at least some reports suggesting hyperoxemia in T-2 dosed rats.

As in swine (see Section V), the hemodynamic changes that occur in rats following T-2 toxin administration may be partly explained by the associated pathologic changes in the myocardium. Myocardial degeneration with foci of cellular infiltration and fibrosis were observed in rats given oral doses of 0.2 to 0.4 mg T-2 toxin/kg body weight.[47] Cardiac lesions in rats that were injected i.p. with T-2 toxin at 3 mg/kg body weight and which died 8 to 20 h later included focal myocardial hemorrhage, marked interstitial edema, and infiltration of mononuclear cells.[66] No definitive cardiac changes were observed in rats killed 6 h after a dose of 2.0 mg/kg, but if the length of time before euthanasia was increased to 1, 2, or 3 d, swelling of myocytes and interstitial edema in both the subendocardial and subepicardial regions were evident.

In vitro work using isolated perfused rat hearts, bathed in a solution containing 2.5 mg T-2 toxin/1, indicated that T-2 toxin has a negative inotropic effect on the heart.[65] The concentrations of T-2 toxin used in this study, however, were comparatively high and would not be expected to frequently occur *in vivo* under conditions of natural exposure.

Dispersed myocytes from 1-d-old rat hearts were cultured and subsequently exposed to T-2 toxin.[67] The rate of spontaneous beating and the relative contractile force of these cells was measured after exposure to T-2 toxin at various concentrations and for various durations. T-2 toxin reduced the rate of beating in a dose-dependent manner. Long exposures (3 h) to comparatively high concentrations of T-2 toxin (5 mg/l) resulted in cell death within 48 h. Shorter exposures (30 min) reduced the rate of spontaneous beating more than 80%. Calcium stimulated increases in contractile force were reduced by more than 100% in cells pretreated with T-2 toxin (2.5 mg/l) when compared to unexposed cells. These results demonstrated direct effects of T-2 toxin on cardiac myocytes.

VIII. GUINEA PIGS

Following i.v. administration of T-2 toxin to guinea pigs at 0.5, 1.0, or 2.0 mg/kg body weight, gradual decreases in both heart rate and blood pressure were reported.[12] In a similar study in which guinea pigs were dosed with T-2 toxin at 2.0 mg/kg body weight, heart rates decreased while blood pressure was maintained near control values for 6 h postdosing, after which blood pressure began to decline.[40] The reductions in heart rate, however, were not preceded by initial increases in heart rate as observed with the rat.

It is interesting that the effects of the trichothecene mycotoxin, fusarenon-X, on guinea pigs seem to be manifested differently than those of T-2 toxin. Ueno et al.[58] reported that i.p. injections of fusarenon-X at 0.5 mg toxin/kg body weight caused heart rates to increase from control values by 145 to 175% at 4 h postdosing. By 10 h postdosing, however, the animals exhibited a significant bradycardia and a concurrent 50% reduction in respiratory rates. Higher i.p. doses of fusarenon-X (5 mg/kg body weight) reduced the period of tachycardia to 2 h. Increased ECG waveform amplitudes were associated with the periods of tachycardia.[58]

Blood gas responses of guinea pigs to trichothecene mycotoxins are similar to those reported for the rat. These are characterized by increases in PaO_2, decreases in $PaCO_2$, and pronounced reductions in arterial pH (i.e., acidosis).[12,40] The data suggest a metabolic acidosis with partial respiratory compensation during an apparent shift from aerobic to anaerobic metabolism. That this occurs despite significant increases in PaO_2 is suggestive of extreme peripheral vasoconstriction and/or decreased oxygen utilization. In view of the cold and cyanotic extremities and the poor capillary refill observed in several species after administration of highly toxic doses of trichothecenes, the vasoconstriction is likely to be a major factor; however, reduced oxygen utilization is also likely as described in the chapter "Effects on the Digestive System and Energy Metabolism".

IX. MICE

Much less cardiovascular work has been done in mice than in rats simply because of the difficulty of instrumentation of the animals and the limited number of blood samples that can be obtained from each animal; however, lesions in mice exposed to trichothecene mycotoxins are similar to those of rats. Tissue damage is evident at both gross and histologic levels. Ueno et al.[56] reported no differences between animals given T-2 toxin whether the mice were dosed by i.v., intragastric, or i.p. routes.

X. SUMMARY

When discussing the cardiovascular effects of any compound in animal models, similarities and differences in response must be analyzed in light of both animal to animal and species to species variations. This is especially true for the trichothecene mycotoxins. The information presented in this chapter indicates that although animal to animal differences appear to be minimal for most parameters, unexplained variations in cardiovascular response to trichothecene toxicosis do occur.

The common features of the cardiovascular dysfunctions include tachycardia followed by hypotension and bradycardia (in the latter stages of toxicosis). These progress until the test animal becomes comatose and subsequently dies.

The cardiovascular effects can be subdivided into two main categories: (1) direct effects on the cardiovascular system and (2) neurogenically mediated (i.e., indirect) effects on the cardiovascular system. Direct effects seem to include a depression in myocardial contractility and a concomittant decline in CO, probably accompanied by a reduction in myocardial ATP. The reduction in CO then leads to hypotension and eventually a life-threatening shock-like syndrome. It also appears that many of the trichothecene mycotoxins have a direct effect on the vasculature of many tissue types, including the heart. Another direct effect of trichothecenes, the suppression of cardiac electrical conduction, may be reflected as atrioventricular conduction abnormalities in a variety of species including horses, dogs, and rats. Anesthetized dogs developed irreversible atrioventricular block when infused with roridin-A, which was not responsive to sympathetic or parasympathetic blocking agents. The hyperpolarizatoin observed in sinus node cells perfused with roridin-A suggests that trichothecenes alter transmembrane ion fluxes in cells of the cardiac conduction system. As would be expected with reduced ion gradients, the myocytes in culture responded to T-2 toxin with reduced automaticity and reduced force of contractions.

The most prevalent neurogenic or indirect effect of trichothecene toxicosis is the intense tachycardia observed in most species. It appears that this significant increase in heart rate is a compensatory response brought about by hypotension and tissue hypofusion. In addition, with sufficiently high doses, endogenous catecholamine concentrations increase, capillaries become plugged, bone marrow immunocytes become depleted, hematocrits increase, the spleen atrophies, and the mucosa and lymphoid tissues of the intestines become necrotic. Clearly, there is a sympathetic stimulation in acute trichothecene toxicosis. The fact that tachycardia and hypertension failed to develop in pithed rats dosed with T-2 toxin, and that trichothecene-induced tachycardias can be somewhat impeded by the administration of the β-blocker propranolol, further substantiate the idea of neurogenic mechanisms.

An acutely toxic intravascular dose among all species reported here ranged from 1 to 3 mg T-2 toxin/kg body weight. At these concentrations, the cardiovascular effects described earlier were observed in most species.

The analyses of blood gases of most test animals suggests that oxygen is available in the primary arterial vasculature (maintained or increased PO_2), but is underutilized or (more likely) inadequately distributed to the periphery as the autonomic nervous system causes a peripheral vasospasm or as the body attempts to maintain blood pressure and blood flow to the vital organs. A decrease in oxygen utilization and a need for ATP may perhaps result from generalized inhibition of protein synthesis, but although mitochondria exposed to trichothecenes exhibit reduced oxygen consumption, a direct connection between protein synthesis inhibition and this mitochondrial effect has not been demonstrated.

The information presented in this chapter indicates that acute T-2 toxicosis involves a complex interaction of multiple organ systems. Most animal species studied to date have exhibited classic signs of circulatory shock which include hypotension, tissue hypoperfusion, and reduced cardiac output. The ultimate cause of death in animals given acutely lethal doses of trichothecene mycotoxins appears to be the development of generalized hemodynamic derangements that are incompatible with life. The sequence of events in many test species suggests that the nervous and immune systems become directly affected early in the course of the toxicosis.

REFERENCES

1. **Bamburg, J. R., Marasas, W. F. O., Riggs, M. V., Smalley, E. B., and Strong, F. M.,** Toxic spiro-epoxy compounds from *Fusaria* and other Hyphomycetes, *Biotechnol. Bioeng.,* 10, 445, 1968.
2. **Beasley, V. R.,** Toxicodynamics of T-2 Toxin in Swine and Cattle, Ph.D. dissertation, University of Illinois, Urbana, 1983.
3. **Beeler, G. W. and Reuter, H.,** Reconstruction of the action potential of ventricular myocardial fibers, *J. Physiol. (London),* 268, 177, 1977.
4. **Belt, R. J., Hass, C. D., Joseph, U., Goodwin, W., Moore, D., and Hoogstraten, B.,** Phase I study of anguidine administered weekly, *Cancer Treat. Rep.,* 63, 11, 1985.
5. **Bubien, J. K. and Woods, W. T., Jr.,** Differential effects of trichothecenes on the canine cardiac action potential, *Toxicon,* 24(5), 467, 1986.
6. **Bubien, J. K. and Woods, W. T., Jr.,** Direct and reflex cardiovascular effects of trichothecene mycotoxins, *Toxicon,* 25(3), 325, 1987.
7. **Bukowski, R., Vaughn, C., Bottombley, R., and Chen, T.,** Phase II study of anguidine in gastrointestinal malignancies: a southwest oncology group study, *Cancer Treat. Rep.,* 66(2), 381, 1982.
8. **Brunner, D. L., Wannemacher, R. W., Neufeld, H. A., Hassler, C. R., Parker, G. W., Cosgriff, T. M., and Dinterman, R. E.,** Pathophysiology of acute T-2 intoxication in the cynomolgus monkey and rat models, in *Trichothecenes and Other Mycotoxins,* Lacey, J., Ed., John Wiley & Sons, New York, 1985, 411.
9. **Carmeliet, E. and Vereecke, J.,** Electrogenesis of the action potential and automaticity, in *Handbook of Physiology. Section 2: The Cardiovascular System,* Berne, R. M., Sperelakis, N., and Geiger, S. R., Eds., American Physiological Society, Bethesda, MD, 1979, 315.
10. **DeNicola, D. B., Rebar, A. H., and Carlton, W. W.,** T-2 toxin mycotoxicosis in the guinea pig, *Food Cosmet. Toxicol.,* 16, 601, 1978.
11. **DeSimone, P. A., Greco, F. A., and Lessner, H. F.,** Phase I evaluation of a weekly schedule of anguidine, *Cancer Treat. Rep.,* 63, 2015, 1979.
12. **Feuerstein, G., Goldstein, D. S., Ramwell, P. W., Zerbe, R. L., Lux, W. E., Jr., Faden, A. I., and Bayorh, M. A.,** Cardiorespiratory, sympathetic, and biochemical responses to T-2 toxin in the guinea pig and rat, *J. Pharmacol. Exp. Ther.,* 232, 786, 1985.
13. **Forgacs, J.,** Strachybotryotoxicosis and moldy corn toxicosis, in *Mycotoxicosis in Foodstuffs,* Wogan, G. N., Ed., MIT Press, Cambridge, MA, 1965.
14. **Forgacs, J. and Carll, W. B.,** Mycotoxicosis, *Adv. Vet. Sci.,* 7, 273, 1962.

15. **Gadjusek, D. C.,** Acute Infectious Hemorrhagic Fevers and Mycotoxicosis in the Union of Soviet Socialist Republics, Army Medical Service Graduate School, Walter Reed Army Medical Center, Washington, D.C., 1958, 82.

16. **Ganong, W. F.,** Circulation through special regions, in *Review of Medical Physiology,* 10th ed., Lange Medical Publications, Los Altos, CA, 1981, 476.

17. **Gilgan, M. W., Smalley, E. B., and Strong, F. M.,** Isolation and partial characterization of a toxin from *Fusarium tricinctum* on moldy corn, *Arch. Biochem. Biophys.,* 114, 1, 1966.

18. **Harrach, B., Mirocha, C. J., Pathre, S. V., and Palyusic, M.,** Macrocyclic trichothecene toxins produced by a strain of *Strachybotrys atra* from Hungary, *Appl. Environ. Microbiol.,* 41, 1428, 1981.

19. **Hassler, C. R.,** Acute and Subchronic Toxicology of T-2 in Monkeys. A Pilot Study, Final report to U.S. Army Medical Research of Infectious Diseases, 1983.

20. **Hayes, M. A., Bellamy, J. E. C., and Schiefer, H. B.,** Subacute toxicity of dietary T-2 toxin in mice: morphological and hematological effects, *Can. J. Comp. Med.,* 44, 203, 1980.

21. **Joffe, A. Z.,** Alimentary toxic aleukia, in *Microbial Toxins,* Academic Press, New York, 1971, 139.

22. **Joffe, A. Z.,** *Fusarium poae* and *F. sporotrichiodes* as principle causal agents of alimentary toxic aleukia, in *Mycotoxic Fungi, Mycotoxins, Mycotoxicoses: Encyclopedic Handbook,* Vol. 3, Wyllie, T. D. and Morehouse, L. G., Eds., Marcel Dekker, New York, 1978, 21.

23. **Joffe, A. Z. and Yagen, B.,** Comparative study of the yield of T-2 toxin produced by *Fusarium poae, F. sporotrichiodes,* and *F. sporotrichiodes* var. *trinchinctum* strains from different sources, *Mycopathology,* 60(2), 93, 1977.

24. **Kosuri, N. R., Ph.D.** dissertation, University of Wisconsin, Madison, 1969.

25. **Kosuri, N. R., Grove, M. D., Yates, S. G., Tallent, W. H., Ellis, J. J., Wolff, I. A., and Nichols, R. E.,** Response of cattle to mycotoxins of *Fusarium tricinctum* isolated from corn and fescue, *J. Am. Vet. Med. Assoc.,* 157, 938, 1970.

26. **Kosuri, N. B., Smalley, E. B., and Nichols, R. E.,** Toxicologic studies of *Fusarium tricinctum* from moldy corn, *Am. J. Vet. Res.,* 32, 1843, 1971.

27. **Lorenzana, R. M., Beasley, V. R., Buck, W. B., Ghent, A. W., Lundeen, G. R., and Poppenga, R. H.,** Experimental T-2 toxicosis in swine. I. Changes in cardiac output, aortic mean pressure, catecholamines, 6-keto-PFG1alpha, thromboxane B2, and acid-base parameters, *Fundam. Appl. Toxicol.,* 5, 879, 1985.

28. **Lundeen, G. R., Poppenga, R. H., Beasley, V. R., Buck, W. B., Tranquilli, W. J., and Lambert, R. J.,** Systemic distribution of blood flow during T-2 toxin-induced shock in swine, *Fundam. Appl. Toxicol.,* 7, 309, 1986.

29. **Matsumoto, H., Ito, T., and Ueno, Y.,** Toxicological approaches to the metabolites of *Fusaria, Jpn. J. Exp. Med.,* 48, 393, 1978.

30. **Matsuoka, Y., Kubota, K., and Ueno, Y.,** General pharmacological studies of fusarenon-X, a trichothecene mycotoxin from *Fusarium* species, *Toxicol. Appl. Pharmacol.,* 50, 87, 1979.

31. **McAllister, R. E., Noble, D., and Tsien, R. W.,** Reconstruction of the electrical activity of cardiac Purkinje fibers, *J. Physiol. (London),* 251, 1, 1975.

32. **McLaughlin, C. S., Vaughn, M. H., Campbell, I. M., Wei, C. M., Strafford, M. E., and Hansen, B. S.,** in *Mycotoxins in Human and Animal Health,* Rodricks, J. V., Hesseltine, C. W., and Mehlman, M. A., Eds., Pathotox Publishers, Park Forest South, IL, 1977, 263.

33. **Mirocha, C. J.,** Trichothecene mycotoxins in farm animals, in *Trichothecenes: Chemical, Biological, and Toxicological Aspects,* Ueno, Y., Ed., Elsevier, New York, 1983, 177.

34. **Mortimer, P. H., Campbell, J., DiMenna, M. E., and White, E. P.,** Experimental myrotheciotoxicosis and poisoning in ruminants of verrucarin-A and roridin-A, *Res. Vet. Sci.,* 12, 508, 1971.

35. **Murphy, W. K., Burgess, M. A., Valdivieso, M., Livingston, R. B., Bodey, G. P., and Freireich, E. J.,** Phase I clinical evaluation of anguidine, *Cancer Treat. Rep.,* 62, 1497, 1978.

36. **Osweiler, G. D., Hook, B. S., Mann, D. D., Buening, G. M., and Rottinghause, G. E.,** Effects of T-2 toxin in cattle, *Proc. U.S. Anim. Health Assoc.,* 214, 1981.

37. **Pace, J.,** Effect of T-2 mycotoxin on rat liver mitochondria electron transport system, *Toxicon,* 21, 675, 1983.

38. **Pang, V. F., Adams, J. H., Beasley, V. R., Buck, W. B., and Haschek, W. M.,** Myocardial and pancreatic lesions induced by T-2 toxin, a trichothecene mycotoxin in swine, *J. Vet. Pathol.,* 23, 310, 1986.

39. **Parker, G. W.,** Acute and subacute effects of T-2 mycotoxin on electrocardiographic and hemodynamic indices in F344 rats, *Fed. Proc.,* 44(5), 1651, 1985.

40. **Parker, G. W., Wannemacher, R. W., and Gilman, F. J.,** The effect of T-2 mycotoxin on the cardiovascular system in the guinea pig, *Fed. Proc.,* 43(3), 578, 1984.

41. **Rafai, P. and Tubolz, S.,** Effect of T-2 toxin on adrenocortical function and immune response in growing pigs, *Zentralbl. Vet. Med. B,* 29, 558, 1982.

42. **Reuter, H.,** Calcium channel modulation by neurotransmitters, enzymes, and drugs, *Nature,* 301, 569, 1983.
43. **Rona, G., Chappel, C. I., Balaze, T., and Gaudry, R.,** An infarct-like myocardial lesion and other toxic manifestations produced by isoproterenol in the rat, *Arch. Pathol.,* 67, 443, 1959.
44. **Rukmini, C., Prasad, J. S., and Rao, K.,** Effects of feeding T-2 toxin to rats and monkeys, *Food Cosmet. Toxicol.,* 18, 267, 1980.
45. **Saito, M., Enomoto, M., and Tatsuno, T.,** Radiometric biological properties of the new scirpene metabolites of *Fusarium nivale, Gann,* 60, 599, 1969.
46. **Schneider, J. A. and Sperelakis, N.,** The demonstration of energy dependence of the isoproterenol-induced transcellular Ca^{++} current in isolated perfused guinea pig hearts. An explanation for mechanical failure of ischemic myocardium, *J. Surg. Res.,* 16, 389, 1974.
47. **Schoental, R., Joffe, A. Z., and Yagen, B.,** Cardiovascular lesions and various tumors found in rats given T-2 toxin, a trichothecene metabolite of *Fusarium, Cancer Res.,* 39, 2179, 1979.
48. **Scott, P. M., Van Walbeek, W., Kennedy, B., and Anyeti, D.,** Mycotoxins (ochrotoxin-A, citrinin, and sterigmatocystin) and toxigenic fungus in grains of agricultural products, *J. Agric. Food Chem.,* 20, 1103, 1972.
49. **Siren, A. and Feuerstein, G.,** Effect of T-2 toxin on regional blood flow and vascular resistance in the conscious rat, *Toxicol. Appl. Pharmacol.,* 83, 438, 1986.
50. **Smalley, E. E.,** T-2 toxin, *J. Am. Vet. Med. Assoc.,* 163, 1278, 1973.
51. **Smalley, E. B., Marasas, W. F. O., Strong, F. M., Bamburg, J. R., Nichols, R. E., and Kosuri, N. R.,** Mycotoxicosis associated with moldy corn, in *Proc. 1st Japan-USA Conference on Toxic Microorganisms,* Herzberg, M., Ed., University of Hawaii, Honolulu, 1970, 163.
52. **Sperelakis, N.,** Origin of the cardiac resting potential, in *Handbook of Physiology, Section 2: The Cardiovascular System,* Vol. 1, Berne, R. M., Sperelakis, N., and Geiger, S. R., Eds., American Phsyiological Society, Bethesda, MD, 1979, 187.
53. **Stahelin, V. H., Kalberer-Rusch, M. E., Singer, E., and Lazary, S.,** Uber einige biologischewirkungen des cytostaticum diacetoxyscirpenol, *Arzneimittel-Forsch,* 18, 989, 1968.
54. **Talmage, D. W.,** (chairman). Protection Against Trichothecene Mycotoxins. Committee on Protection Against Mycotoxins. National Research Council, National Academy Press, Washington, D.C., 1983, 93.
55. **Tsunoda, H., Toyazaki, N., Morooka, N., Nakano, N., Yoshiyama, H., Okubo, K., and Isoda, M.,** *Rep. Food Res., Inst.,* 23, 89, 1968.
56. **Ueno, Y., Ueno, I., Saito, N., Iitoi, Y., Saito, M., Enomoto, M., and Tsunoda, H.,** Toxicological approaches to (+ −)rugulosin, an anthraquinoid mycotoxin of *Penicillium rugulosum, Jpn. J. Exp. Med.,* 41, 177, 1971.
57. **Ueno, Y., Ueno, I., Iitoi, Y., Tsunoda, H., Enomoto, M., and Gkubo, K.,** Toxicological approaches to the metabolites of *Fusaria.* II. Isolation of fusarinon-X from the culture filtrates of *Fusarium nivale, Jpn. J. Exp. Med.,* 41, 507, 1971.
58. **Ueno, U., Ueno, I., Iitoi, Y., Tsunoda, H., Enomoto, M., and Ohtsubo, K.,** Toxicological approaches to the metabolites of *Fusarium.* III. Acute toxicity of fusarenon-X, *Jpn. J. Exp. Med.,* 41, 521, 1971.
59. **Ueno, Y., Ishii, K., Sakai, K., Kanaeda, S., Tsunoda, H., Tanaka, T., and Enomoto, M.,** Toxicological approaches to the metabolites of *Fusarium.* IV. Microbial survey "bean-hulls poisoning of horses" with isolation of toxic trichothecenes, neosolaniol, and T-2 toxin of *Fusarium solani* M-1-1, *Jpn. J. Exp. Med.,* 42, 187, 1972.
60. **Ueno, Y., Sato, N., Ishil, K., Sakai, K., Tsunoda, H., and Enomoto, M.,** Biological and chemical detection of trichothecene mycotoxins of *Fusarium* species, *Appl. Microbiol.,* 25, 699, 1973.
61. **Ueno, Y., Ishil, K., Saito, N., and Ohtsubo, K.,** Toxicological approaches to the metabolites of *Fusaria.* V. Vomiting factor from moldy corn infected with *Fusarium* spp., *Jpn. J. Exp. Med.,* 44, 123, 1974.
62. **Wilson, C. A., Everard, D. M., and Shoental, R.,** Blood pressure changes and cardiovascular lesions found in rats given T-2 toxin, a trichothecene secondary metabolite of certain *Fusarium* microfungi, *Toxicol. Lett.,* 10, 35, 1982.
63. **Wilson, D. J. and Gentry, P. A.,** T-2 toxin can cause vasoconstriction in an *in vitro* bovine ear perfusion system, *Toxicol. Appl. Pharmacol.,* 79, 159, 1985.
64. **Yap, H. Y., Murphy, W. K., DiStefano, A., Blumenschein, G. R., and Bodey, G. P.,** Phase II study of anguidine in advanced breast cancer. Cancer *Treat. Rep.,* 63(5), 789, 1979.
65. **Yarom, R., More, R., Raz, S., Shimoni, Y., Sarel, O., and Yagen, B.,** T-2 toxin effect on isolated perfused rat hearts, *Basic Res., Cardiol.,* 78, 623, 1983.
66. **Yarom, R., More, R., Sherman, Y., and Yagen, B.,** T-2 toxin-induced pathology in the hearts of rats, *Br. J. Exp. Pathol.,* 64, 570, 1983.
67. **Yarom, R., Hasin, Y., Raz, S., Shimoni, Y., Fixler, R., and Yagen, B.,** T-2 toxin effect on cultured myocardial cells, *Toxicol. Lett.,* 31, 1, 1986.

Chapter 5

EFFECTS OF TRICHOTHECENE MYCOTOXINS ON THE NERVOUS SYSTEM

G. Feuerstein, R. M. Lorenzana, and V. R. Beasley

TABLE OF CONTENTS

I. EFFECTS ON HUMANS

Symptoms reported for humans suggest that a toxic effect on the nervous system follows trichothecene exposure. Persons allegedly exposed to "yellow rain" complained of nausea, headache, confusion, decreased memory, anxiety, decreased visual and auditory acuity, decreased sense of balance and libido, anorexia, fever, and seizures.[1,2] Patients with alimentary toxic aleukia (ATA) demonstrated impaired nervous reflexes, depression, hyperesthesia, disorientation, delirium, hallucinations, headaches, hypalgesia, paresis, and loss of taste, smell, vision, hearing, and/or memory.[3]

Headaches and occasional convulsions occurred in persons with severe ATA, even in the first stage of the disease.[4] Although the second stage was generally symptomless, some affected persons developed weakness, fatigue, vertigo, headache, and mydriasis. Surprisingly, in the third stage, neurologic signs were apparently less of a problem, and in spite of serious illness, affected persons generally remained rational. Sometimes, however, various neuropsychiatric manifestations including psychasthenia and states of depression were encountered. An additional reported sign was meningism, which has been defined as pain in the meningocortical region of the brain coincident with marked excitation and subsequent depression of the cortex with vomition, constipation, and thermoregulatory disorders.

Cerebral hemorrhages, encephalitis, and disturbance of the central and autonomic (or the parasympathetic) nervous systems were also reported for humans with ATA. Lesions in the brain included hemorrhages and destruction of neurons at the levels of the third ventricle, in the diencephalon, and in the sympathetic ganglia.

Sometimes vertigo, tachycardia, slight cyanosis and possibly a cold feeling in the extremities were also observed.[5] Overall, circulatory failure and convulsions were rarely encountered.

In the phase I clinical evaluation of diacetoxyscirpenol (Anguidine) to establish the maximum tolerated dose and determine toxic effects for anticancer trials, rapid i.v. infusion produced immediate neurotoxicity. These effects included headache, mild confusion, short periods of coma, hallucinations, somnolence, and ataxia.[6,7] Slow infusions of DAS in cancer patients were successful, however, in reducing the severity of neurologic manifestations seen after bolus injections.[8] When Anguidine was infused over a 3- to 8-h period, clinical signs among patients given high doses included slight confusion, ataxia, dizziness, headaches, fatigue, malaise, depression, hallucinations, and psychomotor seizures.[8,9] In patients given doses greater than 3.5 mg/m^2 (approximately 0.09 mg/kg), a "neurasthenic syndrome" of fatigue, malaise, and depression was common and in some cases disabling. These symptoms were uniformly present in patients receiving 8 and 10 mg/m^2 (approximately 0.21 to 0.26 mg/kg) doses. The central nervous manifestations of DAS administered by infusion over a 3-h period were associated with concurrent hypotension.[9] At a dose of 7.5 mg/m^2 (approximately 0.19 mg/kg), however, signs, including psychomotor seizures, hallucinations, and confusion, lasted as long as 36 h.

Phase II clinical trials initiated after the phase I trials, which screen for activity against various types of neoplasia, indicated doses that gave maximum tolerable side effects. At these lower doses, central nervous system toxic effects in the form of hallucinations, somnolence, confusion, and/or lethargy were observed in 6 to 22% of patients.[10,11] Nausea and vomiting were frequently noted during the clinical trials of Anguidine.

II. NONHUMAN PRIMATES

Rhesus monkeys given repeated oral doses of T-2 toxin at 1 mg/kg/d developed apathy and weakness of the lower limbs.[12]

III. EFFECTS ON OTHER ANIMALS

A. Introduction

Clinical signs of trichothecene toxicosis in animals include effects on posture, locomotion, behavior, and rarely seizure activity, suggesting alterations in the integrity of nervous system function. The signs, however, cannot always be distinguished from similar signs that occur with other primary physiologic disorders induced by trichothecenes. In general, high doses of trichothecenes are required to produce obvious neurologic effects. Unfortunately, few studies in animals have attempted to specifically characterize the neurologic toxicity of trichothecene mycotoxins.

B. Birds

Neurologic disturbances have been noted during studies in which birds were fed diets containing T-2 toxin; however, neurologic effects have not been consistently observed, and there has seemed to be variation between species and between ages within species. When geese were fed grain that had caused ATA in people, rigidity, ataxia, and death occurred.[3,13] Head and leg tremors developed and death occurred in young mature geese that were force-fed barley contaminated with 25 ppm T-2 toxin.[14] In contrast, mature ducks that ate the same grain *ad libitum* became clinically ill, but none died or developed neurologic signs.[15] Unlike the findings of Greenway and Puls,[15] young mallard ducks fed diets containing purified T-2 toxin at concentrations of 20 or 30 ppm for 2 or 3 weeks developed bilateral paresis or dropping of the wings.[16]

Within 4 h after oral administration of T-2 toxin in an LD_{50} study, chickens developed asthenia.[17] The affected birds held their wings with the tips touching the floor. Chickens given high doses became comatose and did not respond to external tactile stimuli. Convulsions usually preceded death.

When chicks were fed a commercial ration containing T-2 toxin at 5 ppm (equivalent to an approximate daily dose of 0.5 mg/kg) from hatching to 26 d of age, electroretinograms revealed no differences from control birds.[18] In contrast, neurologic disturbances which included abnormal wing positioning, loss of the righting reflex, and induction of seizures by rough handling or a loud noise were observed when day-old chicks were fed diets containing 4, 8, or 16 ppm (equivalent to an approximate daily dose of 0.5 to 2.25 mg/kg) of T-2 toxin for 21, 17, or 13 d, respectively.[19] The seizures were perceived as more hysteroid than epileptiform. Neither abnormal wing positioning nor seizures could be stimulated to reoccur until after a rest period of 3 to 6 h. The apparent loss of righting reflexes, however, was present at all times. The nervous signs were not as prevalent as the occurrence of oral lesions, since the former were present in only 38% of the birds even at 16 ppm in the feed.

Abnormal righting reflexes were also noted in 7-d-old chicks that had been fed a *Fusarium sporotrichiella* var. *sporotrichiodes* culture for 17 d.[20] The amount of culture consumed provided doses of T-2 toxin at 0.18 mg/kg/d and neosolaniol at 0.018 mg/kg/d. Evidence of increased tolerance with increasing maturation was suggested by the absence of abnormalities in neurologic function when adult laying hens were fed T-2 toxin at a concentration of 20 ppm (approximately 1 mg/kg/d) in the diet for 3 weeks.[21]

After a single oral dose of T-2 toxin at 2.5 mg/kg, 4-week-old chicks had elevated brain dopamine concentrations at 12 and 24 h, while brain norepinephrine concentrations fell below those of the controls.[22] No neural disturbances were noted in this report, and it was suggested that stress induced by the toxicosis may have influenced the turnover rate of norepinephrine or caused some form of inhibition of the metabolic conversion of dopamine to norepinephrine.

C. Mice, Rabbits, Dogs, and Cats

During an LD_{50} study in mice using fusarenon-X, behavioral or nervous signs included inactivity and a lack of response to external stimuli.[23] No gross or histologic lesions were found in brains or pituitary glands of mice which had been given fusarenon-X at 3 mg/kg i.p.[24]

Thermoregulation is believed to be mediated through the hypothalamus. Slight ataxia and a gradually developing hypothermia occurred within the first 3 h after mice were given fusarenon-X i.p. at 0.7, 3, or 15 mg/kg[25] and also was observed in cats given T-2 toxin s.c. at 0.5 or 1.0 mg/kg.[26] Because it was hypothesized that brain protein synthesis was necessary in the activation of central pyrogenic mechanisms, a very high dose of 10 mg of T-2 toxin was injected into the cerebral ventricles of rabbits following infusion of leukocyte pyrogen and [^{14}C] leucine. T-2 toxin prevented the uptake of leucine into hypothalamic protein and inhibited the development of fever, suggesting an ability of such massive amounts of toxin to suppress the febrile response by a central action.[27]

In Beagle dogs given diacetoxyscirpenol (DAS) in either a single dose of 0.23 mg/kg or in 5 daily doses of 0.12 mg/kg, signs included decreased activity and tremors.[6] Lethal doses also caused ataxia.

All 20 cats given T-2 toxin at 0.06 to 0.1 mg/kg every 48 h for up to 24 d developed clinical signs. These included generalized lassitude and weakness, hind leg ataxia, conjunctivitis, weakness of the head and neck muscles, and, in the terminal stages, anorexia and paralysis.[28] Meningeal hemorrhage and brain edema have also been observed along with extensive pulmonary hemorrhage and bone marrow damage in T-2 dosed cats.[26]

D. Horses, Cattle, and Sheep

Horses experiencing "bean-hulls poisoning" had diminished reflexes, mental excitation, clonic spasms, marked perspiration, convulsions, and "involuntary forward rotation and circular movements".[29] Neuronal degeneration was found in the cerebral cortex. Horses with stachybotryotoxicosis display generalized hemorrhage, including hemorrhages in the brain, cerebral meninges, spinal cord, and adrenals.[4]

Signs potentially related to neurologic dysfunction are not frequently reported in trichothecene toxicoses of cattle or sheep, but may be significant when they occur. Sheep dosed orally with cultures of *Myrothecium roridum* or *M. verrucaria* developed severe lethargy, a wide stance, reluctance to move, and droopy ears.[30] At 48 h postdosing with oral verrucarin A at 2 mg/kg, an affected lamb was dull, weak, unsteady on its feet, and disinclined to move. Similarly, apparent progressive weakness was observed in calves given repeated daily doses of *M. roridum* or *M. verrucaria* cultures sufficient to cause lethality by 4 to 8 d.

A cow was given T-2 toxin by stomach tube at 0.44 mg/kg/d for 15 d during the pre- and postpartum period.[31] The calf, born 4 d after the onset of maternal treatment, was given T-2 toxin (p.o.) at 6 mg/kg/d for 7 d. The calf developed ataxia, knuckling of the rear legs, and severe depression that lasted up to 12 h after each of the daily doses. At that point, the recovery was delayed, and 24 h later, at the time of the next dosing, the animal was still affected. Dosing was thereafter performed every 48 h, but the animal was still depressed after each 2-d interval. During the 2nd week, the calf was anorexic and repeatedly submersed his entire head in a water bucket for 15 s or more and would loudly grind his teeth. This would suggest that at sufficient dosage calves may eventually accumulate toxin, sustain cumulative damage, and/or develop diminished metabolic or excretory capacity.

Older calves given T-2 toxin at 0.6 or 1.2 mg/kg i.v. or 2.4 or 3.6 mg/kg p.o. exhibited decreased alertness at approximately 90 min postdosing that progressed in intensity for 3 to 5 h.[32] By 7 h postdosing, the somnolent calves could be awakened, but would readily assume a recumbent position with their eyes closed. From 3 to 6 h postdosing, the calves appeared weak and unsteady when standing and had leg tremors. Calves at the higher doses were still unsteady at 24 h postdosing with T-2 toxin, while those given lower doses were apparently normal.

E. Swine

Swine given DAS i.v. in doses ranging from 0.3 to 0.5 mg/kg became very lethargic and developed moderate posterior paresis, a staggering gait and reluctance to move.[33] Animals that survived longer than 24 h moved slowly and leaned on the walls on the pen. By the 8th d, the pigs appeared normal. In another study in which swine were given DAS at 0.5 to 1.0 mg/kg i.v., signs included apparent weakness and coma and, in some cases, seizures, and death.[34]

In swine infused with T-2 toxin at 0.6, 2.4, or 4.8 mg/kg via the pulmonary artery, a shock syndrome occurred that was accompanied by significant hemodynamic alterations.[35,36] Evidence that could suggest possible nervous system mediation of this toxic syndrome included the sudden reduction in cardiac output and aortic mean pressure within the first 30 min, the delayed increase in heart rate, the erratic release of catecholamines in the high dose group and the sustained norepinephrine concentrations accompanied by a decrease in blood pressure in the low dose group. The presence of clinical signs referable to cholinergic stimulation (vomiting, diarrhea, flatulence, salivation), signs suggestive of mental depression, and lack of appropriate respiratory stimulation in the presence of metabolic acidosis could be taken as supportive of theory of nervous system mediation.

When T-2 toxin was given to swine as a single i.v. dose varying from 0.13 to 2.3 mg/kg, clinical signs included moderate posterior paresis, staggering gait, and extreme listlessness that progressed to severe posterior paresis, knuckling of the rear feet, and extreme lethargy.[37] The pigs frequently fell due to apparent hindquarter weakness and often dragged both rear legs. In spite of these acute signs, at 24 h postdosing, the surviving pigs reportedly appeared to be normal. Gross examination of swine which expired due to single i.v. doses of T-2 toxin revealed congestion of the meningeal vasculature and infrequently local hemorrhage.[37,38] In some animals, the severity of congestion was sufficient to be grossly indistinguishable from hemorrhage. Otherwise, however, few brain lesions have been observed in swine given acutely toxic doses of trichothecenes. T-2 toxin-induced reductions in brain blood flow of swine are discussed the chapter entitled "Effects on the Circulatory System".

F. Rats and Guinea Pigs

At near lethal doses, clinical signs in rats given T-2 toxin i.p., or *F. tricinctum* cultures p.o., included listlessness, decreased sensitivity to foot-pad pressure, increased irritability to sound, and piloerection.[39] At higher doses, rats appeared to become weak and eventually could not rise. Of rats which survived high doses of T-2 toxin or whole lyophilized cultures of *F. tricinctum*, 60% developed corneal opacities in 40 to 60 d. Some of the rats dying after T-2 toxin was administered by gastric intubation became comatose before death.[40]

Because it was hypothesized that T-2 toxin produced profound, centrally mediated autonomic alterations, a dose of 1.0 mg/kg was given i.v. to rats and concentrations of vasopressin and oxytocin were assayed in the posterior pituitary.[41] The concentrations of vasopressin and oxytocin were decreased 6 to 8 h after toxin administration. Some of the same investigators then demonstrated additional neuroendocrine effects when intact rats and guinea pigs were given a single i.v. dose of T-2 toxin at 0.5, 1.0, or 2.0 mg/kg.[42] Prolonged (6 to 8 h) hypertension and tachycardia were followed by hypotension. Total peripheral resistance was increased and cardiac output declined. Alterations in arterial plasma norepinephrine, epinephrine, and dopamine concentrations are shown in Table 1. These increases suggested strong sympathetic stimulation. The elevations in circulating catecholamines, suggesting sympatho-adrenomedullary activation, were in accord with the profound increase

Table 1
**ALTERATIONS IN BASAL ARTERIAL PLASMA
NOREPINEPHRINE (NE), EPINEPHRINE (EPI) AND DOPAMINE
(DA) IN RATS AND GUINEA PIGS GIVEN T-2 TOXIN I.V.[42]**

Dose		Basal	6 h post-T-2		
(mg/kg)		0	0.5	1.0	2.0
Rat	NE	296 ± 7[a]	1111 ± 174	2050 ± 589	
	EPI	230 ± 33	1565 ± 315	4280 ± 1384	
	DA	135 ± 21	385 ± 52	565 ± 135	
Guinea pig	NE	483 ± 150		3090 ± 1019	5881 ± 2573
	EPI	201 ± 50		1700 ± 538	9224 ± 5911
	DA	483 ± 107		586 ± 136	1079 ± 310

[a]   pg/ml; data are mean ± SEM.

in vascular resistance in the kidneys and peripheral tissues (mesenteric, hindquarters, etc.) which leads to severe reduction of organ blood flow and shock prior to the development of systemic hypotension.[43]

To determine whether the sympathetic outflow was centrally mediated, rats in which the central nervous system was destroyed by pithing but the preganglionic sympathetic nerve trunks remained intact, were given T-2 toxin at 1.0 mg/kg i.v.[42] Two hours after the toxin was given, there were no significant changes in heart rate or blood pressure. While there was a minimal increase in the plasma concentration of norepinephrine (NE) (from about 200 to 400 pg/ml), there were no changes in epinephrine (EPI) or dopamine (DA). The ability of the peripheral sympatho-adrenomedullary system to respond was demonstrated when the spinal cord was electrically stimulated (3 Hz) and the plasma concentration of EPI increased 3-fold, in both saline- and T-2 toxin-treated, pithed rats. It was concluded that the sympathetic effects of T-2 toxin were mediated through a central nervous system mechanism.

More recent studies[51] provide direct evidence for central actions of T-2 in the rat. T-2 toxin, administered directly into the cerebroventricular (ICV) system of the chronically instrumented rat, produced cardiovascular responses at doses which had no effect when administered i.v. (systemically) (Figure 1). While a dose of 33 µg/kg produced no appreciable effects on hemodynamic variables by either route of administration (ICV or systemic), an ICV dose of 100 µg/kg produced definite heart rate and blood pressure elevations not observed after i.v. injection of this same dose of T-2. Furthermore, a dose of 300 µg/kg produced effects by ICV as well as systemic administration. While the systemic administration of T-2 toxin produced only transient tachycardia, however, the ICV administration of this dose of T-2 produced progressive and sustained tachycardia and pressor responses. Also, 50% of the rats given the T-2 by ICV administration at 300 µg/kg did not survive 24 h, while all of the rats given the same dose of T-2 systemically survived 72 h. These studies clearly indicate that T-2 and/or T-2 metabolites have direct effects on the central nervous system, at least in the rat.

It should be pointed out that these studies also demonstrated that the differences between centrally or systemically effective doses of T-2 toxin falls within a narrow dose range, i.e., the ICV dose of T-2 which produced cardiovascular effects is reasonably close to the minimal dose which produces such effects by systemic injection. This phenomenon might be a result of the rapid diffusion of systemically administered T-2 into the central nervous system. This suggestion is supported by recent studies[52] in which ³H-T-2 toxin was administered i.v. to conscious rats; the $T_{1/2}$ of the first (''distribution'') phase of T-2 elimination from the plasma was 1 to 2 min. The limited information available on the fate of T-2 toxin in the nervous system is discussed in a subsequent section of this chapter.

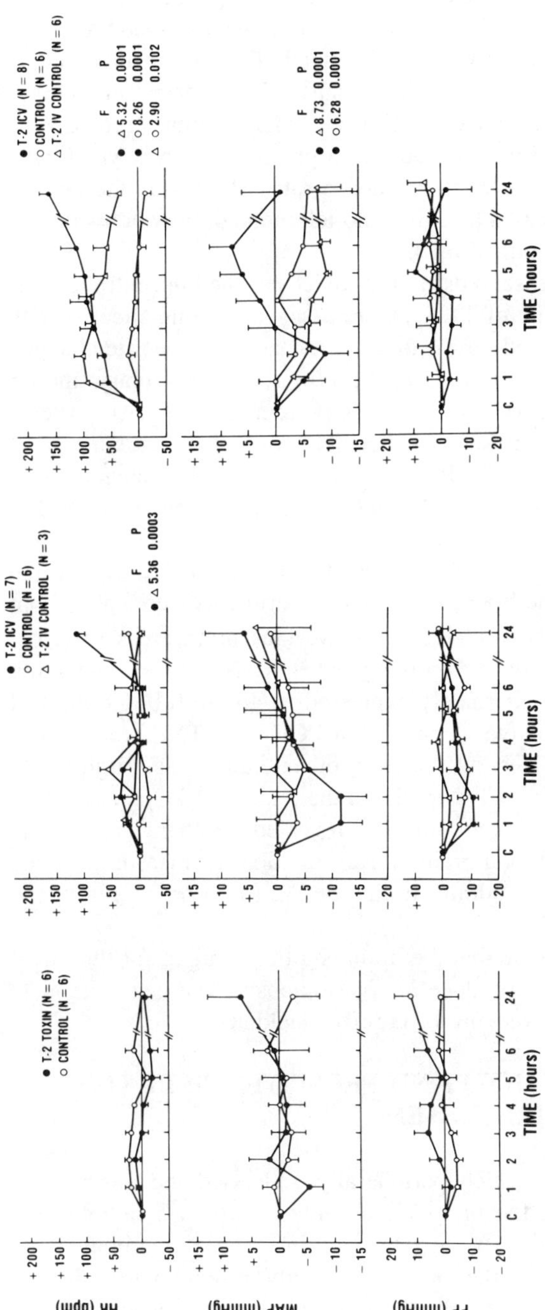

FIGURE 1. Effects of T-2 toxin administered into the cerebral ventricles (ICV) or systemically (i.v.) on hemodynamic variables. (Left) T-2 33 μg/ kg ICV; (middle) T-2 100 μg/kg ICV or i.v.; (right) T-2 300 μg/kg ICV or i.v. F and P values represent statistical analysis by ANOVA with a repeated measures design. All of the data are absolute changes from the control period for which there were no significant differences between the various groups for any of the variables studied. HR = heart rate; MAP = mean arterial pressure obtained via femoral artery catheter; PP = pulse pressure.

Recently, additional biochemical evidence has been raised in support of the involvement of the central nervous system in T-2 toxicosis. These studies (*vide infra*) stemmed from the observations[35] that the circulating levels of prostacyclin and thromboxane (TX) A_2 in swine and prostacyclin in the rat[42] were markedly elevated during the various stages of T-2 toxicosis; however, in none of these studies was the source of these cyclooxygenase metabolites of arachidonate determined. We have postulated that enhanced metabolism of arachidonate to prostaglandins (PGs) might also occur in the brain since many of the central autonomic effects of PGE_2 parallel those found in T-2 toxicosis. That is, PGE_2 administered ICV or directly into the rat hypothalamus (0.5 to 5 nmol) produced a pressor response which was accompanied by tachycardia,[44] effects also seen in T-2 dosed rats. Moreover, the central cardiovascular effects of PGE_2 are accompanied by sympatho-adrenomedullary activation,[44] a phenomenon not found in the T-2-dosed pithed rat.[45]

To further study the potential role of eicosanoids in T-2 toxicosis, the concentrations of various PGs and TXB_2 (the stable metabolite of TXA_2) were assayed in brain slices of rats exposed to T-2 toxin.[46] These studies revealed dose-, time-, site-, and PG-specific changes in the brain of the rats injected with T-2 toxin at 0.75 or 2 mg/kg i.v. The primary finding of this study was marked elevation of PGE_2 (from 0.2 pg/μg protein to 1.2 pg/μg protein) in the cortex of rats several hours after exposure to the high dose of T-2 toxin. Brain prostacyclin concentrations measured as 6-keto-$PGF_{1\alpha}$ were not significantly changed while TXA_2 (measured as TXB_2) showed only temporary changes (2-fold elevation 2 h after T-2 toxin administration).[46]

In order to examine whether the changes in brain prostaglandins of T-2 intoxicated rats were a direct result of T-2 action on the brain, additional experiments were carried out *in vitro*.[46] In these experiments, brain slices obtained from various brain areas (cerebral cortex, hypothalamus, brain stem) were incubated in oxygenated Kreb's buffer containing different concentrations (10^{-3} to 10^{-10} M; alternately expressed as 463 to 0.0463 ppm) of T-2 toxin. These experiments showed selective elevations in PGE_2 and TXB_2 release (by 50 and 25%, respectively) from cortical slices but not from other brain areas. High (10^{-3} to 10^{-4} M; 463 to 46.3 ppm) concentrations of T-2 inhibited the release of PGE_2 and TXB_2 in the cortex as well as other brain areas. Recent studies[53] revealed no changes in whole brain water content and no impairment of blood brain barrier function (as measured by the Evans blue method) at 2, 6, or 24 h after i.v. administration of T-2 (0.25 or 0.5 mg/kg) to conscious rats.

These studies taken together clearly indicate that the brain is a target organ for the direct actions of T-2 toxin at concentrations which produce *in vivo* toxicosis. The neurochemical effects of T-2 toxin on the CNS, however, remain to be fully elucidated.

IV. TRICHOTHECENE ENTRY INTO AND PERSISTENCE IN THE NERVOUS SYSTEM

The authors are aware of three studies which peripherally addressed the question of trichothecene access to and persistence in the brain. In a study in which a radiolabeled unesterified trichothecene skeleton was given i.v. to rats[47] and in which the animals were monitored at time points from 10 min to 24 h, the total radioactivity in brain at 10 min was greater than that in the heart or spleen, but was only 4.7% of that of the liver and 27% of that in the kidneys. The brain radioactivity declined at every time point thereafter, so that at 24 h post-administration the label was present at only 0.005% of the 10-min value. Spleen values were approximately $^1/_2$ those of brain at each time point.

Studies of radiolabeled T-2 toxin administered orally to mice[48] demonstrated that the quantity of label present in the brain at 3.5 h was equivalent to that present at 24 and 48

h. The situation was similar in splenic tissue, whereas the radioactivity of the liver showed a gradual decline and the kidney showed an initial decline from 3.5 to 24 h and then a similar value at 48 h. The total amount of radioactivity expressed as dpm per organ was very similar for brain, spleen, and kidney at both 24 and 48 h. In spite of the apparently flat trend for brain, spleen, and kidney between 24 and 48 h, the radiolabel had declined such that no measurable counts were detected at 72 h in any organ.

When pigs were killed 4 h after being given tritium-labeled T-2 toxin intravascularly at a dose of 0.15 mg/kg, the concentrations of total metabolite residues in brain, spleen, liver, and heart averaged 10.5, 35.5, 73.0, and 24.5 ng/g of tissue, respectively.[49] The brain concentration was less than that present in skeletal muscle (18.5 ng/g), suggesting a lack of selective delivery to the brain. When specific metabolites were quantitated in the brain, an unknown metabolite, PM-XV, later tentatively identified as 3'OH deepoxy HT-2, was present at the highest concentration (0.56 ng/g) followed by deacetyl T-2 tetraol and in turn by 3'OH HT-2, while the parent T-2 toxin was present at a far lower concentration of 0.04 ng/g. In contrast, spleen contained 3'OH HT-2, PM-XV, HT-2, parent T-2, and deacetyl T-2 tetraol at concentrations of 3.09, 2.28, 2.21, 1.89, and 1.22 ng/g, respectively. Concentrations of toxin and metabolites in mesenteric lymph nodes paralleled those in spleen. By virtue of its deepoxidation, 3'OH deepoxy HT-2 is likely to be of substantially reduced toxicity. Overall, therefore, because of the higher concentrations of the parent compound and some of the more toxic metabolites of T-2 toxin in the spleen and muscle, it would appear that as compared to these tissues, a relative degree of protection of the brain may exist.

When one evaluates rat "i.v. trichothecene skeleton study" of Nakano et al.,[47] the mouse oral T-2 data of Matsumoto et al.,[48] and the swine intravascular T-2 experiment of Corley,[49] it would appear that T-2 may have some affinity for the brain, but it probably has a somewhat greater affinity for the spleen, an accepted target organ for the trichothecenes. One must bear in mind, however, that a substantial volume of the brain is comprised by myelinated fibers which may not contain T-2 binding proteins, because of the absence of ribosomes. To date, no information is available on the uptake of T-2 toxin into either neurons or glial cells. It is also suggested that the toxin probably has a greater tendency to accumulate in these organs than does the unmodified trichothecene skeleton which, in view of its structure, is very likely to be far less toxic than T-2 toxin.

In summary, it is clear that additional studies of the distribution of T-2 toxin into various areas of the brain after oral and i.v. administration are needed. Particularly valuable would be determination of the concentrations of toxin and toxic metabolites actually reaching critical neurons of the brain when the various doses are given into the cerebroventricular system as well as when the toxin is given systemically. The resultant information could be used to determine whether the toxin and/or its active metabolites have a significant tendency to be retained in specific areas of the brain and to assess whether such tendencies, if they exist, are correlated with the functional alterations associated with trichothecene mycotoxin exposure.

Of course, a toxicant dose need not have selective uptake by a tissue for that tissue to be a particularly sensitive target.

V. CONCLUSION

T-2 toxicosis is a multisystem disorder which affects every organ and tissue. The scope of effects of T-2 may be related to a primary mechanism of action-inhibition of protein synthesis and its very high penetration coefficient through biological membranes. A degree of accumulation of T-2 toxin occurs in the CNS, but evidence of selective uptake is lacking. Nevertheless, the possible direct actions of T-2 on the brain deserve further investigation.

Hemorrhage into the meninges or brain seems to occur primarily in association with either massive exposure or concurrent with a generalized coagulopathy after repeated exposure of susceptible species. Usually, however, clinical effects, potentially referable to the nervous system, are observed in the absence of hemorrhage.

Much of the evidence in favor of central effects of T-2 toxin is from observations made of exposed humans and animals; these observations consist of motor, sensory, and autonomic (sympathetic and parasympathetic) signs and symptoms. In most of the studies, however, the CNS-related signs were associated with signs of toxicosis and dysfunction of major organs such as those of the cardiovascular, respiratory, and endocrine systems. Therefore, it is likely that some of the neurologic/motor abnormalities seen during T-2 toxicosis are due to the failure of other organs and the development of shock (through reflexive, hypoxic, and endocrine responses).

The evidence in support of a direct action of T-2 toxin in the brain is extremely scarce due to the limited number of experimental studies to date. Nevertheless, while peripheral organ failure no doubt plays an important role in T-2 toxicosis, the more recent data indicate that genuine centrally mediated phenomena also occur. The best example to support such a hypothesis is the absence of sympathetic activation in the T-2 dosed pithed rat (where the CNS is destroyed). The central activation of the sympathetic nervous system by T-2 toxin is in accord with the observation that T-2 toxin stimulates arachidonate metabolism to prostaglandins, since several eicosanoids (e.g., PGE_2) acting in the brain are potent stimulators of the sympatho-adrenomedullary axis. One might hypothesize that the enhanced metabolism of arachidonate may be a result of the inhibition of the synthesis of lipocortin, the potent inhibiting regulatory peptide of phospholipase A_2. Inhibition of the synthesis of lipocortin would result in a "release phenomenon" where phospholipid breakdown to free fatty acids, especially arachidonic acid, is enhanced. Since the release of arachidonate from phospholipids is the rate-limiting reaction in eicosanoid production, a T-2 toxin-induced inhibition of protein synthesis could perhaps ultimately result in rapid activation of eicosanoid production. A seemingly paradoxical phenomenon of enhanced biochemical activity produced by protein synthesis inhibition was also shown by Efrat et al.,[50] who found marked elevation of interleukin-2 production by lymphocytes exposed to T-2 toxin as well as other protein synthesis inhibitors.

The hypothesis regarding the key role of eicosanoids in T-2 toxicosis also gains support from peripheral phenomena associated with T-2 toxicosis. Thus, the rapid development of hemoconcentration could well be a result of the conversion of arachidonate, through the 5-lipoxygenase pathway, to cysteinyl leukotrienes, which together with PGs (e.g., PGI_2, PGE_2) may increase vascular permeability. This results in the leakage of plasma from the intra- to the extravascular compartment. Furthermore, leukotrienes are potent vasoconstrictors, a phenomenon well described in T-2 toxicosis; coronary vasoconstriction and possibly direct cardiac effects might underlie the low cardiac output. Thus, central and peripheral activation of eicosanoid production might play a key role in T-2 toxicosis; however, extensive experimental work is still necessary to elucidate these mechanisms.

ACKNOWLEDGMENTS

This work was supported in part by USAMRIID contracts. The opinions or assertions contained herein are the private ones of the authors and are not to be construed as official or reflecting the views of the Department of Defense or the Uniformed Services University of the Health Sciences or the University of Illinois. The experiments reported herein for our laboratories were conducted according to the principles set forth in the "Guide for the Use and Care of Laboratory Animals," Institute of Laboratory Animal Resources, National Research Council (DHEW Publ. No. NIH 80-23, 1980). The authors wish to thank Ms.

Wanda D. Patterson and the staff of the University of Illinois College of Veterinary Medicine, Word Processing Center, for their help in the preparation of this manuscript.

REFERENCES

1. **Haig, A. M.,** Chemical Warfare in Southeast Asia and Afghanistan: Report to Congress from Secretary of State Haig, March 22, 1982. Spec. Rep. No. 98, U.S. Government Printing Office, Washington, D.C., 1982.
2. **Townsend, A.,** personal communication, 1984.
3. **Cholodenko, M. I.,** Changes in the nervous system in toxic alimentary aleukia (so-called septic angina), *Nevropatol. Psykhiatr.,* 16, 67, 1947.
4. **Forgacs, J., Mycotoxicosis,** in *Advanced Veterinary Sciences,* Brandly, C. A. and Jungherr, E. L., Eds., Academic Press, New York, 1962, 273.
5. **Gadjusek, D. C.,** Acute Infectious Hemorrhagic Fevers and Mycotoxicoses in the Union of Soviet Socialist Republics Army Medical Service Graduate School, Walter Reed Army Medical Center, 1953, 82.
6. **Murphy, W. K., Burgess, M. A., Valdivieso, M., Livingston, R. B., Bodey, G. P., and Freioreich, E. J.,** Phase I clinical evaluation of anguidine, *Cancer Treat. Rep.,* 62, 1497, 1978.
7. **Goodwin, W., Haas, C. D., Fabian, C., Betting, I., and Hoogstraten, B.,** Phase I. Evaluation of anguidine (diacetoxyscirpenol NCS-141537), *Cancer,* 42, 23, 1978.
8. **Belt, R. J., Haas, C. D., Joseph, U., Goodwin, W., Moore, D., and Hoogstraten, B.,** Phase I study of anguidine administered weekly, *Cancer Treat. Rep.,* 63, 1993, 1979.
9. **DeSimone, P. A., Greco, F. A., and Lessner, H. F.,** Phase I evaluation of a weekly schedule of anguidine, *Cancer Treat. Rep.,* 63, 2015, 1979.
10. **Bukowski, R., Vaughn, C., Bottomley, R., and Chen, R.,** Phase II study of anguidine in gastrointestinal malignancies: a south-west oncology group study, *Cancer Treat. Rep.,* 66, 381, 1982.
11. **Yap, H. Y., Murphy, W. K., DiStefano, A., Blumenschein, G. R., and Bodey, G. P.,** Phase II study of anguidine in advanced breast cancer, *Cancer Treat. Rep.,* 63, 789, 1979.
12. **Rukmini, C., Prasad, J. S., and Rao, K.,** Effects of feeding T-2 toxin to rats and monkeys, *Food Cosmet. Toxicol.,* 18, 267, 1980.
13. **Forgacs, J.,** Mycotoxicosis: the neglected disease, *Feedstuffs,* 34, 124, 1962.
14. **Puls, R. and Greenway, J. A.,** Fusariotoxicosis from barley in British Columbia. II. Analysis and toxicity of suspected barley, *Can. J. Comp. Med.,* 40, 16, 1976.
15. **Greenway, J. A. and Puls, R.,** Fusariotoxicosis from barley in British Columbia. I. Natural occurrence and diagnosis, *Can. J. Comp. Med.,* 40, 12, 1976.
16. **Hayes, M. A. and Wobeser, G. A.,** Subacute toxic effects of dietary T-2 toxin in young mallard ducks, *Can. J. Comp. Med.,* 47, 180, 1983.
17. **Chi, M. S., Mirocha, C. J., Kurtz, H. J., Weaver, G., Bates, F., Shimoda, W., and Burmeister, H. R.,** Acute toxicity of T-2 toxin in broiler chicks and laying hens, *Poult. Sci.,* 56, 103, 1977.
18. **Coulter, D. B., Wyatt, R. D., and Stewart, R. G.,** Electroretinograms from broilers fed aflatoxin and T-2 toxin, *Poult. Sci.,* 56, 1435, 1977.
19. **Wyatt, R. D., Colwell, W. M., Hamilton, P. B., and Burmeister, H. R.,** Neural disturbances in chickens caused by dietary T-2 toxin, *Appl. Microbiol.,* 26, 757, 1973.
20. **Hoerr, F. J., Charlton, W. W., Tuite, J., Vesonder, R. F., Rohwedder, W. K., and Szigetti, G.,** Experimental trichothecene mycotoxicosis produced in broiler chickens by *sporotrichiella* var. *sporotrichioides, Avian Pathol.,* 11, 385, 1982.
21. **Wyatt, R. D., Doerr, J. A., Hamilton, P. B., and Burmeister, H. R.,** Egg production, shell thickness and other physiological parameters of laying hens affected by T-2 toxin, *Appl. Microbiol.,* 29, 641, 1975.
22. **Chi, M. S., El-Halawani, M. E., Waibel, P. E., and Mirocha, C. J.,** Effect of T-2 toxin on brain catecholamines and selected blood components in growing chickens, *Poult. Sci.,* 60, 137, 1981.
23. **Ueno, Y., Ueno, I., Iitoi, Y., Tsunoda, H., Enomoto, M., and Ohtsubo, K.,** Toxicological approaches to the metabolites of *Fusaria.* III. Acute toxicity of fusarenon-x, *Jpn. J. Exp. Med.,* 41, 521, 1971.
24. **Shimizu, T., Nakano, N., Matsui, T., and Aibara, K.,** Hypoglycemia in mice administered with fusarenon-x, *Jpn. J. Exp. Med.,* 32, 189, 1979.
25. **Matsuoka, Y., Kubota, K., and Ueno, Y.,** General pharmacological studies of fusarenon-x, a trichothecene mycotoxin from *Fusarium* species, *Toxicol. Appl. Pharmacol.,* 50, 87, 1979.
26. **Sato, N., Ueno, Y., and Enomoto, M.,** Toxicological approaches to the toxic metabolites of *Fusaria.* VIII. Acute and subacte toxicities of T-2 toxin in cats, *Jpn. J. Pharmacol.,* 25, 263, 1975.

27. **Cannon, M., Cranston, W. I., Hellon, R. F., and Townsend, Y.,** Inhibition by trichothecene antibiotics of brain protein synthesis and fever in rabbits, *J. Physiol.*, 322, 447, 1982.
28. **Lutsky, I., Mor, N., Yagen, B., and Joffe, A. Z.,** The role of T-2 toxin in experimental alimentary toxic aleukia: a toxicity study in cats, *Toxicol. Appl. Pharmacol.*, 43, 111, 1978.
29. **Ueno, Y., Ishii, K., Sakai, K., Kanaeda, S., Tsunoda, H., Tanaka, T., and Enomoto, M.,** Toxicological approaches to the metabolites of *Fusaria*. IV. Microbial survey on "bean hulls poisoning of horses" with the isolation of toxic trichothecenes, neosolaniol and T-2 toxin of *Fusarium solani* M-1-1, *Jpn. J. Exp. Med.*, 42, 187, 1972.
30. **Mortimer, P. H., Campbell, J., DiMenna, M. E., and White, E. P.,** Experimental myrotheciotoxicosis and poisoning in ruminants by verrucarin A and roridin A, *Res. Vet. Sci.*, 12, 508, 1971.
31. **Weaver, G. A., Kurtz, H. J., Mirocha, C. J., Bates, F. Y., Behrens, J. C., Robinson, T. S., and Swanson, S. P.,** The failure of purified T-2 mycotoxin to produce hemorrhaging in dairy cattle, *Can. Vet. J.*, 21, 210, 1980.
32. **Beasley, V. R.,** Toxicodynamics of T-2 Toxin in Swine and Cattle, Ph.D. thesis, University of Illinois, Urbana, 1983.
33. **Weaver, G. A., Kurtz, J. H., Mirocha, C., Bates, F. Y., Behrens, J. C.,** Acute toxicity of the mycotoxin diacetoxyscirpenol in swine, *Can. Vet. J.*, 19, 267, 1978.
34. **Coppock, R. W.,** Studies on the Pharmacokinetics and Toxicopathy of Diacetoxyscirpenol and Deoxynivalenol in Swine, Cattle and Dogs, Ph.D. thesis, University of Illinois, Urbana, 1984.
35. **Lorenzana, R. M., Beasley, V. R., Buck, W. B., Ghent, A. W., Lundeen, G. R., and Poppenga, R. H.,** Experimental T-2 toxicosis in swine. I. Change in cardiac output, aortic mean pressure, catecholamines, 6-keto-PGF$_{1\alpha}$, thromboxane B$_2$ and acid-base parameters, *Fundam. Appl. Toxicol.*, 5, 879, 1985.
36. **Lundeen, G. R., Poppenga, R. H, Beasley, V. R., Buck, W. B., Tranquilli, W. J., and Lambert, R. J.,** Systemic distribution of blood flow during T-2 toxin-induced shock in swine, *Fundam. Appl. Toxicol.*, 7, 309, 1986.
37. **Weaver, G. A., Kurtz, H. J., Bates, F. Y., Chi, M., Mirocha, C., Behrens, J. C., and Robinson, T. S.,** Acute and chronic toxity of T-2 mycotoxin in swine, *Vet. Res.*, 103, 531, 1978.
38. **Pang, F. V.,** T-2 Mycotoxicosis in Swine following Topical Application, Intravascular Administration and Inhalation Exposure, Ph.D. thesis, 1986.
39. **Kosuri, N. R., Smalley, E. B., and Nichols, R. E.,** Toxicologic studies of *Fusarium tricinctum* (Corda) Snyder et Hansen from moldy corn, *Am. J. Vet. Res.*, 32, 1843, 1971.
40. **Schoental, R., Joffe, A. Z., and Yagen, B.,** Cardiovascular lesions and various tumors found in rats given T-2 toxin, a trichothecene metabolite of *Fusarium, Cancer Res.*, 39, 2179, 1979.
41. **Zamir, N., Zamir, D., Eiden, L. E., Palkovits, M., Brownstein, M. J., Eskay, R. L., Weber, E., Faden, A. I., and Feuerstein, G.,** Methionine and leucine enkephalin in rat neurohypophysis: different responses to osmotic stimuli and T-2 toxin, *Science,* 228, 606, 1985.
42. **Feuerstein, G., Goldstein, D. S., Ramwell, P. W., Zerbe, R. L., Lux, W. E., Faden, A. I., and Bayorh, M. A.,** Cardiorespiratory, sympathetic and biochemical responses to T-2 toxin in the guinea pig and rat, *J. Pharmacol. Exp. Ther.*, 232, 786, 1985.
43. **Siren, A. L. and Feuerstein, G.,** Effect of T-2 toxin on regional blood flow and vascular resistance in the conscious rat, *Toxicol. Appl. Pharmacol.*, 83, 438, 1986.
44. **Feuerstein, G., Adelberg, S. A., Kopin, I. J., and Jacobowitz, D. M.,** Hypothalamic sites for cardiovascular and sympathetic modulation by prostaglandin E$_2$, *Brain Res.*, 231, 335, 1982.
45. **Feuerstein, G. and Kopin, I. J.,** Effect of PGD$_2$, PGE$_2$, PGF$_{2\alpha}$ and PGI$_2$ on blood pressure, heart rate and plasma catecholamine responses to spinal cord stimulation in the rat, *Prostaglandins,* 21, 189, 1981.
46. **Shohami, E. and Feuerstein, G.,** T-2 toxemia and brain prostaglandins, *Prostaglandins,* 31, 307, 1986.
47. **Nakano, N., Nagahara, A., Shimizu, T., Aibara, K., Fujimoto, Y., Morooka, N., and Tatsuno, T.** The tissue distribution and the pattern of excretion of [^{34}C]-labeled 12, 13-epoxytrichothec-9-ene in mice and rats, *Jpn. J. Med. Sci. Biol.*, 32, 269, 1979.
48. **Matsumoto, H., Ito, T., and Ueno, Y.,** Toxicological approaches to the metabolites of *Fusaria*. XII. Fate and distribution in mice, *Jpn. J. Exp. Med.*, 48, 393, 1978.
49. **Corley, R. A., Swanson, S. P., Gullo, G. J., Johnson, L., Beasley, V. R., and Buck, W. B.,** Distribution of T-2 toxin, a trichothecene mycotoxin, in intravascularly-dosed swine, *J. Agric. Food Chem.*, 34, 868, 1986.
50. **Efrat, S., Zelig, S., Yagen, B., and Kaempfer, R.,** Superinduction of human interleukin-2 messenger RNA by inhibitors of translation, *Biochem. Biophys. Res. Commun.*, 123, 842, 1984.
51. **Feuerstein, G.,** unpublished data.
52. **Hunter, J. and Feuerstein, G.,** unpublished data.
53. **Kempski, J. and Feuerstein, G.,** unpublished observation.

Chapter 6

EFFECTS ON THE INTEGUMENTARY SYSTEM

V. F. Pang, H. B. Schiefer, and V. R. Beasley

TABLE OF CONTENTS

I. INTRODUCTION

Trichothecene mycotoxins are highly irritating to the skin and mucous membranes. This activity may be responsible for the cutaneous and oral inflammatory lesions observed in fusariotoxicosis of chickens,[1] stachybotryotoxicosis,[2,3] and alimentary toxic aleukia (ATA).[4] Long before trichothecenes were incriminated in the diseases above, "stachybotryotoxin"[5,6] and "poaefusarin"[4] were recognized as irritant extracts of toxic food.

The cutaneous irritation potential of trichothecene mycotoxins has long been used as the basis for a bioassay for the detection of these mycotoxins after extracts of *F. sporotrichioides* and related fungi associated with ATA were found to be dermally toxic;[7] however, interest in systemic effects of topically administered trichothecene mycotoxins did not come into focus until recently, following allegations that they might have been used as chemical warfare agents in Southeast Asia and Afghanistan.[8-10]

II. SKIN BIOASSAY AND COMPARISONS BETWEEN TRICHOTHECENE MYCOTOXINS

Several versions of a skin-irritation bioassay have been described for the detection of trichothecene mycotoxins.[11-15] The published methods are simple to perform and highly sensitive; for instance, as little as 10 ng T-2 toxin can be detected in this way.[16]

The dermal toxicity bioassay has also been used to confirm the detection of trichothecene mycotoxins by other methods such as thin-layer chromatography (TLC).[17] In some cases, the effects of extracts in the skin bioassay were found to be closely correlated with T-2 toxin content as determined by gas-liquid chromatography (GLC).[18] A simple skin bioassay is neither quantitative nor specific for any of the trichothecene mycotoxins;[19] however, by application of a series of standard solutions as internal control, test reactions can be appraised in units of concentration of toxin, rather than as subjective measurements of intensity of inflammation, thus providing for an operable, semiquantitative assay.[20]

The degree of dermal toxicity of trichothecene mycotoxins is dependent on their chemical structures, as is their cytotoxicity to cultured cells. To determine the minimum effective doses capable of causing dermal toxicity, 9 type A, 6 type B, 1 type C, and 2 type D trichothecene mycotoxins were investigated recently.[21] All of the test compounds, dissolved in acetone and painted on the shaved backs of guinea pigs, induced redness at the application site within 2 to 10 h after application, but the effective doses ranged widely, from 10^{-11} (5 ng) to 10^{-7} mol. T-2 toxin was most toxic, followed by HT-2 toxin, diacetoxyscirpenol (DAS), verrucarin A, and roridin A. Nivalenol, deoxynivalenol, and their esters were found to be weak dermal irritants.[21]

III. LOCAL LESIONS IN TOPICALLY DOSED ANIMALS

When ATA isolate-originated *Fusarium tricinctum* crude extracts in 20% ethanol were applied in single graded doses to the shaved skin of mice and rats, the treated areas became red and edematous within 24 to 48 h.[22] Keratinization followed, the scabs fell off within 2 to 3 weeks, and hair usually regrew on the healed areas. When the extracts were applied weekly or less often, some hair follicles became atrophic, ulcerated lesions were slower to heal, and treated areas remained depilated for longer intervals. The treated skin had areas of desquamation and regeneration, and the underlying muscle was at times edematous or infiltrated with inflammatory cells. After cessation of treatments, the necrotic lesions healed, but epidermal hyperplasia persisted.

Topical application of purified trichothecene mycotoxins, mainly T-2 toxin, has been studied in a variety of animal species, including rabbits, rats, mice, guinea pigs, pigs, cattle, and cynomolgus monkeys.[20,23-26] In general, the morphologic changes associated with topically applied T-2 toxin were similar among these species. The gross alterations in the applied areas were characterized initially by hyperemia, swelling, serous exudation, and necrosis, and subsequently by formation of scabs which would fall off. At this time, the newly formed skin covering the dosed regions was hairless, but the hair eventually regrew, leaving these areas unnoticeable.[12,14,20,25,26] Microscopically, there was vascular dilation, congestion, edema, and infiltration of neutrophils, and mononuclear and mast cells in the dermis and even in the subcutis with varying degrees of necrosis in the epidermis.[12,20,25,27]

A. Rats

Topical application of 1.3 mg of T-2 toxin dissolved in ethyl acetate to the partially shaved skin of 50 g rats produced extensive coagulative necrosis of the dermis and sloughing of the overlying epidermis with neutrophilic infiltration at the perimeter of the lesion.[12] Walls of arteries in the area of inflammation and adjoining tissues were either "smudged" in appearance or had undergone hyalinization. Although application of two lower doses, 0.12 and 0.47 mg, also caused extensive necrosis of the dermis which extended into the subcutis and was accompanied by neutrophilic infiltration at the margins, there was no complete coagulative necrosis of the dermal tissue.

B. Pigs

In a 2-week study, pigs were treated topically with T-2 toxin at a dose of 15 mg/kg in dimethylsulfoxide (DMSO) on an approximately 10 × 15 cm clipped area on the back that was protected by a nonocclusive foam pad device and were killed sequentially on days 1, 3, 7, and 14.[25] Gross changes in the skin at the site of toxin application consisted of swelling and discoloration, changing gradually from light red to dark purple. The exposed area became scaly on day 3 and became ulcerated and hemorrhagic at the margins on days 7 and 14. The histologic changes began in the epidermis and upper dermis on day 1 and progressively extended into the deep dermis and subcutaneous fat after day 3. The epidermal changes on day 1 consisted on ballooning degeneration and cellular dissociation of individual or groups of epithelial cells in the strata spongiosum and basale, along with formation of vesicles and mild infiltration of neutrophils and eosinophils. These changes were then followed by extensive epithelial necrosis, marked neutrophilic infiltration, pseudoepitheliomatous hyperplasia, and parakeratosis. The changes in the dermis on day 1 were localized mainly around vessels and consisted of edema, fibrin deposition, infiltration of neutrophils and eosinophils, and disruption of collagen. Vascular damage characterized by fibrinoid degeneration and formation of fibrin thrombi occurred in some capillaries. These changes became more apparent and extensive in the dermis with time and extended into subcutaneous fat as well. Fibroplasia began to appear in the dermis on day 7 of exposure. Although fibroplasia became more evident on day 14, extensive necrosis was still present in the dermis.

C. Cattle

Application of 1.5 to 6.0 mg of T-2 toxin in DMSO to the clipped withers or 3 mg of the toxin in 0.2 ml of acetone to the shaved coronary bands and interdigital skin of cattle produced locally inflamed, encrusted lesions which gradually healed.[24] No lesions similar to "fescue foot" occurred after topical application or intramuscular and intermittent oral administration (in a total of 5 doses ranging from 18 to 72 mg in ethanol and propylene glycol) of T-2 toxin.

IV. TOXIN INTERACTIONS AND THE EFFECTS OF A REPEATED DOSE

When administered in mice, either dimethylbenzanthracene or aflatoxin B_1 "initiation" followed by T-2 "promotion" at 25 μg/dose caused extensive skin damage and subsequent tolerance of the treated skin to elevated topical doses of T-2 toxin.[28] In T-2 "promoted" mice, sloughing of skin and subsequent scarring were more pronounced after "initiation" with dimethylbenzanthracene or aflatoxin than after "initiation" with T-2 toxin.

V. EFFECTS OF DOSAGE ON LOCAL INJURY

The severity of the cutaneous lesions is dependent on the dose of T-2 toxin applied to the skin. T-2 toxin in ethyl acetate was topically applied to rats and rabbits at 2-fold serial increases in dose from 0.02 to 0.64 μg and Draize scores were calculated at 24, 48, and 72 h by adding the individual scores for hyperemia and edema.[20] The mean Draize scores for both rabbits and rats increased with increasing concentrations of T-2 toxin, except for rabbits when the scores were calculated at 24 h.[20] Similar dose-dependent reactions were also seen by Marasas et al.[12] who found that topical appplication of 0.12, 0.47, or 1.3 mg of T-2 toxin, dissolved in ethyl acetate, to the partially shaved skin of young rats produced necrosis of both epidermis and dermis. The 1.3 mg T-2 toxin caused complete necrosis of the dermis and sloughing of the covering epidermis with some neutrophilic infiltration at the margin of necrosis, while the two lower doses caused extensive but incomplete necrosis of the dermis, more evident suppurative inflammation, and no sloughing of the epidermis.[12]

VI. VEHICLE COMPARISONS

The cutaneous response to T-2 toxin is affected by the vehicle. Using rats, Hayes and Schiefer[20] found variation in both the intensity of the cutaneous reactions and the percentage of rats developing cutaneous reactions in each group treated with 2 μl of a T-2 solution at a concentration of 100 μg/ml in ethyl acetate, methanol, DMSO, or maize oil. The reaction intensity and percentage of rats affected were similar when T-2 was dissolved in ethyl acetate or methanol, but much less when dissolved in maize oil or DMSO.[20] Similar results with rats were also described by Wannemacher et al.[26] who found that the LD_{50} of topically applied T-2 toxin dissolved in methanol was 12.5 mg/kg, but in DMSO was only 0.5 to 1.0 mg/kg. The LD_{50} dose of T-2 toxin in DMSO caused very mild dermal necrosis; however, the systemic lesions of lymphoid and intestinal epithelium necrosis were prominent.[26] In contrast, the major lesion caused by the LD_{50} of T-2 toxin in methanol was skin necrosis with few detectable systemic effects.[26]

The above results are in agreement with the findings of a study in guinea pigs using radiolabeled T-2 toxin. When 0.1 ml of solution containing 0.5 mg of unlabeled and 10 μCi of [^{3}H] T-2 toxin in either methanol or DMSO was painted on the shaved backs of the guinea pigs, there was an initial 50% disappearance of dermal radioactivity over 1 d for DMSO but only 25% over 7 d for methanol with little additional absorption through day 14.[29] It is suggested that although solvents have an impact, in general, T-2 toxin is slowly absorbed through the skin of guinea pigs and the dermal layer may act as a reservoir for T-2 toxin.

VII. SPECIES COMPARISONS AND TOXIN FATE IN THE SKIN

There is an apparent variation in the cutaneous sensitivity to T-2 toxin between different animal species. In general terms, the upper layer of the epidermis, namely the stratum corneum, is the main barrier to percutaneous permeation and absorption of drugs and toxic compounds. The thickness[30,31] and structural differences[31] of the stratum corneum, and the skin appendages (hair follicles, sweat glands, and sebaceous glands)[30] may contribute substantially to species differences in the penetration rate of a given compound. It has been shown that the skin of densely haired animals (rabbits, rats, guinea pigs, mice) tends to be highly permeable, while the lower permeability of the skin of pigs, monkeys, and dogs is more comparable to that of man.[32-34]

The species differences among laboratory animals appear to hold true in dermal exposure to trichothecene mycotoxins. Hayes and Schiefer[20] observed that rabbits had more prominent erythema and edema in the dosed area of skin than did rats when exposed to the same concentration of T-2 toxin. Moreover, Wannemacher et al.[26] showed that rabbits were the most sensitive to T-2 toxin, while the cynomolgus monkeys were the least sensitive, with rats and guinea pigs of intermediate sensitivity. Furthermore, an apparent variation in the intensity of the cutaneous reaction to a given dose of T-2 toxin was noted not only among individual rabbits and rats, but also within the same individual.[20] The variation from one animal to another was greater in rabbits than in rats.[20]

In spite of the generalizations provided above, skin penetration studies comparing isolated guinea pig and human skin have indicated a comparatively high degree of absorption through human skin. The penetration of [³H] T-2 toxin adsorbed onto corn dust has been studied *in vitro* with diffusion cells covered by excised human epidermis, human whole skin, and guinea pig whole skin.[35] The applied dose was 3.27 to 4.76 mg of corn dust containing 18.2 ppm [³H] T-2 toxin. The total penetration (expressed as percentage dose) through isolated human epidermis, human whole skin, and guinea pig whole skin was $1.12 \pm 0.26\%$, $0.33 \pm 0.07\%$, and $0.13 \pm 0.07\%$, respectively. In consideration of the basis of differences between the human epidermis and human whole skin, it was hypothesized that there was a reservoir for T-2 toxin in the dermis of excised skin. Further, the radioactive compounds in the receptor fluid bathing the human whole skin were composed of 69% T-2 toxin and 25% HT-2 toxin, suggesting that HT-2 was probably formed as result of enzymatic reactions in the skin.[35]

Further evidence of T-2 metabolism by the skin was drawn from *in vivo* studies in which a dose of 15 mg/kg was topically applied to swine.[25,36] The T-2 toxin was dissolved in 0.75 ml of DMSO and applied to an approximately 10×15 cm clipped area on the back. The mean concentrations of free T-2 toxin in the skin at the site of application on days 1, 3, 7, and 14 after dosing were 220, 247, 224, and 41 ppm, respectively.[25] In addition to the parent compound, the following deacetylated metabolites were also detected in the skin: HT-2, neosolaniol, 4-deacetylneosolaniol, T-2 triol, and T-2 tetraol.[25] Significant amounts of T-2 toxin were also detected in the subcutaneous fat up to 14 d after topical administration. Although the lower layers of the epidermis and the dermis generally offer little resistance to penetration of drugs, these regions may bind substances in a manner analogous to protein binding.[30] It has been suggested that the dermis may provide a significant barrier or reservoir for lipid soluble compounds.[37] T-2 toxin is a somewhat lipophilic compound.[38] Therefore, it has been suggested that T-2 toxin and its metabolites are slowly absorbed from the skin and subcutaneous fat which themselves may act as a depot and site of metabolism for the toxin.[25] The amount of adipose tissue present in the subcutis varies not only between species, but also between individuals of the same species and between different regions of the body. These factors may result in a variable rate of toxin absorption between topically exposed individual animals.

VIII. MECHANISM OF LOCAL INJURY

The mechanism of cutaneous injury by T-2 toxin as well as other trichothecene mycotoxins is still unknown. The morphologic changes observed in T-2 treated skin are rather nonspecific[20] and are consistent with those described in the cutaneous reactions to a variety of physical[39] and chemical agents.[40-42] Hayes and Schiefer[20] further demonstrated that in rats the sequential reaction to topically applied croton oil, a well-recognized primary cutaneous irritant,[43] was very similar to that induced by T-2 toxin, although croton oil produced a more severe reaction and more pronounced epidermal hyperplasia. In addition, Hayes and Schiefer[20] observed that T-2 toxin was capable of causing dermal inflammation without necessarily causing epidermal necrosis. Topical application of 0.24 μg of T-2 toxin in ethyl acetate to the clipped backs of rats or rabbits could cause intense dermal inflammation characterized by hyperemia, edema, and neutrophilic infiltration. The epidermis, however, either was only slightly damaged or showed focal coagulative necrosis.

It has been suggested that vascular injury plays a role in the induction of the cutaneous reaction by T-2 toxin and other trichothecene mycotoxins.[21,27] Ueno[21] found that vascular permeability in rabbits was biphasically increased at 5 and 24 h following a subcutaneous injection of 10 μg of fusarenon-X. The first fusarenon-X-induced increment in vascular permeability occurred at 5 h and was not inhibited by pretreatment with either promethazine (an antihistaminic) or indomethacin (a prostaglandin synthetase inhibitor). In addition, no effect on the morphology of rat peritoneal mast cells was found following incubation with 1 μg/ml of T-2 toxin or 10 μg of fusarenon-X for 1 to 2 h nor on the stability of rat liver lysosomes in the presence of 4 μg/ml of fusarenon-X or 5 μg/ml T-2 toxin.[21] It was thus concluded that the increase in vascular permeability induced by trichothecene mycotoxins was due to a direct effect on the capillary vessels instead of being produced by mediators such as histamine released from mast cells or prostaglandins.[21]

Following topical application of 1, 2, 5, 20, or 100 μg of T-2 toxin in either DMSO or ethyl alcohol, rats developed a delayed cutaneous reaction characterized by vascular dilation, stasis, edema, and mononuclear cell infiltration, rich in degraulating mast cells, with a dose-dependent latent period of 4 to 12 h.[27] These changes appeared initially and were most severe in the subcutis and then were seen in the dermis. Epidermal necrosis occurred 1 to 2 d later and was accompanied by neutrophilic infiltration. Both light and electron microscopic studies showed that small vessels were sites of initial change. Ultrastructurally, the endothelial cells were characterized by swelling, decreased pinocytosis, and swollen mitochondria with disorganized cristae, but had tightly closed intercellular junctions. In contrast to the results reported by Ueno,[21] partial degranulation, followed by complete degranulation, was noted in mast cells obtained from peritoneal washes and incubated with 20 μg/ml of T-2 toxin for 30 and 60 min, respectively.[27] Although the cause and effect of the small vessel changes and concomitant mast cell degranulation could not be determined, it was suggested that chemical mediators of inflammation may contribute to these changes and that the epidermal change might simply be a secondary ischemic necrosis due to a significant decrease in blood flow following microvascular injury induced by T-2 treatment.[27] Regardless of the degree of primary vs. secondary effects, these are clearly effects on the dermal vasculature of animals treated topically with trichothecenes.

IX. LOCAL EFFECTS IN HUMANS

In geographical locations where equine stachybotryotoxicosis was enzootic, people developed dermatitis after handling moldy fodder.[2] Occasionally, persons who used straw for fuel or slept on straw mattresses were also affected. Dermatitis developed on the scrotum, axillae, and sometimes the hands.

Five workers involved in processing or dosing sheep and calves with toxic cultures of *Myrothecium roridum* and *M. verrucaria* developed dermatitis.[44] The most commonly affected area was the face, especially eyelids and orbital areas. The lesions were composed of edema, inflammation, and a brief period of desquamation which responded well to corticosteroids.

Workers, manipulating large batch cultures of a *F. tricinctum* strain known to be a T-2 producer, developed facial inflammation followed by desquamation and considerable local inflammation.[45] In a separate incident, laboratory workers were accidentally in contact with crude ethyl acetate extracts containing approximately 200 ppm T-2 toxin. The toxin had been spilled inside their plastic gloves and the exposure lasted 2 min before washing in mild detergent.[15] Those exposed experienced burning sensations on their fingers approximately 4 h later, increasing in severity until 8 h. By 24 h, the burning sensation was replaced by numbness. All sensitivity was lost in the exposed areas by 72 h, after 4 to 5 d the affected skin had become hard and somewhat white. The skin peeled off in 1 to 2 mm thick pieces during the 2nd week, and the underlying skin regained normal sensitivity by the 18th d.

The necrotic lesions in the nose, jaws, fingers, and lips of ATA patients were thought to be compatible with local effects resulting from contact, while the internal hemorrhages were more suggestive of systemic effects of the ingested toxins.[5] Similarities between ATA of man and experimental T-2 toxicosis of animals include dermal inflammation about the mouth and nose and cutaneous hyperemia.[46]

Although localized integumentary effects of trichothecene mycotoxins cannot be considered life-threatening in themselves, they need to be recognized as a significant diagnostic feature and a genuine laboratory hazard.

X. SYSTEMIC EFFECTS AFTER DERMAL ADMINISTRATION

Pigs treated with T-2 toxin topically at a dose of 15 mg/kg showed anorexia, lethargy, and posterior weakness during the first 2 to 3 d, and had persistently elevated body temperature during the first 2 weeks,[25,36] but none of the T-2 treated pigs died. When compared to control pigs, the T-2 treated pigs had prominent neutrophilia, lower serum albumin, higher serum globulin, and lower serum alkaline phosphatase activities as well as significantly decreased body weight gain.[36] Although severe local skin damage was present at the site of application, there were few lesions in the internal organs.[25] These consisted of minimal lymphocytic necrosis in the lymphoid organs and scattered individual cell degeneration and necrosis in the exocrine pancreas.

Death of experimental animals occurred after topical application of crude *Fusarium* spp. extracts.[47] Application of "too high a concentration of a scirpene compound" led to death of rats in 48 to 72 h with "little or no noticeable skin response".[45] T-2 toxin at a dose of 0.25 mg/rat in ethyl acetate applied topically induced death within 60 to 100 h, preceded by anorexia, lethargy, and paresis.[48] Ghosal et al.[49] found that rats given a single dose of 0.1 or 0.2 mg of a T-2 toxin-containing extract form *F. oxysporum* on their skin died within 6 d. Male Sprague Dawley rats given T-2 toxin in DMSO at a dose of 8 mg/kg were dead within 16 h; all those given 4 mg/kg died within 24 h. About 50% of the rats given a dose of 2.5 mg/kg died within 24 h, and a dose of 1.0 mg/kg still caused noticeable effects.[50] These findings are in contrast to those with regard to female White Porton strain rats which tolerated 10.0 mg/kg.[51] Whether a sex-related ability to handle such toxins remains to be established, but species differences exist. Male mice appear to be less sensitive than male rats when T-2 toxin in DMSO is applied topically. When groups of male mice were topically dosed with T-2 toxin in DMSO at 20, 30, or 40 mg/kg deaths occurred in 20/20 of the test animals of each group within 4 to 6 d after application, whereas 17/20 and 5/20 animals died in the 10 and 5 mg/kg groups, respectively, within 7 d.[52]

Different trichothecenes vary in systemic toxicity after topical administration. When various trichothecene mycotoxins were tested using mice under similar conditions, it was found that T-2 toxin was the most potent toxin, followed, in descending order, by DAS, HT-2 toxin, verrucarin-A, and roridin-A. No deaths occurred after application of 3-acetyl-deoxynivalenol (3ac-DON); however, application of mixtures of T-2 toxin, DAS, and 3ac-DON resulted in accelerated death, suggesting a synergistic mode of action.[53] Histologic examination of the internal organs revealed the characteristic T-2 toxin-induced cellular injury at 6 h after topical administration.[52,53]

As in the case of local toxicity, the vehicle or "absorption enhancer" may play an important role in the systemic effects of trichothecene mycotoxins. A new absorption enhancer, 1-dodecylazacycloheptan-2-one ("azone"),[54] accelerated the systemic and lethal toxicity of topically applied T-2 toxin in mice to a considerable degree, whereas the reverse was true for rats.[55] Thus, toxin species and the solvent or "absorption enhancer" differences have to be considered with regard to both local and systemic effects of topical applied trichothecenes.

XI. DERMAL EFFECTS AFTER SYSTEMIC ADMINISTRATION

The frequently observed perioral dermatitis, or the dermatitis on legs, during or after feeding of trichothecene-contaminated feed to rodents cannot be ascribed to a systemic effect, and is probably nothing more than a local dermatitic reaction due to contact with the toxin. The often reported observation of piloerection, or "ruffled" hair coats, in experimental animals after systemic administration of trichothecene mycotoxins, however, has to be interpreted as a trichothecene-related reaction, attributable to general illness.

The daily oral administration of T-2 toxin at 1.5, 2.0, 2.5, or 3.0 mg/kg or DAS at 2.5, 3.0, or 3.5 mg/kg to 7-d-old broiler chicks caused gross and histologic feather lesions from 12 through 24 h after treatment.[56] Feather loss was associated with necrosis of the layer of the ramus and the basilar layer of barb ridges. Only DAS caused necrosis of the stratum germinativum at the neck of the feather follicle. Feathers from chickens given either toxin and killed at 72 or 168 h were considered normal.

When T-2 toxin was given at concentrations of 1 to 16 ppm in the feed of chickens from hatching to 3 weeks of age, growth inhibitory concentrations of 4, 8, and 16 ppm T-2 toxin caused dose-related abnormal feathering.[57] Feather tips were frequently constricted and some quills had a reverse curve. Based on the similarity of the T-2 toxin-induced abnormal feathering to those induced by arginine or other specific amino acid deficiency, it was suggested that T-2 toxin might cause this effect through a nutritional imbalance.

Dermographism, in which scratching of the skin with a dull instrument provokes a linear raised pale streak bordered by hyperemia, occurred in some persons with ATA.[58] This may have been the reflection of a primarily vascular effect.

The best-known systemic effects of trichothecene mycotoxins in man are the observations made on cancer patients receiving i.v. treatments with anguidine (DAS). Erythema and a burning sensation were frequently encountered; loss of hair occurred in some instances.[59,60]

Acute T-2 toxicosis induced in swine after oral, intravascular, or inhalation administration causes a distinct pattern of changes in the skin which progresses over time. Initially, there may be, within 1 to 2 h after dosing, a generalized reddening of the skin. As circulatory disturbance becomes evident, numerous irregularly shaped areas of purple discoloration are observed on the skin of the body, most strikingly on the ventral abdomen. In addition, capillary refill is slowed so that digital pressure on the skin causes blanching which may persist for 30 s or more. The ear margins also become purplish to black and cold with poor capillary refill in the later stages of the shock syndrome.

XII. CONCLUSIONS

Effects of the trichothecene mycotoxins on the integumentary system are neither unique nor of life-threatening significance. Nevertheless, their irritant and dermonecrotic effects after local contact and, to a lesser degree, their cutaneous effects after systemic administration are of substantial importance. As mentioned herein, not only can integumentary effects be used for diagnostic purposes with laboratory animals, but such lesions should be anticipated in a significant fraction of natural outbreaks, but only when the more highly toxic trichothecene mycotoxins are involved. Because of its lower cytotoxicity, the commonly encountered trichothecene, deoxynivalenol, should not be expected to cause cutaneous lesions.

More importantly, the local effects on the skin from topical exposure to trichothecene mycotoxins seem to be a manifestation of a primary vascular insult as well as direct cytotoxic effects. The same may be true for several of the effects of trichothecenes in other organs and systems.

REFERENCES

1. **Wyatt, R. D., Harris, J. R., Hamilton, P. B., and Burmeister, H. R.,** Possible outbreaks of fusariotoxicosis in avians, *Avian Dis.,* 16, 1123, 1972.
2. **Forgacs, J.,** Stachybotryotoxicosis, in *Microbial Toxin,* Vol. 8, Kadis, S., Ciegler, A., and Ajl, S. J., Eds., Academic Press, New York, 1972, 95.
3. **Rodricks, J. V. and Eppley, R. M.,** Stachybotrys and stachybotryotoxicosis, in *Mycotoxins,* Purchase, I. F. H., Ed., Elsevier, Amsterdam, 1974, 181.
4. **Joffe, A. Z.,** Foodborne diseases: alimentary toxic aleukia, in *Foodborne Diseases of Biologic Origin,* Rechcigl, M., Ed., CRC Press, Boca Raton, FL, 1983, 353.
5. **Frogacs, J. and Carll, W. T.,** Mycotoxicoses, *Adv. Vet. Sci.,* 7, 273, 1962.
6. **Palyusik, M.,** Biological test for the toxic substance of *Stachybotrys alternans, Acta Vet. Acad. Sci. Hung.,* 20, 57, 1970.
7. **Joffe, A. Z.,** Biological properties of some toxic fungi isolated from overwintered cereals, *Mycopathol. Mycol. Appl.,* 16, 201, 1962.
8. **Holden, C.,** Unequivocal evidence of Soviet toxin use, *Science,* 216, 154, 1982.
9. **Rosen, R. T. and Rosen, J. D.,** Presence of four *Fusarium* mycotoxins and synthetic material in "Yellow Rain", *Biomed. Mass Spectrom.,* 9, 443, 1982.
10. **Schiefer, H. B.,** Study of the Possible Use of Chemical Warfare Agents in Southeast Asia. A Report to the Department of External Affairs, Canada, Document A/37/308 United Nations General Assembly, New York, 1982.
11. **Gilgan, M. W., Smalley, F. B., and Strong, F. M.,** Isolation and partial characterization of a toxin from *Fusarium tricinctum* on moldy corn, *Arch. Biochem. Biophys.,* 114, 1, 1966.
12. **Marasas, W. F. O., Bamburg, J. R., Smalley, E. B., Strong, F. M., Ragland, W. L., and Degurse, P. E.,** Toxic effects on trout, rats, and mice of T-2 toxin produced by the fungus *Fusarium tricinctum* (Cd.) Snyd. et Hans, *Toxicol. Appl. Pharmacol.,* 15, 471, 1969.
13. **Ueno, Y., Ishikawa, Y., Amakai, K., Nakajima, M., Saito, M., Enomoto, M., and Ohtsubo, K.,** Comparative study on skin-necrotizing effect of scirpene metabolities of *Fusaria, Jpn. J. Exp. Med.,* 40, 33, 1970.
14. **Wei, R. D., Smalley, E. B., and Strong, F. M.,** Improved skin test for detection of T-2 toxin, *Appl. Microbiol.,* 23, 1029, 1972.
15. **Bamburg, J. R. and Strong, F. M.,** 12, 13-Epoxytrichothecenes, in *Microbial Toxins,* Vol. 7, Kadis, S., Ciegler, A., and Ajl, S. J., Eds., Academic Press, New York, 1971, 207.
16. **Chung, C. W., Trucksess, M. W., Giles, A. L., Jr., and Friedman, L.,** Rabbit skin test for estimation of T-2 toxin and other skin-irritating toxins in contaminated corn, *J. Assoc. Off. Anal. Chem.,* 57, 1121, 1974.
17. **Puls, R. and Greenway, J. A.,** Fusariotoxicosis from barley in British Columbia. II. Analyses and toxicity of suspected barley, *Can. J. Comp. Med.,* 40, 16, 1976.
18. **Yagen, B. and Joffe, A. Z.,** Screening of toxic isolates of *Fusarium poae* and *Fusarium sporotrichioides* involved in causing alimentary toxic aleukia, *Appl. Environ. Microbiol.,* 32, 423, 1976.
19. **Eppley, R. M.,** Methods for the detection of trichothecenes, *J. Assoc. Off. Anal. Chem.,* 58, 906, 1975.
20. **Hayes, M. A. and Schiefer, H. B.,** Quantitative and morphological aspects of cutaneous irritation by trichothecene mycotoxins, *Food Cosmet. Toxicol.,* 17, 611, 1979.
21. **Ueno, Y.,** Toxicological features of T-2 toxin and related trichothecenes, *Fundam. Appl. Toxicol.,* 4, S124, 1984.
22. **Schoental, R. and Joffe, A. Z.,** Lesions induced in rodents by extracts from cultures of *Fusarium poae* and *F. sporotrichioides, J. Pathol.,* 112, 37, 1974.
23. **Beasley, V. R.,** The Toxicokinetics and Toxicodynamics of T-2 Toxicosis in Swine and Cattle, Ph.D. thesis, University of Illinois, Urbana, 1983.

24. **Kosuri, N. R., Grove, M. D., Yates, S. G., Tallent, W. H., Ellis, J. J., Wolff, I. A., and Nichols, R. E.,** Response of cattle to mycotoxins of *Fusarium tricinctum* isolated from corn and fescue, *J. Am. Vet. Med. Assoc.,* 157, 938, 1970.

25. **Pang, V. F., Swanson, S. P., Beasley, V. R., Buck, W. B., and Haschek, W. M.,** The toxicity of T-2 toxin in swine following topical application. I. Clinical signs, pathology and residue concentrations, *Fundam. Appl. Fund.,* 9, 41 1987.

26. **Wannemacher, R. W., Jr., Bunner, D. L., Pace, J. G., Neufeld, H. A., and Brennecke, L. M.,** Dermal toxicity of T-2 toxin in guinea pigs, rats, and cynomolgus monkeys, in *Trichothecenes and Other Mycotoxins,* Lacey, J., Ed., John Wiley & Sons, New York, 1985, 423.

27. **Yarom, R., Bergmann, F., and Yagen, B.,** Cutaneous injury by topical T-2 toxin: involvement of microvessels and mast cells, submitted.

28. **Lindenfelser, L. A., Lillehoj, E. B., and Burmeister, H. R.,** Aflatoxin and trichothecene toxins: skin tumor induction and synergistic acute toxicity in white mice, *J. Natl. Cancer Inst.,* 52, 113, 1974.

29. **Wannemacher, R. W., Jr., Bunner, D. L., Pace, J. G., and Dinterman, R. E.,** Dermal absorption of T-2 mycotoxin in guinea pigs, *Toxicologist,* 5, 246, 1985.

30. **Shaw, J. E., Chandrasekaran, S. K., Michaels, A. S., and Taskovich, L.,** Controlled transdermal delivery, *in vitro* and *in vivo,* in *Animal Models in Dermatology with Relevance to Human Dermatopharmacology and Dermatotoxicology,* Maibach, H., Ed., Churchill Livingstone, Edinburgh, 1975, 138.

31. **Bronaugh, R. L., Stewart, R. F., and Congdon, E. R.,** Methods for *in vitro* percutaneous absorption studies. II. Animal models for human skin, *Toxicol. Appl. Pharmacol.,* 62, 481, 1982.

32. **Marzulli, F. N., Brown, D. W. C., and Maibach, H. I.,** Techniques for studying skin penetration, *Toxicol. Appl. Pharmacol. Suppl.,* 3, 76, 1969.

33. **McCreesh, A. H.,** Percutaneous toxicity, *Toxicol. Appl. Pharmacol. Suppl.,* 2, 20, 1965.

34. **Tregear, R. T.,** The permeability of skin to molecules of widely differing properties, in *Progress in Biological Science in Relation to Dermatology,* Vol. 2, Rook, A. J., Ed., Cambridge University Press, London, 1964.

35. **Kemppainen, B. W., Riley, R. T., and Pace, J. G.,** Penetration of [³H] T-2 toxin through excised human and guinea-pig skin during exposure to [³H] T-2 toxin absorbed to corn dust, *Food Chem. Toxicol.,* 22, 893, 1984.

36. **Pang, V. F., Felsburg, P. J., Beasley, V. R., Buck, W. B., and Haschek, W. M.,** The toxicity of T-2 toxin in swine following topical application. II. Effects on hematology, serum biochemistry and immune response, *Fundam. Appl. Fund.,* 9, 50, 1987.

37. **Reifenrath, W. G., Chellquist, E. M., Shipwash, E. A., and Jederberg, W. W.,** Evaluation of animal models for predicting skin penetration in man, *Fundam. Appl. Toxicol.,* 4, S224, 1984.

38. **Ueno, Y., and Shimada, N.,** Reconfirmation of the specific nature of reticulocytes bioassay system to trichothecene mycotoxins of *Fusarium* spp., *Chem. Pharm. Bull.,* 22, 2744, 1974.

39. **Logan, G. and Wilhelm, D. L.,** The inflammatory reaction in ultraviolet injury, *Br. J. Exp. Pathol.,* 47, 286, 1966.

40. **Rostenberg, A.,** Primary irritant and allergic eczematous reactions, *Arch. Dermatol.,* 75, 547, 1957.

41. **Steele, R. H. and Wilhelm, D. L.,** The inflammatory reaction in chemical injury. I. Increased vascular permeability and erythema induced by various chemicals, *Br. J. Exp. Pathol.,* 47, 612, 1966.

42. **Steele, R. H. and Wilhelm, D. L.,** The inflmmatory reaction in chemical injury. III. Leucocytes and other histological changes induced by superficial injury, *Br. J. Exp. Pathol.,* 51, 265, 1970.

43. **Houck, J. C.,** Chemistry of inflammation, *Ann. N.Y. Acad. Sci.,* 105, 765, 1963.

44. **Mortimer, P. H., Campbell, J., DiMenna, M. E., and White, E. P.,** Experimental myrotheciotoxicosis and poisoning in ruminants by verrucarin A and roridin A, *Res. Vet. Sci.,* 12, 508, 1971.

45. **Bamburg, J. R., Marasas, W. F., Riggs, N. V., Smalley, E. B., and Strong, F. M.,** Toxic spiroepoxy compounds form *Fusaria* and other hyphomycetes, *Biotechnol. Bioeng.,* 10, 445, 1968.

46. **Wyatt, R. D., Doerr, J. A., Hamilton, P. B., and Burmeister, H. R.,** Egg production, shell thickness, and other physiological parameters of laying hens affected by T-2 toxin, *Appl. Microbiol.,* 29, 641, 1975.

47. **Joffe, A. Z.,** *Fusarium poae* and *F. sporotrichioides* as principal causal agents of alimentary toxic aleukia, in *Mycotoxic Fungi, Mycotoxins, Mycotoxicoses,* Vol. 3, Wyllie, T. D.and Morehouse, L. G., Eds., Marcel Dekker, New York, 1978, 21.

48. **Bamburg, J. R., Strong, F. M., and Smalley, E. B.,** Toxins from moldy cereals, *J. Agric. Food Chem.,* 17, 443, 1969.

49. **Ghosal, S., Chakrabarti, D. K., and Basu Chaudhary, K. C.,** Toxic substances produced by *Fusarium.* I. Trichothecene derivatives from two strains of *Fusarium oxysporum,* f. sp. carthami., *J. Pharm. Sci.,* 65, 160, 1976.

50. **Schiefer, H. B., Hancock, D. S., and Bhatti, A. R.,** Systemic effects of topically applied trichothecenes. II. Studies with rats and T-2 toxin, *J. Vet. Med.,* A33, 384, 1986.

51. **Crone, H. D.,** The Response of Rats to Cutaneous Dosing with Trichothecene Mycotoxins, Report MRL-R-902, Department of Defence, Materials Research Laboratories, 1983.

52. **Schiefer, H. B. and Hancock, D. S.,** Systemic effects of topical application of T-2 toxin in mice, *Toxicol. Appl. Pharmacol.,* 76, 464, 1984.
53. **Schiefer, H. B., Hancock, D. S., and Bhatti, A. R.,** Systemic effects of topically applied trichothecenes. I. Comparative study of various trichothecenes in mice, *J. Vet. Med.,* A33, 373, 1986.
54. **Stoughton, R. B.,** Enhanced percutaneous penetration with 1-dodecylazacycloheptan-2-one, *Arch. Dermatol.,* 118, 474, 1982.
55. **Schiefer, H. B., Hancock, D. S., and Bhatti, A. R.,** Systemic effects of topically applied trichothecenes. III. The role of absorption enhancers, *J. Vet. Med.,* A33, 390, 1986.
56. **Hoerr, F. J., Carlton, W. W., Yagen, B., and Joffe, A. Z.,** Mycotoxicosis produced in broiler chickens by multiple doses of either T-2 toxin or diacetoxyscirpenol, *Avian Pathol.,* 11, 369, 1982.
57. **Wyatt, R. D., Hamilton, P. B., and Burmeister, H. R.,** Altered feathering of chicks caused by T-2 toxin, *Poult. Sci.,* 54, 1042, 1975.
58. **Wyatt, R. D., Colwell, W. M., Hamilton, P. B., and Burmeister, H. R.,** Neural disturbances in chickens caused by dietary T-2 toxin, *Appl. Microbiol.,* 26, 757, 1973.
59. **Murphy, W. K., Burgess, M. A., Valdivieso, M., Livingston, R. B., Bodey, G. P., and Freireich, E. J.,** Phase I clinical evaluation of anguidine, *Cancer Treat. Rep.,* 62, 1497, 1978.
60. **Yap, H. Y., Murphy, W. K., DiStefano, A., Blumenschein, G. R., and Bodey, G. P.,** Phase II study of anguidine in advanced breast cancer, *Cancer Treat. Rep.,* 63, 789, 1979.

Chapter 7

TREATMENT AND PROPHYLAXIS FOR TRICHOTHECENE MYCOTOXICOSIS

Robert F. Fricke and Robert H. Poppenga

TABLE OF CONTENTS

I. INTRODUCTION

Although there are many effective therapeutic agents for treatment of various fungal diseases, specific therapies against the toxins produced by these fungi are, at present, not readily available. Historically, naturally occurring trichothecene mycotoxicoses have affected both humans and livestock as a result of ingestion of fungal contaminated food or grain. These natural disease outbreaks are most effectively controlled by either avoidance or removal of the source of contamination.

Naturally occurring mycotoxicoses, such as alimentary toxic aleukia (ATA) in humans and various syndromes affecting livestock, have been attributed to the consumption of trichothecene-contaminated food or grain. In humans, ATA is a sometimes lethal disorder affecting the gastrointestinal (GI) tract, hematopoietic system, and major autonomic functions. Therapy for persons with ATA is largely supportive, with the intensity of the treatment increasing with the severity of the disease. In the milder, initial stages of the disease, treatment has consisted of blood transfusions with the administration of sulfonamides, vitamins C and K, and mixtures of nucleic acids and calcium.[1-3] The single most important countermeasure, however, was termination of exposure to contaminated grains.

In addition to the adverse human health effects, livestock losses as a result of consumption of trichothecene mycotoxins may also be significant. Historically, naturally occurring livestock disease syndromes associated with trichothecenes have included syndromes referred to as moldy corn toxicosis in the U.S. and Canada, bean-hull poisoning and red-mold toxicosis in Japan, and dendrochiotoxicosis and stachybotryotoxicosis in the U.S.S.R. Again, the most effective treatment has been removal of the source of the toxin coupled with symptomatic and supportive therapy.

Renewed interest in the effects of trichothecene mycotoxins developed with the alleged use of toxic fungal extracts in warfare.[4] Because of the potential medical risk that mycotoxins might pose to exposed civilian and military personnel, evaluation of currently available therapy for acute mycotoxin exposure was recently undertaken. A National Academy of Science (NAS) report[5] dealing with protection against and treatment for trichothecene mycotoxicosis concluded that no specific approaches, other than supportive or symptomatic care were known and, further, that the only known prophylactic measure was avoidance of exposure. Treatment for trichothecene mycotoxicosis following deliberate exposure is clearly not as simple as removal of the source of contamination and represents a more complex medical problem. To deal with this threat, recent efforts have been directed toward defining effective medical countermeasures.

Several factors complicate the formulation of effective therapies for mycotoxicoses. The disease syndromes which occur following acute exposure to high levels of mycotoxins do not necessarily mimic those that result from chronic exposure to lower levels of toxin. The most recent efforts have focused on the acute effects of trichothecene mycotoxins, particularly T-2 toxin and diacetoxyscirpenol (DAS). Possible chronic effects on the immune or hematopoietic systems are not as easily recognized, but may have a bearing on therapeutic intervention. In addition, whether as a result of natural occurrence or use in biological warfare, exposure to trichothecenes may often involve combinations of toxins whose interactions have not been clearly defined.

II. TREATMENT OF TRICHOTHECENE MYCOTOXICOSIS

A. Overview of Potential Therapy

The current treatment for trichothecene mycotoxicosis is based upon available data, as well as research conducted in the authors' laboratories. Classes of therapeutic agents evaluated as potential therapy include: (1) GI-adsorbing agents, (2) antioxidants, (3) microsomal

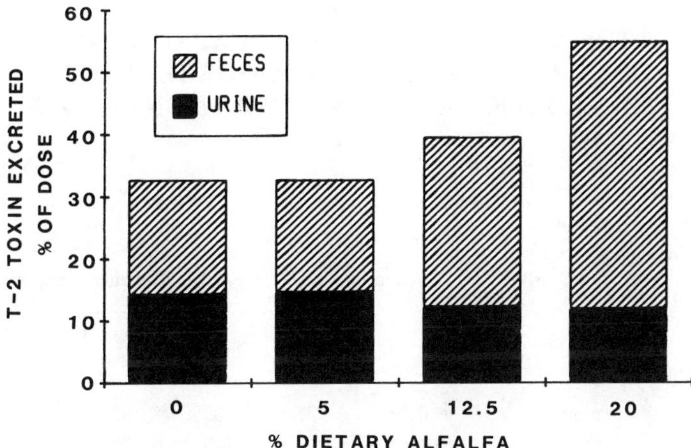

FIGURE 1.   Effect of dietary alfalfa roughage on urinary and fecal excretion of T-2 toxin. Rats were fed diets containing from 0 to 20% alfalfa for 2 weeks before being challenged with 7.5×10^7 dpm (^{3}H) T-2 toxin (0.172 mCi/mg). Urine and fecal samples were collected for 21 h after exposure and the amount of radioactivity was determined. (Adapted from Reference 7 and Table 7.)

inducing agents, (4) anti-inflammatory agents, (5) multiple drug therapy, and (6) miscellaneous drugs. The rationale for using these agents stems largely from review of the biochemical, clinical, and pathophysiologic effects of trichothecene mycotoxins. For certain agents with documented protective effects, further studies were conducted to verify and expand the findings.

B. GI-Adsorbing Agents
1. Rationale for Use of Adsorbing Agents and Osmotic Cathartics
The potential efficacy of GI-adsorbing agents for treatment of mycotoxin poisoning is supported by several observations. First, after exposure to crude T-2 toxin, fasted animals, when compared to fed controls, showed increased lethality.[6] Further, available data suggested that intestinal roughage and GI adsorbents may play a role in altering both the toxicity and excretion of mycotoxins. Animals fed diets supplemented with either high fiber[7,8] or bentonite[9] showed decreased lethality and improvement in both weight gain and feed consumption after exposure to either T-2 toxin or zearalenone. By increasing the amount of dietary alfalfa, the fecal, but not urinary, elimination of T-2 toxin was increased (Figure 1).[10,11] Similar results were also obtained with bentonite.[9] The effectiveness of crude dietary fiber or bentonite in decreasing the lethality of mycotoxins indicated that other adsorbing agents in the GI tract might also be efficacious.

Activated charcoal and cholestyramine, an ion exchange resin, have been used effectively as oral antidotes for treatment of animals after both systemic and oral exposure to a wide variety of toxicants.[12-15] Activated charcoal decreased the toxicity and mortality of aflatoxin after acute oral exposure of goats[16] or chronic oral exposure of chickens.[17] Cholestyramine has been used to decrease the toxicity of the insecticide, chlordecone (Kepone®), by short-circuiting its extensive enterohepatic recirculation.[14] Since T-2 toxin and its conjugated metabolites appear in the bile,[18,19] enterohepatic circulation may play a role in the reabsorption of parent compound and especially metabolites, contributing to overall toxicity. Adsorbing agents, such as activated charcoal and cholestyramine, were therefore worthy of evaluation for the treatment of animals after either oral or systemic exposure to T-2 toxin.

Cathartics are used in conjunction with activated charcoal to shorten the intestinal transit time of toxicants.[20] Because adsorbing agents traditionally have been used in conjunction

Table 1
THE *IN VITRO* ADSORPTIVE CAPACITY OF DIFFERENT AMOUNTS OF ADSORBENTS FOR THREE DIFFERENT CONCENTRATIONS OF T-2 TOXIN

Conc of adsorbent (mg/ml) (vol = 2.5 ml)	Brand	Conc of T-2 toxin (vol = 1 ml)		
		1 mg/ml	2 mg/ml	3 mg/ml
		Mean % of T-2 toxin adsorbed		
52	Calgon	100	82	72
	Amoco PX-21	100	88	77
	Norit A	100	70	66
	SuperChar	100	95	92
104	Calgon	100	82	79
	Amoco PX-21	100	85	84
	Toxiban	60	60	58
	Norit A	100	78	68
	SuperChar	100	95	92
	SuperChar + sorbitol	100	100	89
	Cholestyramine	10	5	3
	SuperChar + sorbitol + preservatives	100	92	92
250	Calgon	100	98	97
	Amoco PX-21	100	100	95
	Norit A	100	97	95
	SuperChar	100	100	100

Calgon and Norit A: activated charcoal; Amoco PX-21 and SuperChar: super-activated charcoal; Toxiban: activated charcoal + kaolin; Cholestyramine: ion-exchange resin.

with osmotic cathartics, such as sorbitol, magnesium sulfate, or sodium sulfate, the efficacy of adsorbents alone and with cathartics has been evaluated. These agents are not well absorbed from the GI tract. Due to their resultant osmotic effect, water is attracted to and retained within the lumen of the GI tract. This fluid accumulation causes increased peristalsis which, in turn, promotes evacuation from the GI tract to reduce the possibility of desorption of the toxicant from the activated charcoal.[21]

2. Efficacy of Adsorbing Agents Alone and In Combination with Cathartics

The potential value of adsorbing agents for the treatment of T-2 toxin-exposed animals was initially assessed by measuring the *in vitro* binding of T-2 toxin to different adsorbing agents. Highly activated charcoal (Super-A X-21®, Anderson Development Company, Adrian, MI or SuperChar®, Gulf Bio-Systems, Dallas) and cholestyramine (Questran®, Mead Johnson, Evansville, IL), both bound T-2 toxin *in vitro*. The *in vitro* adsorptive capacities of several different activated charcoals and cholestyramine for T-2 toxin were recently evaluated by Bratich.[22] As shown in Table 1, highly activated charcoal at various concentrations was more effective in binding T-2 toxin than the other adsorbing agents tested.

The efficacy of oral administration of either activated charcoal[23] or cholestyramine[24] for the treatment of animals with parenterally produced T-2 toxicosis has been assessed. Fasted mice were challenged with an s.c. toxin dose of 2.8 mg/kg and then treated orally with 7 g/kg of either activated charcoal or cholestyramine. After 72 h, the mice treated with the adsorbents showed significantly improved survival. The respective percentage of lethalities for control, charcoal-treated, and cholestyramine-treated groups were 50, 10, and 20%.

The LD_{50} values of T-2 toxin for charcoal-treated[23] and cholestyramine-treated[24] mice were determined. Varying doses of T-2 toxin were administered s.c., followed immediately by either water (control) or adsorbing agent (7 g/kg, p.o.). The control LD_{50} value decreased from 3.2 mg/kg at 24 h to 1.1 mg/kg after 96 h. LD_{50} values for the charcoal-treated group remained essentially the same throughout the experiment, with a 24-h LD_{50} value of 4.5 mg/kg, decreasing only slightly to a 96-h value of 4.2 mg/kg. The cholestyramine-treated mice had a 24-h LD_{50} value approximately equal to the charcoal-treated group, but after 96 h, the value decrease to 3.6 mg/kg.

To further evaluate the ability of activated charcoal to improve survival after parenteral exposure to T-2 toxin, various charcoal-dosing regimens were tested in T-2 toxin-treated rats.[25]

In preliminary studies with rats, the administration of super-activated charcoal (1 g/kg, p.o.) either in 3 doses (immediately, 4, and 8 h) or in 2 doses (immediately and 6 h) after the administration of T-2 toxin i.v. at 0.6 or 0.75 mg/kg, respectively, was ineffective in decreasing toxin-induced lethality. In control rats not given T-2 toxin, the super-activated charcoal was evenly distributed throughout the GI tract and had a transit time of about 12 h. However, as a result of T-2 intoxication, apparent stasis occurred which resulted in the retention of charcoal in the stomach and proximal small intestine for as long as 24 h after toxin administration. Inhibition of intestinal peristalsis following acute trichothecene exposure has been noted to occur in rats given T-2 toxin orally[26] and in guinea pigs given fusarenon-X i.v.[27] It has also been reported, however, that the intestinal propulsion of a charcoal containing meal was enhanced in mice given fusarenon-X at 1 mg/kg.[27] Effects on GI motility, which clearly are sometimes contradictory, are discussed further in the chapter "Effects on the Digestive System and Energy Metabolism".

Due to these findings, the efficacy of super-activated charcoal was assessed using rats in a pretreatment dosing protocol.[25] The administration of super-activated charcoal (1 g/kg, p.o.) 13 and 1 h before and 4 h after the administration of T-2 toxin i.v. at 0.8 mg/kg resulted in significant improvement in survival (Figure 2).

Based upon these studies, it appears that activated charcoal following parenteral toxin exposure is efficacious in mice, whereas in rats pretreatment is necessary to ensure that adequate amounts of charcoal reach a greater proportion of the intestine so that maximal adsorption of T-2 toxin and its metabolites can occur. This species difference in efficacy may be due to variation with regard to trichothecene effects on intestinal peristalsis.

The efficacy of activated charcoal for treatment of animals with oral T-2 toxin exposure has also been assessed.[23] Mice were challenged with a 5 mg/kg oral dose of T-2 toxin and then treated with either water (control) or activated charcoal (7 g/kg, p.o.). The activated charcoal was administered either immediately or 1 h after toxin exposure. The number of surviving mice in the control group progressively declined throughout the observation period, reaching 10% survival after 72 h. The percentage of surviving mice in the charcoal-treated groups was significantly higher than the untreated controls, with values of 100 and 70% for immediate and 1 h posttreatment, respectively.

Galey et al.[26] demonstrated the therapeutic efficacy of highly activated charcoal in treating rats with orally induced T-2 toxicosis. The adsorbent, at doses as low as 0.5 g/kg, when given immediately after the administration of T-2 toxin, resulted in 100% survival (Figure 3). Possibly of more importance was the observation that when treatment was delayed up to 5 h, the activated charcoal was still somewhat effective in improving survival.

The effect of different cathartics on the efficacy of activated charcoal after oral administration of T-2 toxin has also been evaluated. Highly activated charcoal, with or without

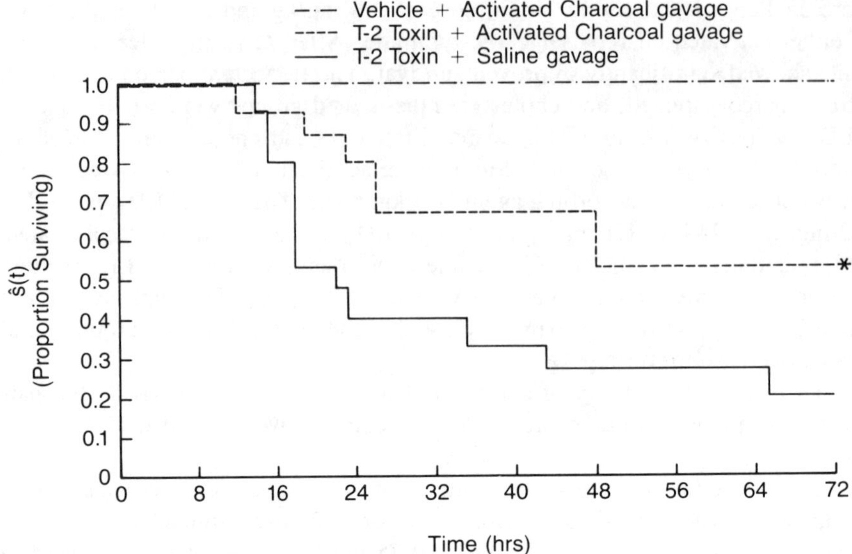

FIGURE 2.   Effect of pre- and postdosing administration of highly activated charcoal on the survival time course of T-2 toxin-dosed rats. Rats were given either saline or highly activated charcoal (1 g/kg, p.o.) 12 h before, immediately, and 4 h after the intravenous administration of 50% ethanol or T-2 toxin (0.8 mg/kg). p-values <0.05 (saline vs. charcoal treatment) are denoted as *.

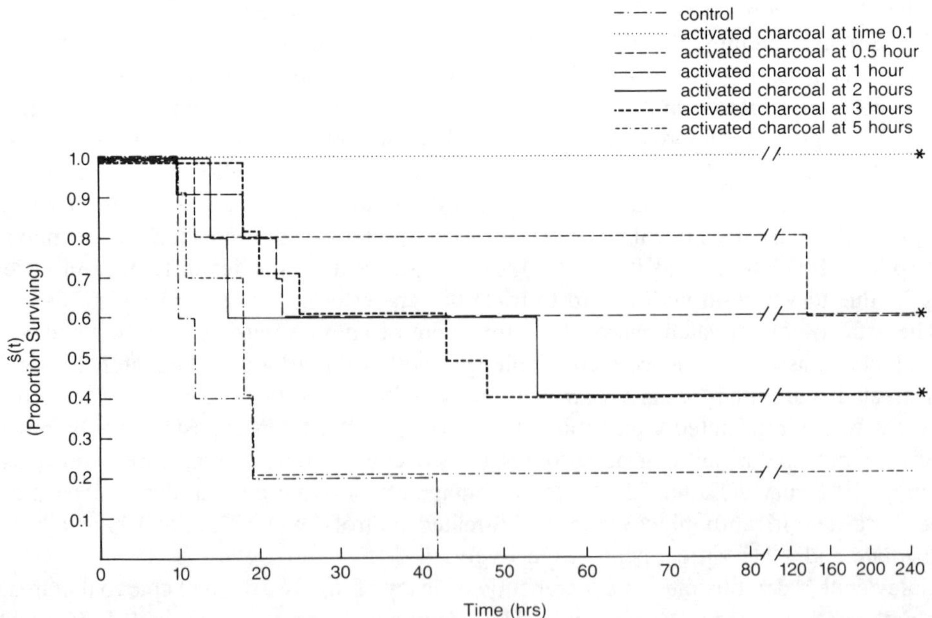

FIGURE 3.   Effect of orally administered activated charcoal (1 g/kg) on the survival time course of rats when given at varying times following the oral administration of T-2 toxin (8 mg/kg). There was a significant improvement in survival for those groups given the activated charcoal immediately, 0.5, 1.0, 2.0, or 3.0 h after the T-2 toxin compared to the control group given only T-2 toxin (p <0.05 denoted by *).

Table 2
EFFECT OF VARIOUS ACTIVATED CHARCOAL
PREPARATIONS (0.9 G/KG, P.O.) ON SURVIVAL
RATES IN RATS WHEN GIVEN AFTER T-2 TOXIN (25
MG/KG, P.O.: 6× THE LD$_{50}$ DOSE)

	T-2 toxin (25 mg/kg)	
	Survivors/animals dosed	Charcoal/T-2 toxin
SuperChar	6/10	37/1
Calgon	0/10	37/1
Toxiban	0/10	37/1
Norit A	0/10	37/1
SuperChar + Sorbitol	7/10	37/1
Control	0/10	—

sorbitol as a cathartic, given immediately after T-2 toxin, significantly improved survival rates when compared to three other charcoal preparations (Table 2).[22]

Galey et al.[26] studied the efficacy of highly activated charcoal in combination with the osmotic cathartics sorbitol, magnesium sulfate, or sodium sulfate in rats given T-2 toxin. The addition of cathartics to the charcoal did not improve survival above that of preparations containing only charcoal (Figure 4). In fact, when rats were given T-2 toxin, followed 3 h later by activated charcoal, alone or in combination with either sorbitol or sodium sulfate, a significant decrease in survival rate occurred in those groups given the activated charcoal-cathartic combinations vs. only the activated charcoal (Figure 5). In the latter study, the decrease in survival of the activated charcoal plus cathartic-treated groups may have been due to an exacerbation of circulatory shock resulting from increased fluid movement into the intestinal tract.

In summary, activated charcoal and cholestyramine were effective for treating mice orally exposed to T-2 toxin. In rats, after oral exposure to high levels of T-2 toxin, highly activated charcoal was superior to other activated charcoal formulations in preventing the onset of clinical signs and the occurrence of death. For treatment of oral toxin exposure in mice, activated charcoal was 100% effective if administered immediately after the toxin. The effectiveness of activated charcoal decreased as the time bewteen toxin exposure and treatment was increased. Nevertheless, some improvement in survival was noted even when treatment was delayed up to 5 h after T-2 toxin administration.

Orally administered activated charcoal and cholestyramine also improved survival in mice after parenteral exposure to T-2 toxin. With rats, activated charcoal pretreatment greatly improved the observed benefit. The efficacy of orally administered activated charcoal for parenterally induced T-2 toxicosis may be explained by either of two hypotheses:

1.   T-2 toxin and its metabolites may undergo enterohepatic recirculation with the reabsorbed toxin contributing to the toxicosis
2.   The severe GI damage which occurs after acute exposure to T-2 toxin may allow for the passage of endotoxin through compromise of the intestinal epithelial barrier.

The activated charcoal may bind with T-2 toxin and its metabolites after secretion in the bile to prevent their reabsorption, and may also bind bacterial endotoxins.

C. Efficacy of Antioxidants
1. Rationale for Use

The mechanism of toxicity of sporidesmin, a nontrichothecene mycotoxin produced by the saprophytic fungus, *Pithomyces chartarum*, involves the formation of superoxide radi-

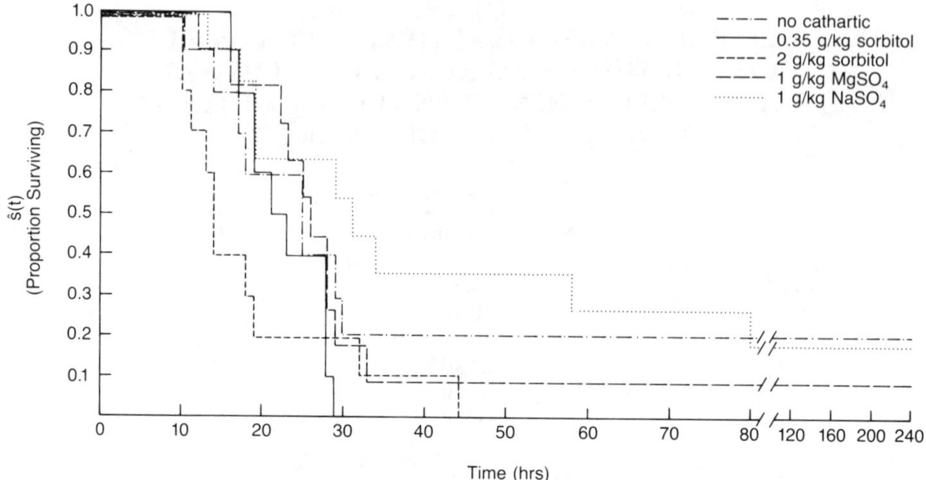

FIGURE 4.   Effect on survival time course in rats of orally administered activated charcoal (1 g/kg), given either alone or in combination with sorbitol (0.35 or 2 g/kg), magnesium sulfate (1 g/kg), or sodium sulfate (1 g/kg) immediately after the oral administration of T-2 toxin (8 mg/kg, p.o.). There was no significant difference in survival between any of the groups.

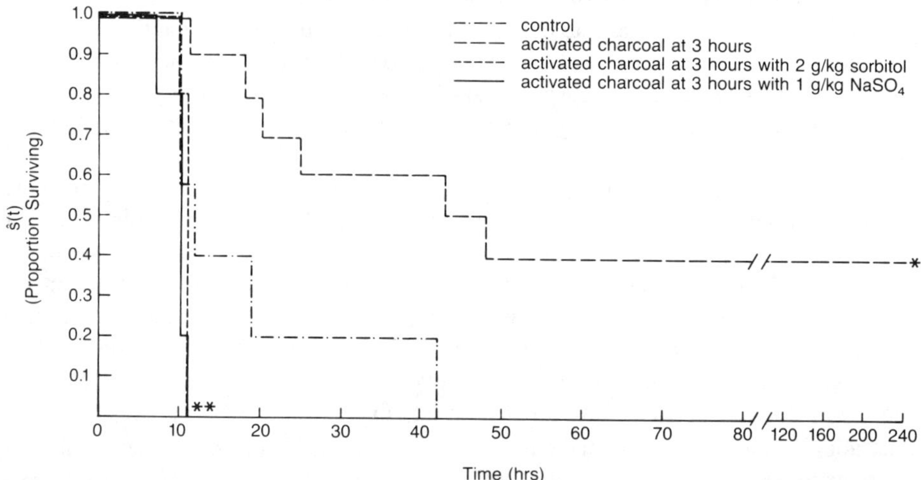

FIGURE 5.   Effect of activated charcoal (1 g/kg) either alone or in combination with sorbitol (2 g/kg) or magnesium sulfate (1 g/kg) on the survival time course of rats given T-2 toxin p.o. (8 mg/kg) 3 h previously. When compared to the control group (denoted by *), there was a significant increase in survival for the group given activated charcoal alone at 3 h after T-2 toxin administration. In contrast, there was a significant reduction in survival in the 2 groups given the activated charcoal-cathartic combinations 3 h after the administration of T-2 toxin (denoted by **) when compared to the positive control group ($p < 0.05$).

cals.[28] A disulfide bridge in this mycotoxin undergoes a cyclic reduction/autoxidation process, which is thought to be responsible for the formation of superoxide radical anion. Experimentally, the formation of superoxide radicals can be detected by measuring the reduction of nitroblue tetrazolium. Various antioxidants were found to inhibit the sporidesmin-induced reduction of nitroblue tetrazolium.

Although the toxic effects of sporidesmin can be directly attributed to the formation of free radicals, there is no direct evidence for trichothecene mycotoxin-induced free radical generation. The indirect measurement of *in vivo* cellular damage resulting from free radical

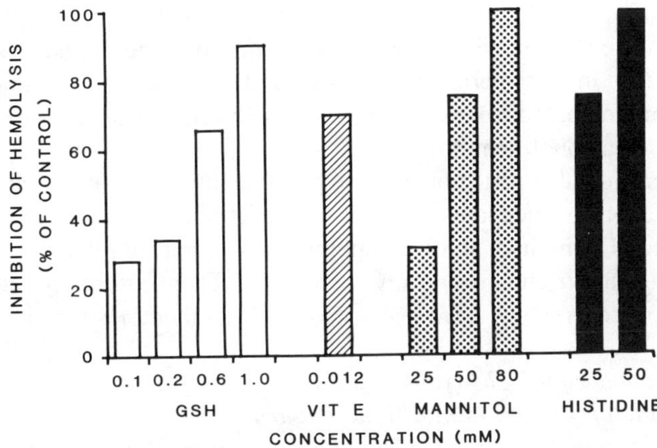

FIGURE 6.   Effect of free radical scavengers on T-2 toxin-induced hemolysis. Erythrocytes were incubated wtih T-2 toxin at a concentration of 0.38 mM in the presence of glutathione (GSH), vitamin E (Vit E), mannitol, or histidine at the indicated concentrations. Amount of hemolysis was determined after 3 (GSH, Vit E), or 3.5 h (mannitol, histidine). (Adapted from Table 3 in Reference 31.)

formation may be the only detection means available. Tapple[29] outlined indirect evidence which would, as a general rule, indicate the involvement of free radical-induced lipid peroxidation in the generation of a nonspecific toxic response. This evidence includes, in part, the measurement of products of lipid peroxidation, such as thiobarbituric acid (TBA)-reactive compounds and the amelioration of toxicosis by exogenously administered antioxidants. Tsuchida et al.[30] reported indirect evidence of free radical formation as a result of T-2 toxin exposure. The amounts of TBA-reactive products in the GI tract, spleen, thymus, lung, heart, kidney, and liver were measured after an acutely toxic oral dose of T-2 toxin (4 mg/kg). Of the tissues examined, only the liver contained significant increases in TBA-reactive substances at 480 to 625% of control values, suggesting increased lipid peroxidation. The concentration of hepatic, TBA-reactive substances remained at the control level for the first 2 to 4 h after toxin administration, but increased significantly after 6 h. The TBA values reached a maximum at 24 h and remained elevated through 48 h.

In vitro studies have focused on the possible membrane-destabilizing effects of T-2 toxin. The increased fragility of certain cell membranes after exposure to T-2 toxin may be due to the generation of reactive intermediates, since antioxidants have been effective in ameliorating cytotoxicity. *At very high concentrations* T-2 toxin caused hemolysis in isolated rat erythrocytes.[31] The amount and time of onset of hemolysis correlated well with toxin concentration. Further, various antioxidants, such as histidine, mannitol, and especially glutathione and vitamin E, when added to the incubation medium, all inhibited T-2 toxin-induced hemolysis in a dose-dependent manner (Figure 6). Moreover, *in vitro* studies demonstrated similar lytic effects of T-2 toxin on isolated mouse thymus cells.[32] The addition of quercetin, a bioflavonoid with antioxidant properties,[33] to the incubation medium protected the thymocytes against the cytotoxic effect of T-2 toxin.

Although evidence suggests that trichothecene mycotoxins may react with cellular macromolecules, definitive linkage of the specific reactions between trichothecene and cellular macromolecules with whole animal pathophysiologic or pathologic effects remains speculative. Ueno and Matsumoto[34-36] provided *in vitro* evidence that suggests the occurrence of covalent binding of trichothecene mycotoxins to reactive sulfhydryl groups of enzymes. The enzymatic activities of creatine kinase, alcohol dehydrogenase, and lactate dehydrogenase, when preincubated without substrate, were all inhibited by *high concentrations* of T-2 toxin, neosolaniol, and fusarenon-X. In contrast, when the toxins were added after preincubation of the enzyme with either enzyme substrate or thiol compounds, such as glutathione or dithiothreitol, no loss in enzymatic activity occurred. Additional experiments showed that incubations with radiolabeled toxins resulted in stoichiometric binding of toxin to reactive sulfhydryl groups of alcohol dehydrogenase.[36]

Thus, at least some data indicate not only the possible involvement of free radical formation and lipid peroxidation as mechanisms of action of trichothecene mycotoxins, but more importantly, potential benefit of thiol compounds and other antioxidants for treatment for and prophylaxis against trichothecene mycotoxicosis. There are many naturally occurring and synthetic antioxidants which have been considered as therapies for mycotoxin exposure.

2. Efficacy in Treatment for T-2 Mycotoxicosis
a. Efficacy of Glutathione and Glutathione Prodrugs

Various thiol compounds have been used to treat animals with experimentally induced aflatoxicosis.[37] Goats pretreated with either cysteine, methionine, or thiosulfate, and then exposed to aflatoxin, all had significantly longer mean survival times when compared to aflatoxin-treated controls. If treatment was delayed until 8 h after aflatoxin exposure, however, the thiol compounds were ineffective. In addition, pretreatment of goats with diethylmaleate, a depletor of hepatic glutathione, potentiated the lethality of aflatoxin.

Of the naturally occurring thiol compounds, glutathione is present at comparatively high intracellular concentrations.[38] Despite this, glutathione can rapidly be depleted after food deprivation[39] or exposure to toxins or other xenobiotics.[40,41] Rats treated wtih aflatoxin B_1 showed a progressive, time-dependent decrease in hepatic glutathione content which was accompanied by a corresponding increase in glutathione-S-transferase activity.[42] Similarly, acute exposure of mice to T-2 toxin resulted in a progressive decrease in hepatic glutathione concentrations, reaching a minimum at 6 to 8 h after dosing.[43] In contrast to the effects of aflatoxin noted earlier, the observed decrease in hepatic glutathione levels as a result of T-2 toxin exposure was not accompanied by changes in the activities of glutathione-S-transferase, glutathione reductase, or glutathione peroxidase.[43]

Acute exposure of mice to T-2 toxin caused decreased feed and water consumption (Figure 7).[43] Because fasting by itself can cause decreased hepatic glutathione concentrations,[39] the observed depletion of hepatic glutathione may have been due to the toxin-induced decrease in feed intake, rather than a direct effect of the toxin. To resolve this point, experiments were conducted in which groups of both control and toxin-treated animals were (1) allowed free access to both feed and water throughout the experiment (group A); (2) fed before, but fasted after toxin administration (group B); or (3) fasted throughout the entire experiment (group C).[42] Glutathione concentrations were determined 6 h after toxin treatment (4 mg/ kg, s.c.) In group A, hepatic glutathione levels decreased from a control value of 9.01 $\pm$ 0.66 to 4.26 $\pm$ 0.41 (μmol/g tissue) after toxin treatment. Similarly, in group B, glutathione levels were 3.76 $\pm$ 0.65 for the T-2 toxin-treated animals, which was much lower than the control value of 7.18 $\pm$ 0.26. If the decreased glutathione concentrations observed with T-2 toxin treatment were entirely a result of anorexia, then the control and toxin-treated values in group B should have been closer. Clearly, even though fasting did decrease hepatic glutathione in the control mice, T-2 toxin caused significant additional depletion. In mice fasted before and after T-2 toxin administration (group C), the trichothecene produced a smaller, but still significant decrease, with values of 4.45 $\pm$ 0.39 and 2.45 $\pm$ 0.26 for control and toxin-treated mice, respectively. These data therefore suggest that T-2 toxin itself, in addition to its anorexic effect, is responsible for decreased hepatic glutathione concentrations.

Despite the aforementioned depletion, experimental evidence indicates that the therapeutic usefulness of glutathione administration may be limited. Glutathione is not transported as

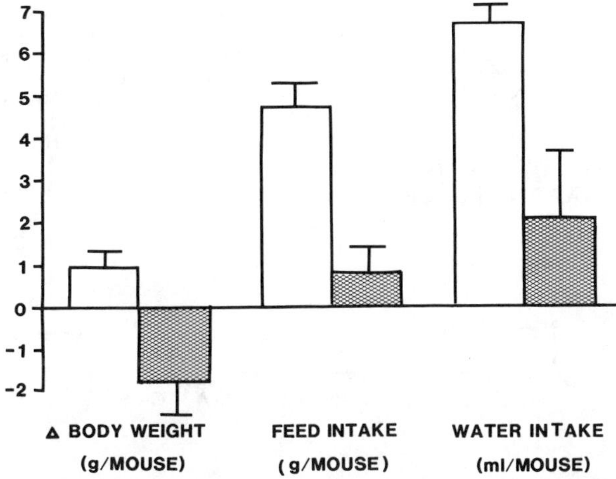

FIGURE 7.   Effect of T-2 toxin on weight gain and feed and water consumption. Mice were injected with either vehicle (control) or T-2 toxin (2 mg/kg, s.c.) and after 24 h, the change in body weights from initial values and the amount of feed and water consumed were determined. Data for control (open bars) and toxin-treated animals (cross-hatched bars) are represented as mean ± S.E. All *p*-values (toxin vs. control) for the measured parameters were <0.001.[42]

an intact molecule; instead it is metabolized before intracellular transport.[38] This may account for the observed ineffectiveness of glutathione given i.p. to mice at 100 mg/kg 2 h before T-2 toxin given s.c. at 1 to 3 mg/kg.[44] A new class of drugs has been developed which act as precursors of intracellular glutathione.[45,46] The glutathione prodrugs, L-2-oxo (OTC) and L-2-methyl (MTCA) derivatives of thiazolidine-4-carboxylate, are known to be readily transported across cellular membranes and converted to free, intracellular cysteine, which is incorporated into glutathione and is the limiting amino acid in glutathione formation (Figure 8). These glutathione prodrugs can therefore maintain cellular glutathione levels, even under conditions of oxidative stress.[46-48]

Further, other thiazolidine-4-carboxylate derivatives have been used as radioprotective agents[49,50] and in geriatric medicine.[51]

To assess the effect of altered glutathione concentrations in changing the toxicity of T-2 toxin in mice, hepatic glutathione was either increased by pretreatment with OTC or MTCA, or depleted by overnight fasting or by pretreatment with buthionine-SR-sulfoximine (BSO), a potent inhibitor of glutathione synthesis.[52] With OTC or MTCA pretreatment, the relative potency values (ratio or treated/control LD_{50} for T-2 toxin) were increased to 1.37, a value significantly higher than the control value of 1.00.[53] Further, after BSO treatment or overnight fasting, the relative potency values were significantly decreased with values of 0.37 and 0.52, respectively.[53] Therefore, it appears that conditions which either increase or decrease hepatic glutathione concentrations either protect against or potentiate the toxicity of T-2 toxin, respectively.

Another precursor of glutathione, *N*-acetylcysteine, has been used successfully in other toxicoses of replenishment of depleted hepatic glutathione;[54] however, in a group of rats given T-2 toxin at an i.v. dose of 1 mg/kg followed immediately by *N*-acetylcysteine (140 mg/kg, i.p.) and again 5 h later (70 mg/kg, i.p.), no improvement in survival was noted when compared to a control group given T-2 toxin alone.[55] The use of *N*-acetylcysteine as a pretreatment drug was not evaluated. This may explain the discrepancy in efficacy when compared to the OTC and MTCA results. Alternatively, it is apparent that i.p. injection of rats with *N*-acetylcysteine actually depletes hepatic glutathione, whereas oral administration

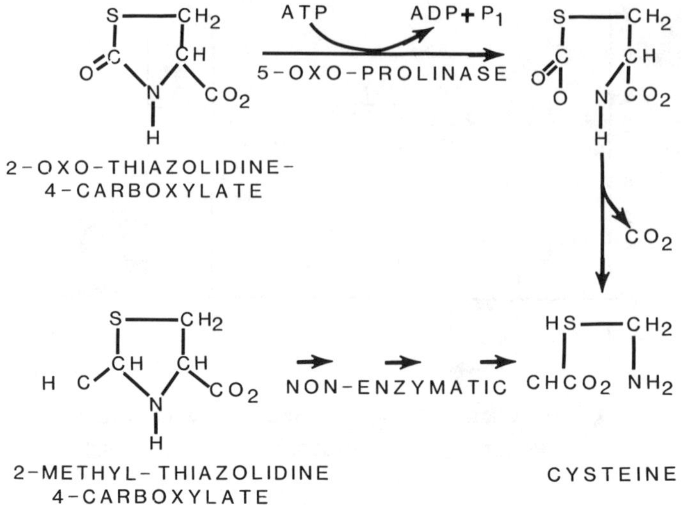

FIGURE 8.   Proposed mechanism of action of glutathione prodrugs: intracellular delivery of cysteine.

does not.[56] Orally administered *N*-acetylcysteine may still be of value, therefore, in the treatment of acute T-2 toxicosis. Nevertheless, *in vitro* experiments indicated that *N*-acetylcysteine was not as effective as either OTC or MTCA in elevating hepatic glutathione levels. In those studies, the ability of primary cultures of rat hepatocytes to synthesize glutathione from *N*-acetylcysteine, OTC, and MTCA was evaluated.[57] OTC and *N*-acetylcysteine increased intracellular glutathione by 204 and 224%, respectively, while *N*-acetylcysteine produced only a 125% increase.

b. Efficacy of Ascorbic Acid in T-2 Toxicosis

Ascorbic acid is an effective water-soluble antioxidant. The effectiveness of ascorbic acid as an antioxidant is, however, dependent upon several factors which may either increase or decrease the formation of free radicals and lipid peroxides. At low doses, in the presence of metal ions (Cu^{2+}, Fe^{2+}), ascorbic acid promotes the formation of free radicals and peroxidation of membranes, but at high doses, ascorbic acid functions as an effective antioxidant.[58] Ascorbic acid is effective in lessening the toxicity of many compounds which are converted to reactive intermediates.[59] *In vitro* ascorbic acid decreased the microsomal binding of benzene[60] which undergoes metabolic activation to reactive free radical intermediates.[61]

The efficacy of ascorbic acid in the treatment of animals for T-2 toxicosis was recently evaluated using mice.[62] The LD_{50} values (mg/kg) for T-2 toxin at 48 h postexposure were 2.59 for control mice and 3.39, 3.61 and 3.19 for mice given ascorbic acid at doses of 400, 800, and 1200 mg/kg, respectively. All were significantly greater than the control value (*p* <0.01).

To further assess the protective effects of ascorbic acid, control and treated mice were given T-2 toxin s.c. at 3.1 mg/kg immediately after ascorbic acid at 0, 400, 800, or 1200 mg/kg i.p. The proportion of surviving mice was determined for each group at approximately 2-h intervals for 176 h (Figure 8). All of the ascorbic acid-treated groups showed an initial decrease in the proportion of surviving animals during the first 24 h after toxin exposure, with delayed deaths occurring at 80 to 100 h in the 400 and 1200 mg/kg treatment groups; however, all groups given ascorbic acid subsequently experienced significantly improved survival compared to the control group in which a progressive decrease in survival occurred.

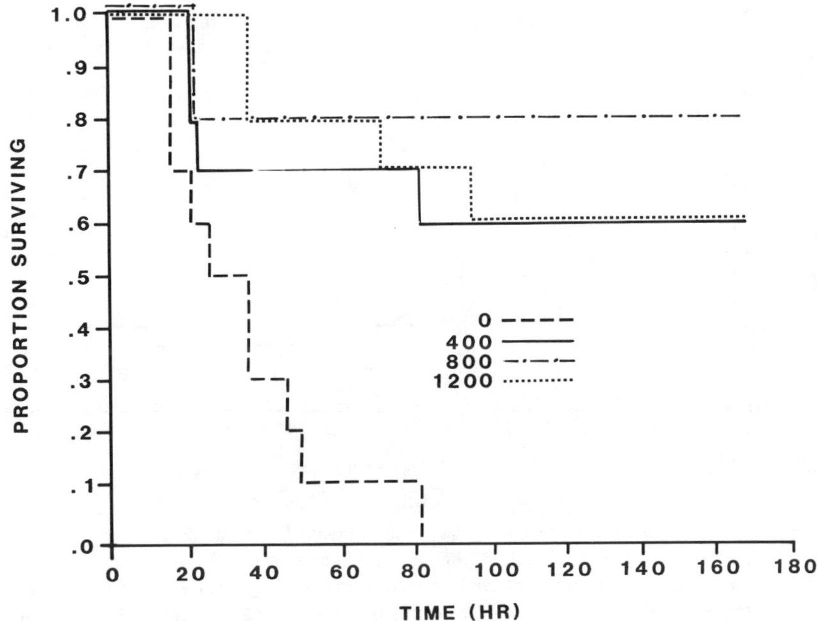

FIGURE 9.   Effect of ascorbic acid on proportion of mice surviving a lethal dose of T-2 toxin. Mice were treated with ascorbic acid (0, 400, 800, or 1200 mg/kg, i.p.) and then immediately exposed to T-2 toxin (3.1 mg/kg, s.c.). The proportion of animals surviving was determined at various times up to 176 h after toxin exposure.

The percent survival (after 176 h), mean time to death, and mean survival time were determined via analysis of survival curves (Figure 9). There was 0% survival (after 80 h) for the untreated positive control mice. Survival values for the ascorbic acid-treated groups were 60% for both 400 and 1200 mg/kg groups and 70% for the 800 mg/kg group. Mean time to death values for the treated mice that died were 36, 51, and 59 h for the 400, 800, and 1200 mg/kg dose groups, respectively. None of these times was significantly longer than the control value of 21 h. Unlike mean time to death, mean survival time considers the data for both dying and surviving mice. The mean survival times for the control and treated groups were estimated using the Kaplan-Meier product limit of the cumulative survival curve.[63] Compared to the mean survival time of 34 h for the positive control group, all of the treated groups had times significantly longer, with values of 115, 132, and 124 h for ascorbic acid doses of 400, 800, and 1200 mg/kg, respectively. In mice, ascorbic acid appears to be effective in decreasing the lethality associated with acute T-2 toxicosis.

Unlike the mouse data, the use of ascorbic acid was unsuccessful in female Sprague-Dawley rats given acutely toxic doses of T-2 toxin.[64] In one study, rats were dosed with T-2 toxin (1 mg/kg, i.v.) followed immediately by sodium ascorbate i.p. at doses of 0, 400, 800, or 1200 mg/kg. The proportion of surviving animals over time is shown in Figure 10. Sodium ascorbate was not effective in improving survival and, in fact, resulted in significantly decreased survival rates in the 400 and 1200 mg/kg treatment groups. The efficacy of ascorbic acid as a pretreatment therapy was also evaluated. Rats were pretreated with ascorbic acid i.p. at 0, 400, 800, or 1200 mg/kg 12 h prior to the administration of T-2 toxin i.v. at 1 mg/kg and a second equivalent dose of ascorbic acid was given immediately after the toxin. No improvement in survival was noted for any group, although there was no significant decrease in survival in contrast to the previous study. Surprisingly, ascorbyl palmitate,[65,66] a more lipid-soluble analog of ascorbic acid, was ineffective in alleviating T-2 toxicosis in mice.

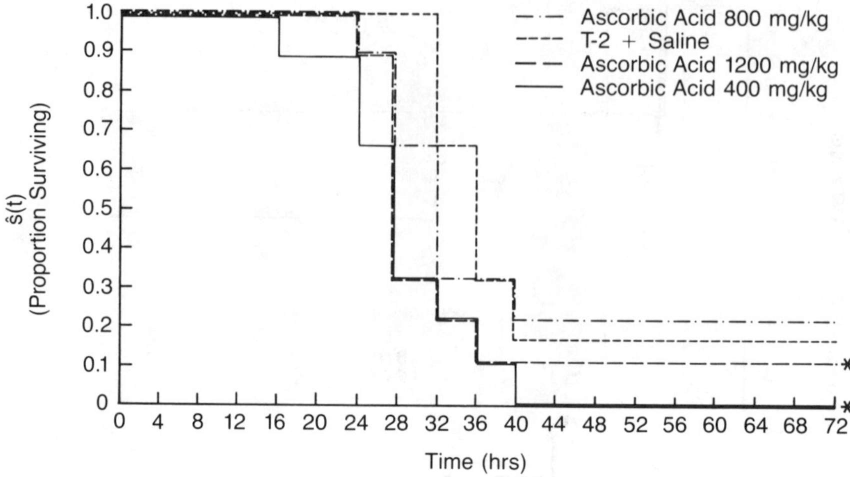

FIGURE 10.   Survival of rats given T-2 toxin (1 mg/kg, i.v.) followed immediately by varying doses of ascorbic acid (400, 800, or 1200 mg/kg, i.p.). There was no improvement in survival noted for any group given ascorbic acid and, in fact, there was a significant decrease in survival between the groups given ascorbic acid at either 400 or 1200 mg/kg (denoted by *) vs. the control group given T-2 toxin and no treatment ($p < 0.05$).

The reason for the difference in response of mice and rats to ascorbic acid therapy is not readily apparent. Although approximately equivalent doses of T-2 toxin were used (LD_{99}), the mice were given the T-2 toxin s.c., whereas the rats were dosed i.v. Because of species differences, additional animal species should be used before reaching a conclusion on the value of ascorbic acid as a therapy for acute T-2 toxicosis.

c. Efficacy of Vitamin E

The role of vitamin E as an antioxidant and free radical scavenger has been extensively reviewed.[67,68] Vitamin E is effective in lessening the severity of various toxicoses when administered either in the form of a dietary supplement or via multiple daily injections. A single bolus injection of vitamin E at high doses was also found to be effective in counteracting the damaging effects of ionizing radiation.[69,70] Of importance as a suggestion of potentially effective therapy was the finding that animals on a vitamin E-deficient diet were more susceptible to the peroxidative effects of T-2 toxin.[29] Further, by supplementing the diet with vitamin E, T-2 toxin-induced, hepatic lipid peroxidation was markedly inhibited.

The efficacy of vitamin E as a pretreatment for T-2 toxicosis was evaluated using mice.[71] As summarized in Figure 11, the positive control LD_{50} values progressively declined from the 24-h value of about 2 to 1.3 mg/kg after 96 h. The LD_{50} values for the vitamin E-pretreated mice, however, remained essentially unchanged throughout the duration of the experiment. Vitamin E, therefore, not only afforded protection against the initial lethal effect of T-2 toxin, but against delayed lethality as well.

Because a bolus injection of vitamin E at high doses was effective in lessening the toxic effects of ionizing radiation,[69] similar experiments were conducted to assess the value of acute vitamin E administration. Mice were treated either immediately or 4 h after toxin exposure with a single i.p. injection of vitamin E at a dose of 1200 mg/kg, a dose which showed effective radiation protection.[69] Compared to the controls, administration of vitamin E either immediately or 4 h postexposure did not afford significant protection against the lethal effects of T-2 toxin. Thus, the data suggest that for treatment of trichothecene mycotoxicosis, vitamin E must be administered before toxin exposure.

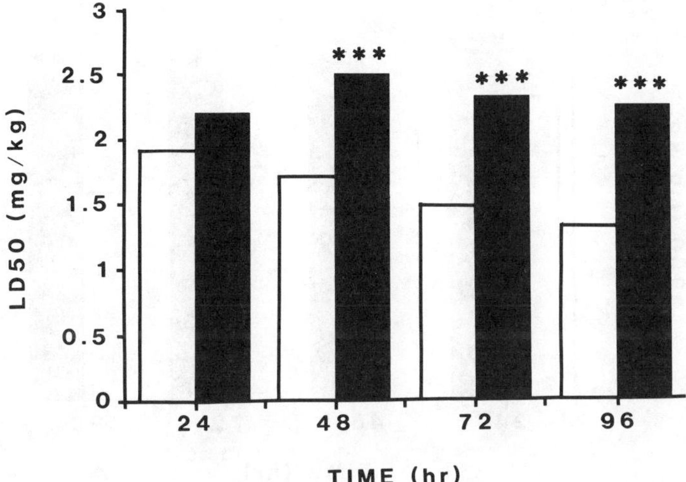

FIGURE 11.   Effect of pretreatment with vitamin E on LD_{50} values for T-2 toxin. Mice were pretreated daily for 3 d with an i.p. injection of either the vehicle (open bars) or vitamin E at 120 mg/kg (solid bars). T-2 toxin was administered 24 h after the final pretreatment and the LD_{50} values determined at 24-h intervals for 96 h. The *p*-values (treated vs. controls) < 0.001 are represented as ***.

d. Efficacy of Antioxidant Food Additives

Many synthetic food additives are effective antioxidants by functioning as effective free-radical scavengers both *in vivo* and *in vitro*.[72] Substituted phenols, such as butylated hydroxytoluene (BHT) and butylated hydroxyanisole (BHA), have been shown to protect experimental animals against the toxicity of various toxins and other xenobiotics. Hepatocytes, isolated from BHT pretreated rats, were less susceptible to genotoxicity from *in vitro* exposure to aflatoxin B_1.[73] The amount of binding of aflatoxin B_1 to DNA and RNA was markedly reduced by BHT pretreatment of the exposed hepatocytes. Pretreatment with BHA also decreased the acute toxicity of the pyrollizidine alkaloid monocrotaline, and that of both acetaminophen and bromobenzene.[74,75]

In addition to the above antioxidants, various pyrogallol derivatives, such as the *n*-propyl ester of gallic acid, and quinolines, such as ethoxyquin (Santoquin®, Monsanto Chemical Co., St. Louis), are also effective antioxidants and may therefore have potential for being effective therapeutic agents. Further, Trolox C®[76] (Hoffman LaRoche, Nutley, NJ), a more water-soluble analog of vitamin E is also an effective antioxidant. Although useful *in vitro* as an antioxidant food additive, the *in vivo* effectiveness of this analog has not been established. *In vitro* Trolox C® is capable of rapidly repairing amino acid free radicals formed in aqueous solution.[77]

To evaluate the potential benefit of BHT for the treatment of animals with T-2 toxicosis, mice were pretreated with BHT and challenged with T-2 toxin.[71] As summarized in Figure 12, the LD_{50} values for the untreated mice declined progressively throughout the observation period, reaching a minimum value of 1.33 mg/kg after 96 h. The BHT-treated mice, however, showed only a small decline, with LD_{50} values of 2.34 and 2.09 mg/kg at 24 and 96 h, respectively. Further experiments, however, determined that as in the case of vitamin E, pretreatment with BHT was necessary for protection against T-2 toxin. When treated with a single bolus injection of BHT 4 h before toxin exposure, the LD_{50} values were not significantly different from untreated controls.[71]

Other antioxidant food additives such as *n*-propyl gallate, ethoxyquin, and Trolox C®

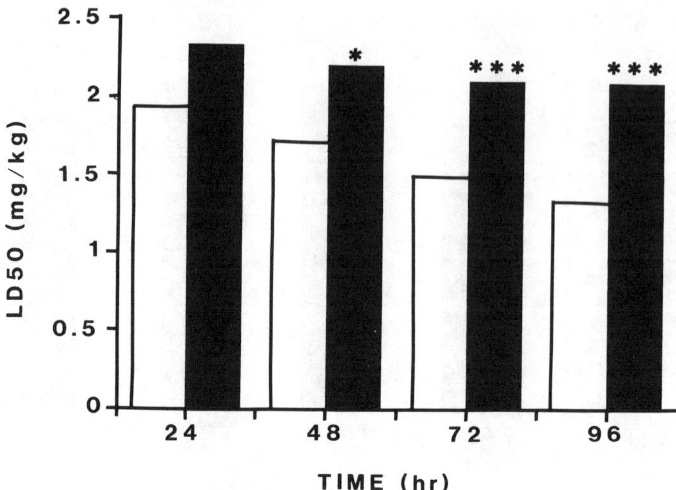

FIGURE 12.   Effect of pretreatment with BHT on LD_{50} values for T-2 toxin. Mice were pretreated daily for 3 d with an i.p. injection of either vehicle or BHT at 120 mg/kg and T-2 toxin was administered 24 h after the final dosing. The LD_{50} values for control (open bars) and BHT-treated (solid bars) groups were determined at 24-h intervals for 96 h. The *p*-values (treated vs. control) of <0.05 and <0.001 are represented as * and ***, respectively.

have been similarly evaluated. None of these compounds was found to be effective in the treatment of mice given T-2 toxin.

3. Effects of Other Antioxidants

Various drugs, in addition to their intended therapeutic uses, act secondarily as effective antioxidants. The phenothiazine drugs phenothiazine, promethazine, and chlorpromazine, are effective therapeutically as antihistamines and tranquilizers[78,79] and commercially as important industrial antioxidants.[72,80] *In vitro*, promethazine, at concentrations equivalent to therapeutically effective doses, decreases carbon tetrachloride-induced lipid peroxidation of rat liver microsomes.[81] Another antioxidant drug of interest in the treatment of trichothecene mycotoxicosis is WR2721, which is used as a radioprotective agent.

Both WR2721 and promethazine were evaluated as potential therapeutic agents for treatment of T-2 toxicosis.[71] Mice were treated with WR2721 at doses of 50, 250, or 500 mg/ kg, followed 45 min later by T-2 toxin at 2 mg/kg. As the dose of WR2721 increased, the percent lethality increased from 10% for the untreated group to 100% for the highest dose group. Also, the mean time to death values were significantly decreased by treatment with WR2721. Thus, although WR2721 is an effective antiradiation agent, it potentiated the toxicity of T-2 toxin. Similarly, promethazine at 50 and 100 mg/kg increased the percent lethality in T-2 toxin-treated mice from 49% for positive controls to 90% for mice given either dose of promethazine.

Dimethylsulfoxide (DMS)) is effective both as an anti-inflammatory drug and as an antioxidant. As an antioxidant, DMSO effectively neutralizes hydroxyl radicals, which may play a role in T-2 toxin-induced lysis of rat erythrocytes *in vitro*.[31] As mentioned above, the lysis of erythrocytes was preventable by adding mannitol, a specific hydroxyl radical quencher, to the media. *In vivo*, however, when compared to rats given only T-2 toxin (1 mg/kg, i.v.), no improvement in survival was noted by immediate treatment with DMSO (1 g/kg, i.p.).[55]

In summary, with the antioxidants tested as therapeutic agents for T-2 mycotoxicoses, pretreatment was necessary to show significant protection, and only vitamin E or BHT were of benefit. Although vitamin E was found to be an effective antiradiation agent when administered acutely at high doses, a similar protective effect in the treatment of T-2 toxicosis was not observed. High doses of ascorbic acid were, however, effective in mice but not rats when administered at the same time as T-2 toxin. Similarly, pretreatment of rats with ascorbic acid was also of no benefit. Two additional food additive antioxidants tested, ethoxyquin and Trolox C®, were also ineffective. DMSO, a specific hydroxyl radical scavenger, was not beneficial. Finally, two antioxidants, promethazine and WR2721, were clearly contraindicated.

D. Role of Microsomal-Inducing Agents in Altering the Lethality and Metabolism of T-2 Toxin

1. Efficacy of Microsomal-Inducing Agents

The activities of enzymes involved in the microsomal metabolism of toxins and other xenobiotics are dependent upon several factors, which include (in part) age, diet, and the inductive and depressant effects of drugs and other exogenous and endogenous substances.[82] Age-related effects in mammals include an increase in the enzymes involved in microsomal metabolism with maturation. Thus, young, immature animals, which may be lacking in some or all of the necessary microsomal enzymes, show increased sensitivity and lethality when exposed to various toxins and xenobiotics.[83] In mice, lethality from fusarenon-X decreased with increasing age. Further, the LD_{50} values for T-2 toxin increased from approximately 0.5 mg/kg at 3 weeks of age to over 3 mg/kg at 6 weeks of age.[84]

Microsomal enzyme-inducing agents have been used experimentally to assess the involvement of increased rates of biotransformation in altering toxicity. Kosuri[85] demonstrated that by either increasing or inhibiting the rates of microsomal metabolism, the lethal effects of T-2 toxin were either decreased or increased, respectively. In recent experiments, however, Ueno[44] presented data indicating that mice pretreated with microsomal inducing agents and then challenged with T-2 toxin had LD_{50} values that were not significantly different from untreated controls. In contrast, further studies of microsomal induction in trichothecene toxicosis have confirmed the efficacy of pretreatment with microsomal enzyme inducers in decreasing the lethality of T-2 toxin.[86] The various reports are described in the following discussion.

In the series of experiments, Kosuri[85] investigated the role of microsomal enzyme activities in altering the toxicity of either crude toxin extracts or purified T-2 toxin. Rats were pretreated with either phenobarbital or diethylaminoethyl diphenylpropylacetate (SKF 525A) to either induce or inhibit, respectively, the activities of microsomal enzymes. After treatment, rats were exposed to T-2 toxin at a sublethal dose of 1 mg/kg or a lethal dose of 3 mg/kg. As summarized in Figure 13, of the animals exposed to the lower toxin dose, there was no lethality for both the toxin-only and phenobarbital-treated groups; however, treatment with SKF 525A potentiated the toxicity of the mycotoxin, resulting in 90% lethality. For animals administered the high dose of toxin, there was 100% lethality for both the control and SKF 525A-treated animals, whereas the phenobarbital-treated rats showed only 10% lethality. These data clearly indicate that increasing or inhibiting the rate of T-2 toxin metabolism results in (respectively) decreased or increased lethality.

Recently, Ueno[44] presented data indicating that microsomal-inducing agents did not alter the lethality of T-2 toxin. In these experiments, mice were pretreated for 4 d with phenobarbital (75 mg/kg) or 3-methylcholanthrene (24 mg/kg) and then exposed to T-2 toxin. The LD_{50} values for the treated mice were not significantly different from the control group.

To clarify the conflicting data on the merits of microsomal inducing agents, mice were pretreated with phenobarbital and challenged with T-2 toxin 24 h after the final phenobarbital dose. For phenobarbital pretreated mice, the LD_{50} value was significantly higher than for

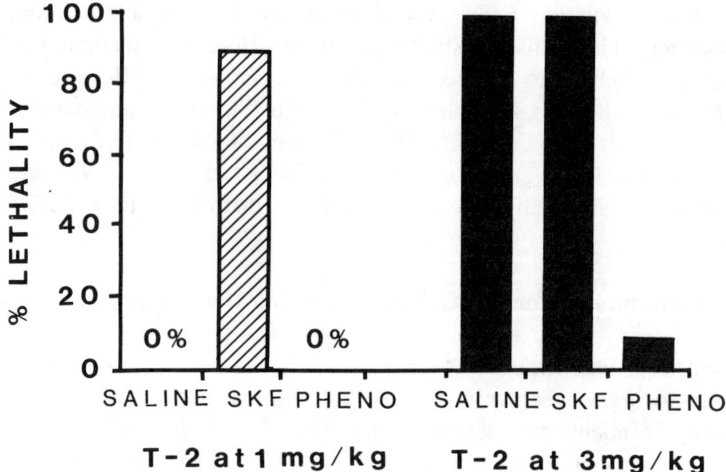

FIGURE 13.   Effect of pretreatment with saline, SKF 525-A, or phenobarbital on percent lethality in T-2 toxin-treated mice. Mice were pretreated with saline (control), SKF 525-A (SKF) (4 d at 30 mg/kg/d i.p.) or phenobarbital (PHENO) (3 d at 75 mg/kg/d, i.p.), and then challenged with T-2 toxin at doses of 1 mg/kg, i.p. (cross-hatched bars) or 3 mg/kg, i.p. (solid bars). (Adapted from Table 8, Reference 85.)

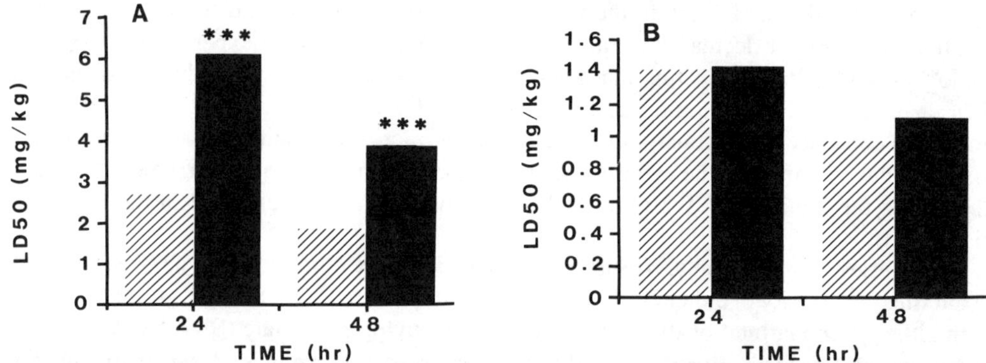

FIGURE 14.   Effect of phenobarbital on LD_{50} values for T-2 toxin. (A) Mice were pretreated for 4 d with phenobarbital (100 mg/kg/d, i.p.), then given varying doses of T-2 toxin at 24 h after the final treatment. LD_{50} values were determined 24 and 48 h later for both control (cross-hatched bars) and phenobarbital-treated (solid bars) groups. All p-values (control vs. treated) were <0.001. (B) The effect of phenobarbital administered at the same time as T-2 toxin on LD_{50} values. Phenobarbital (50 mg/kg, i.p.) was administered at the same time as T-2 toxin. LD_{50} values were determined 24 and 48 h later for both control (cross-hatched bars) and phenobarbital-treated (solid bars) groups. The p-values (control vs. treated) did not reveal significant differences.

the saline-treated controls (Figure 14A). To protect against the lethal effect of T-2 toxin, pretreatment with phenobarbital was necessary. When phenobarbital was administered at the same time as toxin, the LD_{50} values were not significantly different from saline-treated controls (Figure 14B).[87] This finding is interesting because phenobarbital treatment at the same time as toxin administration might have been expected to act as a substrate and inhibitor of mixed function oxidase enzymes to therefore increase the toxicity of T-2 toxin, as in the case of SKF 525A.

To further define the role of microsomal enzyme induction in altering the lethality of T-

2 toxin, other known inducing agents were evaluated. Since T-2 toxin contains an epoxide moiety, agents capable of inducing microsomal epoxide hydrolase activity were evaluated. *trans*-Stilbene oxide[88] and metyrapone[89] are both capable of inducing microsomal epoxide hydrolase, while 3-methylcholanthrene is not.[90]

Mice were pretreated daily for 3 d with 50 mg/kg of either *trans*-stilbene oxide, metyrapone, or 3-methylcholanthrene.[86] A full 24 h after the final dosing with the inducing agent, mice were given T-2 toxin. The relative potency values (ratio of treated/control LD_{50}) were 1.58, 1.84, and 2.69 for metyrapone-, 3-methylcholanthrene-, and *trans*-stilbene oxide-pretreated mice, respectively. All of these values were significantly higher than the control value of 1.0.

Clearly, from the available data, pretreatment with microsomal-inducing agents results in significant protection against the lethal effects of T-2 toxin. The protective effect of microsomal-inducing agents is, in all likelihood, a result of increased metabolism of T-2 toxin to less toxic compounds.

2. Biotransformation of T-2 Toxin

Although it is presumed that the protective effect of microsomal-inducing agents is a result of the increased rate of biotransformation, there are few data to support this contention directly. As discussed in the chapter entitled "The Absorption, Distribution, Metabolism, and Excretion of Trichothecene Mycotoxins", T-2 toxin undergoes a variety of metabolic alterations, eventually leading to the formation of less toxic metabolites.

The effect of *trans*-stilbene oxide, a potent inducer of microsomal enzymes, on *in vitro* microsomal metabolism of ^3H T-2 toxin has been studied.[91] Microsomes from both control and *trans*-stilbene oxide-treated mice were used in initial experiments to assess the effect of T-2 toxin on the activities of several microsomal enzymes. Mice were pretreated with vehicle only (control) or *trans*-stilbene oxide (50 mg/kg/d for 3 d). After pretreatment, mice were then given either T-2 toxin (6 mg/kg, s.c.) or the vehicle alone. Microsomes were prepared 6 h later and assayed for cytochrome P-450, epoxide (styrene oxide) hydrolase, 7-ethoxycoumarin-*O*-deethylase, and NADPH cytochrome *c* reductase. Pretreatment with *trans*-stilbene oxide significantly increased the activities of all the microsomal enzymes. T-2 toxin did not significantly change the activities of either epoxide hydrolase, cytochrome *c* reductase, or 7-ethoxycoumarin-*O*-deethylase, but caused a significant and consistent decrease in cytochrome P-450 levels of both control and induced microsomes. Similar reductions in cytochrome P-450 levels had been previously observed in T-2 toxin-treated rats.[29]

After confirmation that *trans*-stilbene oxide induced several microsomal enzymes, experiments were carried out to determine the effect of microsomal induction on the rate of metabolism of T-2 toxin. Microsomes were isolated from control and *trans*-stilbene oxide-pretreated (50 mg/kg/d for 3 d, i.p.) mice.[92] Microsomes were then incubated with ^3H T-2 toxin, and at various time points, media samples were processed and metabolites were separated by thin layer chromatography (TLC) and scanned for radioactivity. A comparison of the metabolic profiles for the control and induced microsomes revealed that during the first 30 min of incubation, the rate of biotransformation of labeled T-2 toxin was 4 times greater for the induced than for the untreated control microsomes. Further, after 60 min of incubation, there was no detectable T-2 toxin remaining with the induced microsomes, while the control microsomes still had 15% of the initial T-2 toxin remaining. The increased rate of degradation of T-2 toxin by the induced microsomes was also reflected in the higher amount of HT-2 toxin produced after both 30 and 60 min of incubation.

In summary, these data demonstrate that microsomal enzyme inducers increase the *in vitro* rate of metabolism of T-2 toxin. Although similar *in vivo* metabolism studies have not been carried out, the *in vitro* findings would strongly suggest that *in vivo* the decreased lethality of T-2 toxin which follows administration of enzyme inducers is a result of its increased biotransformation to less toxic metabolites.

E. Effectiveness of Anti-Inflammatory Agents
1. Rationale for Use

Trichothecene mycotoxins produce a variety of physiological responses, including profound effects on the cardiovascular system. Acute administration of highly toxic doses of T-2 toxin in several species leads to the development of a state of circulatory shock with characteristic changes in cardiac output, heart rate, and mean arterial blood pressure.[93-95] In swine, the development of shock was also accompanied by increased plasma concentrations of catecholamines, thromboxane (TX) B_2, and 6-keto-$PGF_{1\alpha}$.[96] At lethal doses of T-2 toxin, the release of these vasoactive substances apparently cannot adequately counteract the toxin-induced reductions in blood pressure and cardiac output.

An effective therapy for the treatment of animals experiencing shock is the intensive, short-term use of high doses of several water-soluble glucocorticoid salts.[97-100] Glucocorticoids are effective in increasing survival in hemorrhagic,[101,102] traumatic,[103] experimental endotoxin,[104,105] and snake venom-induced shock.[106]

Mechanisms for the protective effect of steroids during shock are not fully understood. The postulated beneficial actions of glucocorticoids, as summarized by Hankes,[107] include (in part):

1.   A positive inotropic effect
2.   Vasodilation of arterioles and venules
3.   Inhibition of the release of vasoconstrictor substances
4.   Increased lactic acid metabolism
5.   Improved glycolytic flux and increased energy metabolism
6.   Stabilization of lysosomes

Glucocorticoids may, therefore, be effective in the treatment of animals with T-2 toxicosis by attenuating some of the observed pathophysiologic and biochemical effects. These documented effects of acutely toxic doses of trichothecenes include:

1.   The development of a shock-like state[93-95]
2.   Release of vasoactive compounds[96]
3.   Lactic acidosis[93]
4.   Decreased energy metabolism[108]
5.   Release of lysosomal enzymes[109]

Recent experiments revealed that during acute T-2 intoxication in rats, the plasma activities of several lysosomal enzymes increased markedly (Figure 15).[109] These data not only suggest the involvement of lysosomal enzyme release as a cellular response to T-2 toxin, but also suggest possible benefit from glucocorticoids by stabilizing both lysosomal and plasma membranes. Although anti-inflammatory steroids decrease the release of lysosomal enzymes during shock,[110] experiments to determine whether this occurs in T-2 toxin-exposed animals have not been carried out.

There is still some controversy in the literature concerning the beneficial effect of glucocorticoids for use in T-2 toxicosis. Ueno[44] was not able to demonstrate a protective effect using corticosteroids. In this study, daily treatment with prednisolone (50 mg/kg, s.c.) for 3 d did not significantly change the LD_{50} value for T-2 toxin. More recent evidence,[111,112] however, clearly demonstrated a protective effect of several rapidly acting anti-inflammatory glucocorticoids, including dexamethasone, methylprednisolone, prednisolone, and hydrocortisone, in decreasing lethality due to T-2 toxin.

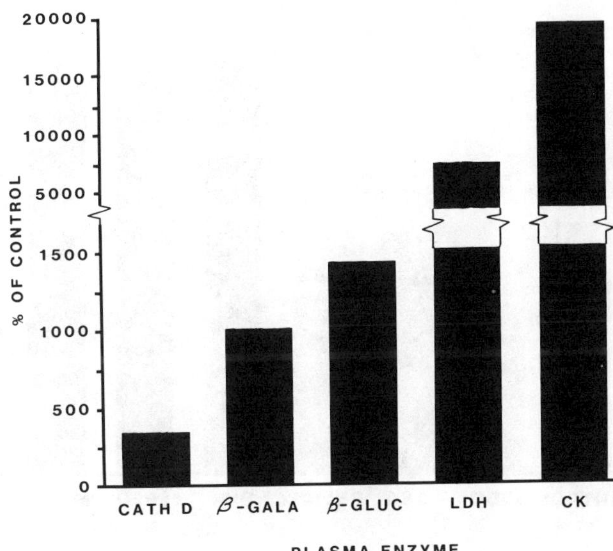

FIGURE 15.   Effect of T-2 toxin on release of lysosomal enzymes. Plasma activities of cathepsin D (CATH D), β-galactosidase (β-GALA), β-glucuronidase (β-GLUC), LDH, and CPK were measured 6 h after dosing rats with T-2 toxin (2 mg/kg, i.v.). Data represent the percent of control activity.

2. Efficacy of Anti-Inflammatory Agents
a. Efficacy of Steroidal and Nonsteroidal Anti-Inflammatory Agents

The effectiveness of steroidal and nonsteroidal anti-inflammatory agents in preventing T-2 toxin-induced lethality has been evaluated using mice[111] (Figure 16). Of the nonsteroidal anti-inflammatory agents evaluated, indomethacin and phenylbutazone increased (relative potency value <1.0) the lethality of T-2 toxin, whereas acetylsalicylic acid was ineffective (relative potency values not significantly different from 1.0). Unlike these nonsteroidal agents, the steroidal anti inflammatory agents showed significant protection (relative potency value >1.0) against the lethal effects of T-2 toxin. At equivalent doses of anti-inflammatory activity, dexamethasone sodium phosphate, prednisolone sodium succinate, methylprednisolone sodium succinate, and hydrocortisone sodium succinate all provided significant protection.

To further assess the efficacy of steroidal anti-inflammatory agents, mice were exposed to an LD_{70} dose of T-2 toxin and treated simultaneously with either the vehicle (control), dexamethasone sodium phosphate, prednisolone sodium succinate, methylprednisolone sodium succinate, or hydrocortisone sodium succinate.[113] The mean survival time was significantly higher in the dexamethasone-treated group, while prednisolone, methylprednisolone, and hydrocortisone were ineffective in increasing mean survival time. The percent lethality in the dexamethasone- and prednisolone-treated groups was significantly lower than in the T-2 toxin positive control group.

In another study using rats, methylprednisolone sodium succinate (30 mg/kg, i.p.), administered immediately after T-2 toxin (1 mg/kg, i.v.), was effective in lessening the clinical signs associated with acute exposure to T-2 toxin.[55] Those animals given the steroid were more alert and active than the untreated controls and did not exhibit the impaired peripheral circulation manifested in the untreated controls by cold, bluish-appearing tails and feet. Moreover, survival was significantly improved with steroid treatment (Figure 17). In this study, no comparisons of efficacy between the various glucocorticosteroids were made.

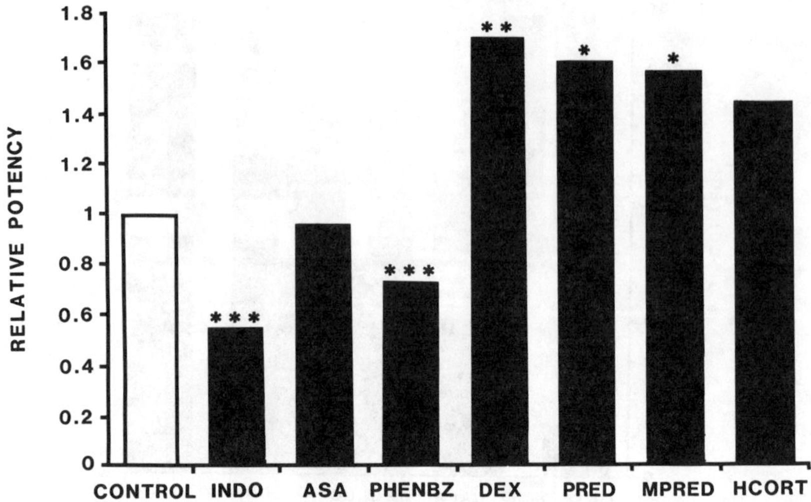

FIGURE 16.   Efficacy of steroidal and nonsteroidal anti-inflammatory agents for the treatment of T-2 toxicosis. Mice were treated wtih saline (control), indomethacin (INDO) (10 mg/kg, i.p.), acetylsalicylic acid (ASA) (300 mg/kg, i.p.), phenylbutazone (100 mg/kg, i.p.), dexamethasone (DEX) (10 mg/kg, i.p.), prednisolone or hydrocortisone (HCORT) (266 mg/kg, i.p.) and immediately challenged with varying doses of T-2 toxin. The relative potency values were determined 48 h after treatment.

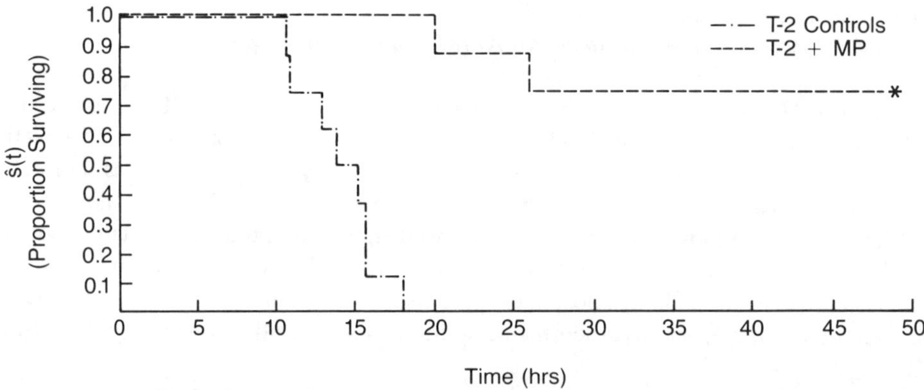

FIGURE 17.   Effect of methylprednisolone sodium succinate (i.p. at 30 mg/kg) on survival of rats when given immediately after T-2 toxin (i.v. at 1 mg/kg). There was significantly greater survival in the group given T-2 toxin plus methylprednisolone (denoted by *) when compared to the group given T-2 toxin alone ($p < 0.05$).

b. Efficacy of Dexamethasone in Decreasing Lethality of T-2 Toxin

Because dexamethasone showed the highest efficacy in mouse studies, further experiments were carried out to determine the effectiveness of pre- and postexposure treatment.[111] Dexamethasone was administered either 1 h before, the same time as, or 1, 2, or 3 h postadministration of a lethal dose of T-2 toxin. Overall, pretreatment with dexamethasone showed the highest efficacy as assessed by mean time to death, mean survival time, and percent lethality (Figure 18). The percent lethality was lowest in the 1-h pretreatment group. A progressive increase in lethality was seen as the time after toxin administration (before dexamethasone treatment) increased. The percent lethality for -1, 0, and $+1$ h treatment times were all significantly less than the positive control values. Dexamethasone also sig-

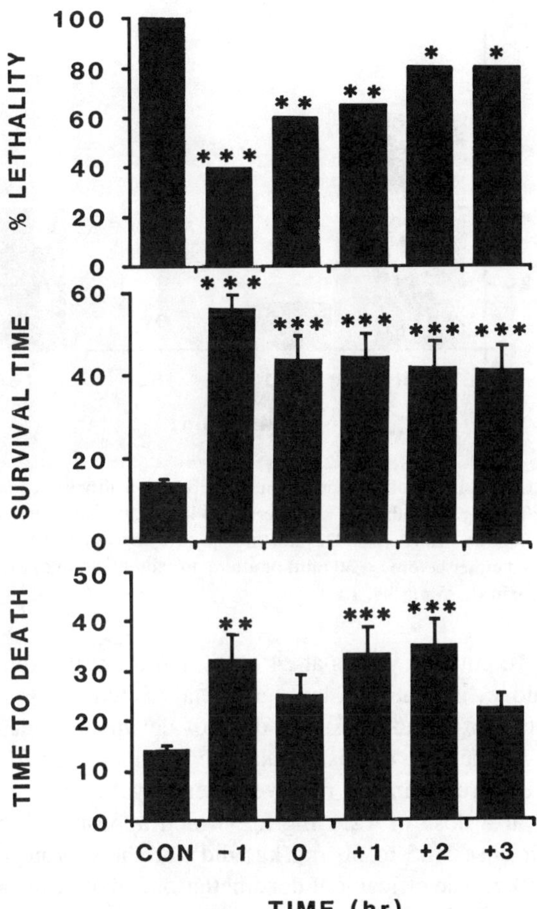

FIGURE 18.   Effect of varying the time of dexamethasone administration on percent lethality, survival time, and time to death of T-2 toxin-treated mice. Mice were treated with saline (control) or dexamethasone (13 mg/kg, i.p.) either prior to (-1 h), the same time (0 h), or at various times after ($+1$, $+2$, or $+3$ h) exposure to T-2 toxin (5 mg/kg, s.c.). The percent lethality, survival time (mean $\pm$ S.E.), and time to death (mean $\pm$ S.E.) were determined over 72 h. The p-values (treated vs. control) of <0.05, <0.01, and <0.001 are represented as *, **, and ***, respectively.

nificantly increased the mean time to death when compared to the control value of 14 h. In the dexamethasone-treated mice, however, there was no correlation between the time of dexamethasone administration and the mean time to death. The mean survival times for the dexamethasone-treated groups were all significantly higher than for the untreated T-2 toxin controls. The 1-h dexamethasone pretreatment resulted in the longest survival time, whereas the mean survival times of the simultaneous and postexposure dexamethasone treatment groups were all approximately the same.

Dexamethasone alone was next compared to combinations of dexamethasone with either prednisolone or methylprednisolone with regard to the ability to prevent death from T-2 intoxication.[114] In this experiment, dexamethasone (16 mg/kg, i.p.) was administered either alone or in combination with an i.p. dose of 125 mg/kg of either prednisolone or methyl-prednisolone. Dexamethasone combined with either prednisolone or methylprednisolone was

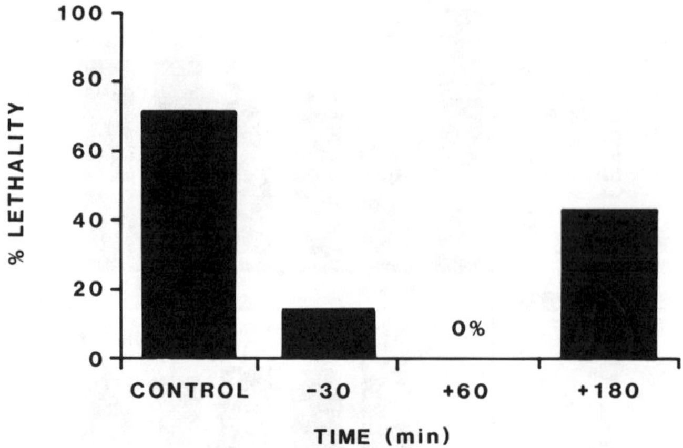

FIGURE 19.   Effect of dexamethasone on percent lethality from T-2 toxin in rats. The percent lethality was determined in control (saline-treated) or dexamethasone-treated rats. Dexamethasone (1.6 mg/kg, i.m.) was administered either before (-30 min) or after ($+60$ or $+180$ min) exposure to T-2 toxin (0.75 mg/kg, i.v.).

effective, but the relative potency values at 24 or 48 h after toxin exposure were lower than with dexamethasone alone, indicating a less beneficial response.

The relationship between the administered dose of dexamethasone and relative potency was also evaluated.[111] As the dose of dexamethasone was increased from 0.125 to 12.5 mg/kg, i.p., a progressive increase in the relative potency value was observed. The highest efficacy was obtained at a dose of 12.5 mg/kg, which appeared to be the optimum. Experiments at very high doses (25 to 50 mg/kg) did not show protection greater than that achieved with 12.5 mg/kg. The efficacy of dexamethasone given i.m. was also evaluated.[111] A similar dose-response relationship was obtained; however, the equivalent effective dose of steroid was less than 1/10 of that found for i.p. administration. The optimum dose for i.m. administration was approximately 0.25 mg/kg and again, higher doses did not increase efficacy.

The efficacy of dexamethasone for treatment of animals with acute T-2 toxicosis was recently confirmed by Tremel et al.[112] Rats were treated with an i.v. injection of dexamethasone sodium phosphate either 30 min before or at 60 to 180 min after being challenged with an approximately LD_{70} dose of T-2 toxin. Compared to untreated controls, dexamethasone reduced lethality when administered either before or after toxin exposure (Figure 19). Treatment 180 min after toxin exposure appeared to be less effective than either 30 min before or 60 min after the toxin. Clearly, these results are consistent with the mouse experiment described above.

In summary, steroidal, but not nonsteroidal, anti-inflammatory agents were effective in reducing the lethality of T-2 toxin as assessed by percent lethality, mean survival time, mean time to death, and relative potency, a function of change in the LD_{50}. Of the steroids tested, hydrocortisone, prednisolone, methylprednisolone, and dexamethasone were all effective in decreasing lethality from T-2 toxin. When tested in mice at equivalent doses of glucocorticoid activity, however, dexamethasone showed the highest efficacy. In both mice and rats, dexamethasone was found to be most effective when given before toxin exposure, with decreased efficacy as the time between the toxin dosing and the administration of steroid increased. Combination of dexamethasone with either prednisolone or methylprednisolone did not increase therapeutic efficacy above that found with dexamethasone alone.

F. Efficacy of Multiple Drug Treatments

1. Dexamethasone Sodium Phosphate in Combination with PGE₁

As previously discussed, dexamethasone is highly efficacious in several animal species for the treatment of acute T-2 toxicosis. PGE_1 is also effective for the treatment of other circulatory shock states.[115,116] Salutary effects of PGE_1 have been hypothesized to include vasodilation, improved cardiac function, and like the glucocorticoids, membrane stabilization with a resultant decrease in the release of lysosomal enzymes.[116] Thus, the combination of dexamethasone and PGE_1 for therapy of acute T-2 toxicosis appeared promising. The slow i.v. infusion of PGE_1 (Alprostadil, courtesy of Upjohn Co.) was assessed in young female Sprague-Dawley rats.[64] PGE_1 was infused via a tail vein over a 2-h period at a total dose of 50 mg/kg. A combination therapy was also evaluated and consisted of the i.v. administration of dexamethasone at 6 mg/kg given immediately and 4 h after T-2 toxin administration and a slow i.v. infusion of PGE_1 at 5, 25, or 50 μg/kg begun immediately after the first dose of dexamethasone. PGE_1 infused alone did not improve survival times. In contrast, the combination of dexamethasone and PGE_1 did improve survival times compared with the control group given T-2 toxin and no therapy. Of significance, however, was the observation that the improvement noted with the combination therapy was no better than that obtained when dexamethasone was given alone.

The lack of efficacy of PGE_1 in combination with dexamethasone may be due to two factors: (1) the infusion of PGE_1 may have been started too early in the course of the toxicosis for its pharmacologic effects to ameliorate clinical symptomatology; (2) the pharmacologic actions of dexamethasone may have precluded the need for the PGE_1. Additional work is necessary in order to evaluate the efficacy of dexamethasone in conjunction with PGE_1 and other potentially effective therapeutic agents.

2. Combined Protocols in Swine

Due to the complex pathophysiologic effects which occur during acute T-2 intoxication, the use of a single therapeutic agent alone might not ensure the maximum probability of survival. Therefore, a study was undertaken to assess multiple drug protocols for their efficacy in alleviating the effects of T-2 toxicosis in swine. The individual therapeutic agents used in this study and their administration protocols are given in Table 3. The doses employed were based on either previously recognized uses of the particular agent and were thus the same for each individual animal on an mg/kg body weight basis, or an attempt to maintain certain physiologic parameters, as in the case of arterial blood pressure or arterial blood pH. In the latter case, the amounts of sodium bicarbonate or normal saline administered varied among individual animals, depending on their particular needs. Metoclopramide was included in each of the therapeutic protocols, including controls, to reduce toxin-induced emesis. Previous studies had demonstrated that metoclopramide could control emesis in dogs following i.v. administration of fusarenon-X.[27] It was hoped that the use of the antiemetic would also facilitate retention of the activated charcoal and magnesium sulfate.

Four different multiple drug protocols were evaluated for efficacy in treating swine during acute T-2 toxicosis. Because of previous evidence demonstrating reliable benefit from glucocorticoids, the therapeutic protocols all included dexamethasone as well as the metoclopramide. The metoclopramide plus dexamethasone therapy was combined with activated charcoal and magnesium sulfate, sodium bicarbonate, and normal saline, or with only two of these three additional agents (Table 4). After the administration of T-2 given by a slow, 2 to 3 min, i.v. infusion, the different therapeutic protocols were started. Animals were observed over 48 h and the individual and groups' survival times were recorded (Table 4).

While the number of animals per group was small, several important observations are worth noting. Two out of three animals in the group given either the complete therapeutic regimen (group 2) or the complete regimen less normal saline (group 5) survived 48 h.

Table 3
SWINE THERAPEUTIC STUDY

Drug	Source	Dosage regimen
Metoclopramide	Injectable form (5 mg/ml) courtesy of A. H. Robins Company	1 mg/kg body weight i.v. immediately prior to T-2 toxin administration and 0.25 and 1.25 h post T-2 toxin
Activated charcoal	SuperChar® courtesy of Gulf BioSystems, Inc.	2 g activated charcoal (dry weight)/kg body weight in 420 ml tap water p.o. 0.5 and 4 h post-T-2
Magnesium sulfate	Epsom salt, magnesium sulfate USP, purchased from Dow Chemical Company	0.5 g/kg body weight p.o. mixed with activated charcoal slurry and administered 0.5 and 4 h post-T-2
Dexamethasone sodium phosphate	Azium S/P® (4 mg dexamethasone sodium phosphate/ml), purchased from Schering Corporation	6 mg/kg body weight i.v. immediately and 4 h post-T-2, then 4 mg/kg 8 and 12 h post-T-2, followed by 2 mg/kg 16 and 20 h post-T-2 and 1 mg/kg 24 h post-T-2
Sodium bicarbonate	5% sodium bicarbonate injection, USP, purchased from Abbott Laboratories	Variable speed i.v. drip based on hourly arterial blood pH measurements; started if pH <7.350 and stopped if pH >7.350
Normal saline	0.9% sodium chloride injection, USP, purchased from Abbott Laboratories	Rapid i.v. drip (gravity flow) as MAP begins decline; administration slowed to maintenance levels if MAP does not respond or if CVP+ >10 mmHg

Note: In this study the various drugs were tested in a multiple drug treatment protocol; their sources and the drug administration protocols followed during the study are given.

One animal given all therapy minus sodium bicarbonate (group 4) also lived for the entire 48-h observation period. All the animals which survived 48 h were alert and active. Whether the surviving animals would have succumbed due to secondary complications is not known, but thorough postmortem examinations of each animal failed to reveal lesions which would have signaled the likelihood of imminent death.

There were no significant differences in survival times for those pigs in groups 2 (all therapy), 4 (no sodium bicarbonate), or 5 (no normal saline). Had the data not been censored due to scheduled euthanasia, a greater difference in survival times compared to the control group would have occurred. The inclusion of sodium bicarbonate may have been helpful in maintaining a more normal arterial blood pH (Figure 20), however, other components of the treatment protocol appeared to promote acid-base balance with equal or greater potency. The i.v. administration of a large volume of normal saline (up to 14 l given over 8 to 10 h) was ineffective in maintaining mean aortic blood pressure.

Interestingly, the group without activated charcoal and magnesium sulfate did perform more poorly than the other three treatment groups. This observation agrees with the protective effect of oral activated charcoal in treating both mice and rats with parenterally induced T-2 intoxications, as discussed earlier.

Only partial success was achieved with the use of metoclopramide as an antiemetic. This may have been due to the use of a suboptimal dosage regimen and further evaluation, particularly of a continuous i.v. infusion, may be warranted.

Table 4
TREATMENT OF SWINE

Group (n = 3)*	Treatment	Mean weight (kg)	Survival time (h)	Mean survival time (h)
1	Control	51.0	9.4, 7.8,	8.6
	T-2 + metoclopramide		8.6	
2	Metoclopramide	53.3	9.5,	+*,**
	Dexamethasone		48.0,	
	Normal saline and NaHCO$_3$		48.0	
	Activated charcoal + MgSO$_4$			
	(All therapy)			
3	Metoclopramide	45.5	15.8,	18.0*
	Dexamethasone		20.1,	
	Normal saline and NaHCO$_3$		18.0	
	(No activated charcoal or			
	MgSO$_4$)			
4	Metoclopramide	47.8	11.3,	+*,**
	Dexamethasone		22.5,	
	Activated charcoal + MgSO$_4$		30.0,	
	Normal saline		48.0	
	(No NaHCO$_3$)			
5	Metoclopramide	53.6	23.5,	+*,**
	Dexamethasone		48.0,	
	Activated charcoal + MgSO$_4$		48.0	
	NaHCO$_3$			
	(No saline)			

Note: All swine were given T-2 toxin i.v. at a dose of 3.6 mg/kg. The various drugs were administered according to the protocols given in Table 3. Since those animals which survived for 48 h were killed, the 48-h survival time was considered to be censored. There was a significant improvement in survival noted for all treatment groups vs. the control group (denoted by *). In addition there was significantly higher survival in those groups given activated charcoal in combination with magnesium sulfate (groups 2, 4, and 5, denoted by **) when compared to the group not given the activated charcoal-magnesium sulfate combination (group 3).

G. Miscellaneous Therapeutic Agents

1. Attempts to Influence Changes in Blood Coagulation

Other therapies have been evaluated in the treatment of animals with acute T-2 toxicosis. Specific treatment intended to counteract the hematologic effects of T-2 toxin met with mixed and conflicting results. Rats given sublethal doses of T-2 toxin showed increased clotting and prothrombin times.[6] As a potential therapy for T-2 toxin-induced coagulopathy, Kosuri[84] found that vitamin K counteracted the increase in prothrombin times caused by T-2 toxin, although treatment did not have any effect in lessening the associated mortality. Calcium gluconate was also tried, but was ineffective. Recent work by Cosgriff et al.[117] demonstrated that T-2 toxin produces significant decreases in all coagulation factors, except fibrinogen. Unlike the results inferred by Kosuri,[84] however, Cosgriff and co-workers found that treatment with vitamin K did not alter the effects of T-2 toxin on coagulation factors.

2. Efforts to Antagonize GI Effects

Studies with guinea pigs showed that inhibition of intestinal peristalsis after fusarenon-X intoxication (1 mg/kg, i.v.) could be antagonized by pilocarpine treatment (0.2 mg/kg, i.v.).[27] Additional studies in dogs revealed that fusarenon-X-induced (0.3 mg/kg, i.v.)

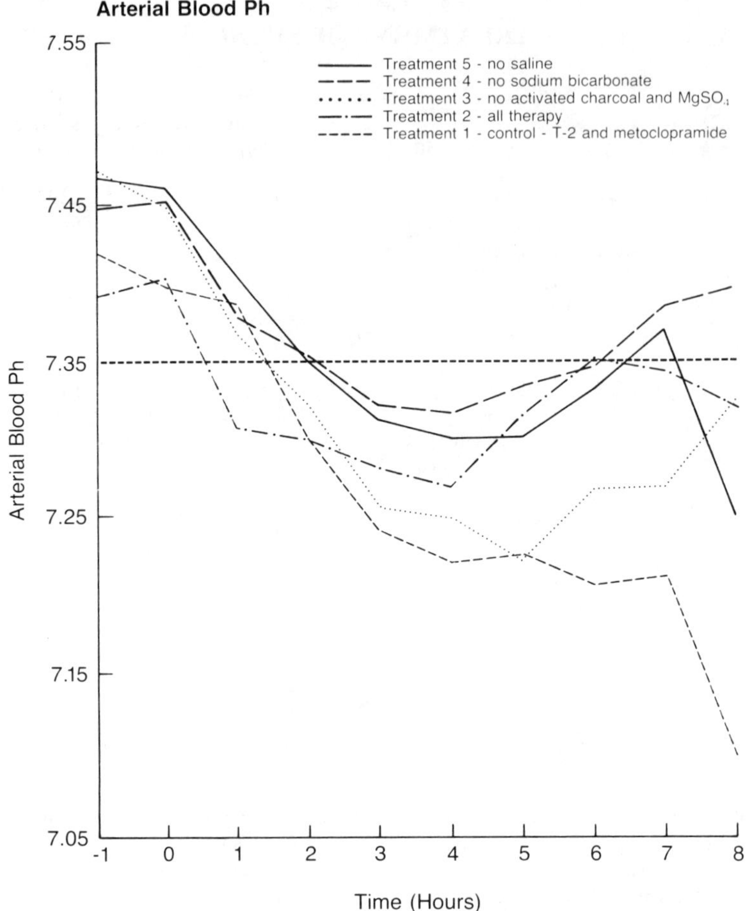

FIGURE 20.   Effect of the various treatment combinations (Table 4) on arterial blood pH through the first 8 h of observation in swine given T-2 toxin i.v. at 3.6 mg/kg. Intravenous sodium bicarbonate therapy was begun when the arterial blood pH fell below 7.35. While similar trends in pH were initially noted for all the groups, the decline began to moderate in the treatment groups as compared to the control group between 4 and 6 h after T-2 toxin administration. The inclusion of sodium bicarbonate in treatment protocols (groups 2, 3, and 5) did not appear to moderate the drop in pH or hasten its return to normal when compared to the treatment group which did not receive sodium bicarbonate (group 4). Thus, other aspects of therapy appear to be at least of equal value in moderating the metabolic acidosis attributable to T-2 toxicosis.

vomiting was attenuated by s.c. injection of either metoclopramide (0.5 mg/kg) or chlorpromazine (1 gm/kg).

3. Trials with Herbal Drugs

Further, the efficacy of Chinese herbal drugs was evaluated in mice given T-2 toxin.[118] After treatment with *Panax ginseng* and *Atractylodes japonica* (500 mg/kg, p.o.) or *Paeonia albiflora typica* (250 mg/kg, p.o.), there was a 30% survival rate. Other herbal drugs, *Glycyrrhiza uralensis*, *Scutellaria baicalensis*, *Rehmannia glutinosa*, and *Plantago asiatica* were not effective.

4. Assessment of a Proposed Competitive Inhibitor

Trichodermin is a trichothecene mycotoxin with a structure and biochemical activity similar to that of T-2 toxin, although trichodermin is much less acutely toxic. Based upon pathophysiologic studies completed to date, the exact mode of action of the trichothecenes as it relates to acute toxicity is unknown; it is conceivable that cell receptors play a role in cellular penetration of the toxin. It has been suggested that complete T-2 toxin cell membrane receptor occupation is a critical first step in the expression of T-2 cytotoxicity.[119] If the difference in toxicity between T-2 toxin and trichodermin was due to different binding affinities for a common cell membrane recpetor, trichodermin might serve to competitively inhibit T-2 toxin entry into the cell and thus decrease its cytotoxicity. In addition, both trichodermin and T-2 toxin competitively bind and inhibit peptidyl transferase, a key enzyme in ribosomal protein synthesis.[120,121]

Despite the proposed potential benefit, trichodermin, when given i.p. to rats at 100 mg/kg either 1 h prior to or 1 h after the i.v. administration of T-2 toxin at 1 mg/kg, caused a significant decrease in mean survival time compared to a positive control group given T-2 toxin alone.[55] Thus, in contrast to a hypothesized inhibitory action of trichodermin on the interaction of T-2 toxin with cell components and a resultant decrease in toxicity, there was an indication of an additive or synergistic effect.

5. Monoclonal Antibodies

Unlike the lack of definitive benefit for most of the other "miscellaneous therapies", the use of a monoclonal anti-T-2 antibody provided significant protection against the lethal effects of T-2 toxin.[122] When the antibody was given 15 min before administration of a lethal dose of T-2 toxin, there was 100% survival. If treatment was delayed until 60 min after toxin exposure, however, the number of surviving animals decreased to 25%; thus, it appears important to bind the toxin before it binds to cellular receptors.

III. CONCLUSIONS AND SUMMARY

The treatment of animals for trichothecene toxicoses represents a complex problem, which is compounded by our presently inadequate understanding of the biochemical and pathophysiologic effects of the toxin. Due to expanded research on trichothecene mycotoxicosis after their alleged use as biological warfare agents,[4] a substantial amount of new information has become available on both the biochemical and physiologic effects of these toxins. Even with this new information, however, ideal therapeutic approaches have not been identified.

Of the different therapies evaluated for trichothecene mycotoxicosis, several have proved effective in decreasing lethality. Other than the use of adsorbents or anti-T-2 toxin monoclonal antibodies, all of the therapeutic agents provide either symptomatic or supportive therapy. The agents found to be clearly effective in experimental animals both before and after toxin administration are glucocorticoids and activated charcoal. The success of glucocorticoid administration in decreasing lethality of T-2 toxin makes these agents and other antishock drugs worthy of further investigation. GI adsorbing agents, such as activated charcoal, were effective in treating experimental animals with either parenterally or orally induced T-2 toxicosis. Overall, conventional supportive therapy for treatment of circulatory shock plus intragastrically administered activated charcoal was of substantial benefit to animals exposed to high doses of T-2 toxin. For treatment of shock, glucocorticoids, especially dexamethasone, have proved to be highly effective. Initial experiments, based on a limited number of swine, suggest that activated charcoal and dexamethasone are effective in conjunction with other supportive therapy; however, the combination of dexamethasone and PGE_1 did not improve survival in rats over that obtained with dexamethasone alone.

While combined therapy is potentially of great benefit to the T-2 toxin-dosed animal (survival of 3 times the LD_{50}), individual therapeutic components may not be highly effective if strictly targeted endpoints are examined rather than general improvement. The rapid intravenous administration of normal saline to swine dosed acutely with T-2 toxin did not reverse the decline in mean arterial blood pressure. The results, however, do indicate areas needing further study. In this instance, it would appear that the use of plasma expanders such as dextran should be investigated.

The value of the therapeutic agents evaluated to date may be limited either because efficacy could not be confirmed in at least two species, or pretreatment over several days was necessary. For example, the antioxidants tested, vitamin E and BHT, were both efficacious but required pretreatment to be fully effective. Similarly, phenobarbital and other microsomal-inducing agents require pretreatment. Neither vitamin E, BHT, nor phenobarbital were effective when administered at the same time as the toxin. Of the other antioxidants evaluated, ascorbic acid was clearly beneficial in treating mice, but was ineffective in rats.

In summary, a great deal of progress has been made in the management of animals with trichothecene mycotoxicoses. Further experiments based on these findings might define the mechanism of the protective action of the various therapeutic agents and hopefully expand the list of protective drugs. The knowledge gained in these studies may provide insight into the therapeutic management of other toxicoses.

REFERENCES

1. **Levin, I. I.,** Treatment of alimentary toxic aleukia with sulfonamide compound preparations, *Clin. Med.,* 7, 54, 1946.
2. **Friedman, M. Yu.,** Prophylaxis of alimentary toxic aleukia (septic angina), in *Alimentary Toxic Aleukia (Septic Angina),* Medical Publishing House, Moscow, 1945, 54.
3. **Joffe, A. Z.,** Alimentary toxic aleukia, in *Microbial Toxins: Algal and Fungal Toxins VII,* Kadis, S., Ciegler, A., and Ajl, S. M., Eds., Academic Press, New York, 1971, 139.
4. U. S. Department of State, Spec. Rep. No. 104: Chemical Warfare in Southeast Asia and Afghanistan: An Update, U.S. Department of State, Washington, D.C., 1982.
5. National Academy of Science, *Protection Against Trichothecene Mycotoxins,* National Academy Press, Washington, D.C., 1983, 158.
6. **Smalley, E. B., Marasas, W. F. O., Strong, F. M., Bamburg, J. R., Nichols, R. E., and Kosuri, N. R.,** Mycotoxins associated with moldy corn, in Proc. 1st U.S.-Japan-Conf. on Toxic Micro-Organisms, Herzberg, M., Ed., UJNR and US Department of the Interior, Washington, D.C., 1970, 163.
7. **Carson, M. S. and Smith, T. K.,** Effect of feeding alfalfa and refined plant fibers on the toxicity and metabolism of T-2 toxin in rats, *J. Nutr.,* 113, 304, 1983.
8. **Smith, T. K.,** Influence of dietary fiber, protein, and zeolite on zearalenone toxicosis in rats and swine, *J. Anim. Sci.,* 50, 278, 1980.
9. **Carson, M. S. and Smith, T. K.,** Role of bentonite in prevention of T-2 toxicosis in rats, *J. Anim. Sci.,* 57, 1498, 1983.
10. **Smith, T. K.,** Effect of dietary protein, alfalfa and zeolite on excretory patterns of 5′, 5′, 7′, 7′-zearalenone in rats, *Can. J. Physiol. Pharmacol.,* 58, 1251, 1980.
11. **James, L. J. and Smith, T. K.,** Effects of alfalfa on zearalenone toxicity and metabolism in rats and swine, *J. Anim. Sci.,* 55, 110, 1982.
12. **Picchioni, A. L.,** Activated charcoal — a neglected antidote, *Pediatr. Clin. N. Am.,* 17, 535, 1970.
13. **Johnson, J. D., Gibson, S. J., and Ober, R. E.,** Cholestyramine-enhanced fecal elimination of carbon-14 in rats after administration of ammonium (^{14}C) perfluorooctanoate or potassium (^{14}C)perfluorooctanesulfonate, *Fundam. Appl. Toxicol.,* 4, 972, 1984.
14. **Cohen, W. J., Boylan, J. J., Lanke, R. V., Fariss, M. W., Howell, J. R., and Guzelian, P. S.,** Treatment of chlordecone (Kepone®) toxicity with cholestyramine, *N. Engl. J. Med.,* 298, 243, 1978.
15. **Cooney, D. O.,** A "superactive" charcoal for antidotal use in poisonings, *Clin. Toxicol.,* 11, 387, 1977.
16. **Hatch, R. C., Clark, J. D., Jain, A. V., and Weiss, R.,** Induced acute aflatoxicosis in goats: treatment with activated charcoal or dual combinations of oxytetracycline, stanozolol, and activated charcoal. *Am. J. Vet. Res.,* 43, 644, 1982.

17. **Dalvi, R. R. and Ademoyero, A. A.**, Toxic effects of aflatoxin B_1 in chickens given feed contaminated with *Aspergillus flavus* and reduction of the toxicity by activated charcoal and some chemical agents, *Avian Dis.*, 28, 61, 1983.
18. **Pace, J. G., Watts, M. R., Burrows, E. P., Dinterman, R. E., Matson, C., Hauer, E. C., and Wannemacher, R. W., Jr.**, Fate and distribution of ^{3}H-labeled T-2 mycotoxin in guinea pigs, *Toxicol. Appl. Pharmacol.*, 80, 377, 1985.
19. **Corley, R. A., Swanson, S. P., and Buck, W. B.**, Glucuronide conjugation of T-2 toxin and metabolites in swine bile and urine, *J. Agric. Food Chem.*, 33, 1085, 1985.
20. **Buck, W. B. and Bratich, P. M.** Activated charcoal: preventing unnecessary death by poisoning, *Vet. Med.*, 81, 73, 1986.
21. **Jenkins, W. L.**, Drugs affecting gastrointestinal function, in *Veterinary Pharmacology and Therapeutics*, 5th ed., Booth, N. H. and McDonald, L. E., Eds., Iowa State University Press, Ames, 1985, 600.
22. **Bratich, P. M.**, Adsorptive capacity of activated charcoals and other adsorbents for nitrate, carbaryl, strychine, chlorpyrifos and T-2 toxin and their efficacy in preventing toxicosis, in press.
23. **Fricke, R. F. and Jorge, J. M.**, Assessment of efficacy of activated charcoal for treatment of acute T-2 toxin poisoning, *J. Toxicol., Clin. Toxicol.*, submitted.
24. **Fricke, R. F.**, unpublished observation.
25. **Poppenga, R. H., Lambert, R. J., Beasley, V. R., and Buck, W. B.**, Therapeutic efficacy of orally administered super activated charcoal in rats exposed to a lethal intravenous dose of T-2 toxin, submitted.
26. **Galey, F. D., Lambert, R. J., Busse, M., and Buck, W. B.**, Therapeutic efficacy of activated charcoal for rats exposed to oral lethal doses of T-2 toxin, *Toxicon*, 25, 493, 1987.
27. **Matsuoka, Y., Kubota, K., and Ueno, Y.**, General pharmacological studies of fusarenon-x, a trichothecene mycotoxin from *Fusarium* species, *Toxicol. Appl. Pharmacol.*, 50, 87, 1979.
28. **Munday, R.**, Studies on the mechanism of toxicity of the mycotoxin, sporidesmin. I. Generation of superoxide radical by sporidesmin, *Chem.-Biol. Interact.*, 41, 361, 1982.
29. **Tappel, A. L.**, Vitamin E and selenium protection from *in vivo* lipid peroxidation, *Ann. N.Y. Acad. Sci.*, 355, 18, 1980.
30. **Tsuchida, M., Miura, T., Shimizu, T., and Aibara, K.**, Elevation of thiobarbituric acid values in the rat liver intoxicated by T-2 toxin, *Biochem. Med.*, 31, 147, 1984.
31. **Segal, R., Milo-Goldzweig, I., Joffe, A. Z., and Yagen, B.**, Trichothecene-induced hemolysis. I. The hemolytic activity of T-2 toxin, *Toxicol. Appl. Pharmacol.*, 70, 343, 1983.
32. **Markham, R. J. F., DiNinno, V. L., Erhardt, N. P., Penman, D., and Bhatti, A. R.**, Investigation of T-2 Mycotoxin-Induced Cytotoxicity *In Vitro* and Protective Effects of Flavonoid Compounds, Suffield Memo. No. 1150, Defence Research Establishment Suffield, Ralston, Alberta, Canada, 1986.
33. **Younes, M. and Siegers, C. P.**, Inhibitory action of some flavonoids on enhanced spontaneous lipid peroxidation following glutathione depletion, *Planta Med.*, 43, 240, 1981.
34. **Ueno, Y.**, Mode of action of trichothecenes, *Pure Appl. Chem.*, 49, 1737, 1977.
35. **Ueno, Y.**, Mode of action of trichothecenes, *Ann. Nutr. Aliment.*, 31, 885, 1977.
36. **Ueno, Y., and Matsumoto, H.**, Inactivation of some thiol-enzymes by trichothecene mycotoxins from *Fusarium* species, *Chem. Pharm. Bull.*, 23, 2439, 1975.
37. **Hatch, R. C., Clark, J. D., Jain, A. V., and Mahaffey, E. A.**, Experimentally induced acute aflatoxicosis in goats treated with ethyl maleate, glutathione precursors, or thiosulfate, *Am. J. Vet. Res.*, 40, 505, 1979.
38. **Meister, A. and Anderson, M. E.**, Glutathione, *Ann. Rev. Biochem.*, 52, 711, 1983.
39. **Leaf, G. and Neuberger, A.**, The effect of diet on the glutathione content of the liver, *J. Biochem.*, 41, 280, 1974.
40. **Lauterburg, B. H. and Mitchell, J. R.**, *In vivo* regulation of hepatic glutathione synthesis: effects of food deprivation on glutathione depletion by electrophilic compounds, *Adv. Exp. Med. Biol.*, 136(Part A), 453, 1981.
41. **Bartoli, G. M. and Sies, H.**, Reduced and oxidized glutathione efflux from liver, *FEBS Lett.*, 86, 89, 1978.
42. **Emerole, G. O., Neskovic, N., and Dixon, R. L.**, The detoxication of aflatoxin B_1 with glutathione in the rat, *Xenobiotica*, 9, 737, 1979.
43. **Fricke, R. F. and Jorge, J. M.**, Effect of T-2 toxin, fasting, and 2-methyl-thiazolidine-4-carboxylate, a glutathione prodrug, on hepatic glutathione levels, *Toxicol. Appl. Pharmacol.*, submitted. 1986.
44. **Ueno, Y.**, Toxicological feature of T-2 toxin and related trichothecenes, *Fundam. Appl. Toxicol.*, 4, S124, 1984.
45. **Williamson, J. M. and Meister, A.**, Stimulation of hepatic glutathione formation by administration of L-2 oxothiazolidine-4-carboxylate, a 5-oxo-prolinase substrate, *Proc. Natl. Acad. Sci. U.S.A.*, 78, 936, 1981.
46. **Nagasawa, H. T., Goon, D. J. W., and Zera, R. T.**, Prodrugs of L-cysteine as liver-protective agents. 2-(RS)-methyl- thiazolidine-4(R)-carboxylic acid, a latent cysteine, *J. Med. Chem.*, 25, 489, 1982.

47. **Williamson, J. M., Boettcher, B., and Meister, A.,** Intracellular cysteine delivery system that protects against toxicity by promoting glutathione synthesis, *Proc. Natl. Acad. Sci. U.S.A.,* 79, 6246, 1982.

48. **Nagasawa, H. T., Goon, D. J. W., Muldoon, W. P., and Zera, R. T.,** 2-Substituted thiazolidine-4(R)-carboxylic acids as prodrugs of L-cysteine. Protection of mice against acetaminophen hepatotoxicity, *J. Med. Chem.,* 27, 591, 1984.

49. **Terol, A., Fernandez, J.-P., Robbe, Y., Chapat, J.-P., Granger, R., and Sentenac-Roumanou, H.,** Activite radioprotectrice et cinetique d'hydrolyse de phenyl-2 thiazolidines, *Eur. J. Med. Chem.,* 13, 153, 1978.

50. **Terol, A., Fernandez, J.-P., Robbe, Y., Chapat, J.-P., Granger, R., Fatome, M., Andrieu, L., and Sentenas-Roumanou, H.,** Recherche d'agents radioprotecteurs derives de la phenyl-2 thiazolidine, *Eur. J. Med. Chem.,* 13, 149, 1978.

51. **Weber, H. U., Fleming, J. F., and Miquel, J.,** Thiazolidine-4-carboxylic acid, a physiologic sulfhydryl antioxidant with potential value in geriatric medicine, *Arch. Gerontol. Geriatr.,* 1, 299, 1982.

52. **Griffith, O. W. and Meister, A.,** Potent and specific inhibition of glutathione synthesis by buthionine sulfoximine (*S-n*-butyl homocysteine sulfoximine), *J. Biol. Chem.,* 254, 7558, 1979.

53. **Fricke, R. F., Beauchamp, B., and Keeling, L.,** Effect of glutathione prodrugs on lethality of T-2 mycotoxin in mice, *Fed. Proc.,* 43, 2175, 1984.

54. **Rumack, B. H.,** Acetaminophen, in *Clinical Management of Poisoning and Drug Overdose,* Haddad, L. M. and Winchester, J. F., Eds., W.B. Saunders, Philadelphia, 1983, 562.

55. **Poppenga, R. H., Beasley, V. R., and Buck, W. B.,** Assessment of potential therapies for acute T-2 toxicosis in the rat, *Toxicon,* 25, 537, 1987.

56. **Estrela, J. M., Saez, G. T., Such, L., and Vina, J.,** The effect of cysteine and *N*-acetyl cysteine on rat liver glutathione (GSH), *Biochem. Pharmacol.,* 32, 3483, 1983.

57. **Fricke, R. F.,** Unpublished observation, 1986.

58. **Kunimoto, M., Inoue, K., and Nojima, S.,** Effects of ferrous ion and ascorbate-induced lipid peroxidation on liposomal membranes, *Biochem. Biophys. Acta,* 646, 169, 1981.

59. **Corcoran, G. B., Mitchell, J. R., Vaishnav, Y. N., and Horning, E. C.,** Evidence that acetaminophen and *N*-hydroxyacetaminophen form a common arylating intermediate, *N*-acetyl-*p*-benzoquinoneimine, *Mol. Pharmacol.,* 18, 536, 1980.

60. **Smart, R. C. and Zannoni, V. G.,** Effect of covalent binding of benzene and phenol metabolites to isolated tissue preparations, *Toxicol. Appl. Pharmacol.,* 77, 334, 1985.

61. **Johansson, I. and Ingelman-Sundberg, M.,** Hydroxyl radical-mediated cytochrome P-450 dependent metabolic activation of benzene in microsomes and reconstituted enzyme systems from rabbit liver, *J. Biol. Chem.,* 258, 7311, 1983.

62. **Fricke, R. F. and Jorge, J.,** Protective effect of asscorbic acid in decreasing T-2 toxin-induced lethality in mice, *Fed. Proc.,* 45, 574, 1986.

63. **Benedetti, J., Yuen, K., and Young, L.,** Life tables and survival K functions, in *BMDP Statistical Software,* Dixon, W. J., Brown, M. B., Engleman, L., Frane, J. W., Hill, M. A., Jennrich, R. I., and Toporek, J. D., Eds., University of California Press, Berkeley, 1984, 555.

64. **Poppenga, R. H., Beasley, V. R., and Buck, W. B.,** Assessment of ascorbic acid and dexamethasone in combination with PGE_1 for the treatment of acute T-2 toxicosis in the rat, submitted.

65. **Klaui, H. and Pongracz, G.,** Ascorbic acid and derivatives as antioxidants in oils and fats, in *Ascorbic Acid (Vitamin C),* 1st ed., Counsell, J. N. and Hornig, D. H., Eds., Applied Science Publishers, Englewood, N.J., 1981, chap. 9.

66. **Pongracz, G.,** Antioxidant activity for use in food, *Int. J. Vit. Nutr. Res.,* 43, 517, 1973.

67. **McKay, P. B. and King, M. M.,** Vitamin E: its role as a biologic free radical scavenger and its relationship to the microsomal mixed-function oxidase system, *Basic Clin. Nutr.,* 1, 289, 1980.

68. **Tappel, A. L.,** Protection against free radical lipid peroxidation reactions, *Pharmacol. Intervention Aging Process,* 97, 111, 1978.

69. **Rostock, R. A., Stryker, J. A., and Abt, A. B.,** Evaluation of high-dose vitamin E as a radioprotective agent, *Radiology,* 136, 763, 1980.

70. **Sakamoto, K. and Sukka, M.,** Reduced effect of irradiation on normal and malignant cells irradiated in mice protected with vitamin E, *Br. J. Radiol.,* 46, 538, 1973.

71. **Fricke, R. F.,** unpublished data, 1985.

72. **Slater, T. F.,** *Free Radical Mechanisms in Tissue Injury,* Vol. 1, Pion, London, 1972, chap. 5.

73. **Salocks, C. B., Hsieh, D. P. H., and Byard, J. L.,** Effects of butylated hydroxytoluene pretreatment on the metabolism and genotoxicity of aflatoxin B_1 in primary cultures of adult rat hepatocytes: selective reduction of nucleic acid binding, *Toxicol. Appl. Pharmacol.,* 76, 498, 1984.

74. **Miranda, C. L., Reed, R. L., Cheeke, P. R., and Buhler, D. R.,** Protective effects of butylated hydroxyanisole against the acute toxicity of monocrotaline in mice, *Toxicol. Appl. Pharmacol.,* 59, 424, 1981.

75. **Miranda, C. L., Henderson, M. C., Schmitz, J. A., and Buhler, D. R.,** Protective role of dietary butylated hydroxyanisole against chemical-induced acute liver damage in mice, *Toxicol. Appl. Pharmacol.,* 69, 73, 1983.
76. **Cort, W. M., Scott, J. W., Araujo, M., Mergens, W. J., Cannalonga, M. A., Osadca, M., Harley, H., Parrish, D. R., and Pool, W. R.,** Antioxidant activity and stability of 6-hydroxy-2,5,7,8-tetramethylchroman-2-carboxylic acid, *J. Am. Oil Chem. Soc.,* 53, 174, 1975.
77. **Bisby, R. H., Ahmed, S., and Cundall, R. B.,** Repair of amino acid radicals by a vitamin E analogue, *Biochem. Biophys. Res. Commun.,* 119, 245, 1984.
78. **Jarvik, M. E.,** Drugs used in the treatment of psychiatric disorders, in *The Pharmacological Basis of Therapeutics,* 4th ed., Goodman, L. S. and Gilman, A., Eds., Macmillan, New York, 1971, 155.
79. **Douglas, W. W.,** Histamine and antihistamines; 5-hydroxytryptamine and antagonists, in *The Pharmacological Basis of Therapeutics,* 4th ed., Goodman, L. S. and Gilman, A., Eds., Macmillan, New York, 1971, 621.
80. **Murphy, C. M., Ravner, H., and Smith, N. L.,** Antioxidant activity and stability of 6-hydroxy-2,5,7,8-tetramethyl-chroman-2-carboxylic acid, *Chem. Ind.,* 42, 2479, 1950.
81. **Slater, T. F.,** The inhibitory effects *in vitro* of phenothiazines and other drugs on lipid-peroxidation systems in rat liver microsomes, and their relationship to the liver necrosis produced by carbon tetrachloride, *Biochem. J.,* 106, 155, 1968.
82. **Mannering, G. J.,** Hepatic cytochrome P-450-linked drug-metabolizing systems, in *Concepts in Drug Metabolism,* Part B, Jenner, P. and Testa, B., Eds., Marcel Dekker, New York, 1981, 53.
83. **Pelkonen, O.,** Developmental drug metabolism, in *Concepts in Drug Metabolism,* Part A, Jenner, P. and Testa, B., Eds., Dekker, New York, 1981, 285.
84. **Fricke, R. F.,** unpublished observations, 1984.
85. **Kosuri, N. R.,** Toxicity of *Fusarium tricinctum* in Rats and Cattle, Ph.D. thesis, University of Wisconsin, Madison, 1969.
86. **Fricke, R. F.,** Decreased toxicity of T-2 mycotoxin in mice pretreated with microsomal inducing agents, *Fed. Proc.,* 42, 626, 1983.
87. **Fricke, R. F.,** unpublished observation, 1985.
88. **Seidegard, J., DePierre, J. W., Morgenstern, R., Pilotti, A., and Ernster, L.,** Induction of drug-metabolizing systems and related enzymes with metabolites and structural analogues of stilbene, *Biochem. Biophys. Acta,* 672, 65, 1981.
89. **Alworth, W. L., Dang, C. C., Ching, L. M., and Viswanathan, T.,** Stimulation of mammalian epoxide hydrase activity by flavones, *Xenobiotica,* 10, 395, 1980.
90. **Hammock, B. D. and Ota, K.,** Differential induction of cytosolic epoxide hydrolase, microsomal epoxide hydrolase, and glutathione S-transferase activities, *Toxicol. Appl. Pharmacol.,* 71, 254, 1983.
91. **Fricke, R.,** Effect of T-2 toxin on activities of *trans-* stilbene oxide-induced hepatic microsomal enzymes, *Toxicologist,* 6, 141, 986.
92. **Fricke, R. F.,** unpublished data, 1983.
93. **Feuerstein, G., Goldstein, D., Ramwell, P., Zerbe, R., Lux, W., Faden, A., and Bayorh, M.,** Cardiorespiratory, sympathetic and biochemical responses to T-2 toxin in the guinea pig and rat, *J. Pharmacol. Exp. Ther.,* 232, 786, 1985.
94. **Lorenzana, R. M., Beasley, V. R., Buck, W. B., and Ghent, A. W.,** Experimental T-2 toxicosis in swine. II. Effect of intravascular T-2 toxin on serum enzymes and biochemistry, blood coagulation, and hematology, *Fundam. Appl. Toxicol.,* 5, 893, 1985.
95. **Ueno, Y., Sato, N., Ishii, K., Sakai, K., Twundo, H., and Enomoto, E.,** Biological and chemical detection of *Fusarium* species, *Appl. Microbiol.,* 25, 699, 1973.
96. **Lorenzana, R. M., Beasley, V. R., Buck, W. B., Ghent, A. W., Lundeen, G. R., and Poppenga, R. H.,** Experimental T-2 toxicosis in swine. I. Changes in cardiac output, aortic mean pressure, catecholamines, 6-keto-PGF$_{1\mathrm{alpha}}$, thromboxane B$_2$, and acid-base balance, *Fundam. Appl. Toxicol.,* 5, 879, 1985.
97. **Rosenthal, R. C. and Wilcke, J. R.,** Glucocorticoid therapy, in *Current Veterinary Therapy VIII,* Kirk, R. W., Ed., W.B. Saunders, Philadelphia, 1983, 854.
98. **McDonald, L. E.,** Hormones influencing metabolism, in *Veterinary Pharmacology and Therapeutics,* 5th ed., Booth, N. H. and McDonald, L. E., Eds., The Iowa State University Press, Ames, 1982, 553.
99. **Adams, H. R. and Parker, J. L.,** Pharmacological management of circulatory shock: cardiovascular drugs and steroids, *J. Am. Vet. Assoc.,* 175, 86, 1979.
100. **Dietzman, R. H., Motsay, G., and Lillehei, R. C.,** The use of corticosteroids in the treatment of septic shock, in *Septic Shock in Man,* Hershey, S. G., Del Guercio, L. R. M., and McConn, R., Eds., Little, Brown, Boston, 1971.
101. **Telivuo, L. and Louchimo, I.,** Experimental haemorrhagic shock in rabbits, *Acta Anaesthesiol. Scand.,* 10, 1, 1965.

102. **Lefer, A. M. and Martin, J.,** Mechanism of the protective effect of corticosteroids in hemorrhagic shock, *Am. J. Physiol.,* 216, 314, 1969.

103. **Vander Vennet, K. and Schneewind, J. H.,** The effect of steroids on mortality in experimental traumatic shock, *Proc. Soc. Exp. Biol. Med.,* 109, 674, 1962.

104. **Thomas, C. S. and Brockmann, S. K.,** The role of aderenal corticosteroid therapy in *Escherichia coli* endotoxin shock, *Surg. Gynecol. Obstet.,* 126, 61, 1968.

105. **Schrauwen, E. M. and Houvenaghel, A. M.,** Endotoxin shock in the pigs beneficial effects of pretreatment with prednisolone sodium succinate, *Am. J. Vet. Res.,* 45, 1650, 1984.

106. **Ogawa, H.,** Studies on protective effects of corticosteroids against habu-venom shock in rats, *Gumma J. Med. Sci.,* 14, 60, 1965.

107. **Hankes, G. H.,** Therapy of shock: the corticosteroid question, *Vet. Clin. N. Am.,* 6, 277, 1976.

108. **Pace, J. G.,** Effect of T-2 mycotoxin on rat liver mitochondria electron transport system, *Toxicon,* 21, 675, 1983.

109. **Fricke, R. F.,** unpublished data, 1986.

110. **Spath, J. A., Jr., Gorczynski, R. J., and Lefer, A. M.,** Possible mechanisms of the beneficial action of glucocorticoids in circulatory shock, *Surg. Gynecol. Obstet.,* 137, 597, 1973.

111. **Fricke, R. F.,** Beneficial effect of dexamethasone in improving survival in acute T-2 toxicosis, *Toxicol. Appl. Pharmacol.,* 1986.

112. **Tremel, H., Strugala, G., Forth, W., and Fichtl, B.,** Dexamethasone decreases lethality of rats in acute poisoning with T-2 toxin, *Arch. Toxicol.,* 57, 74, 1985.

113. **Fricke, R. F.,** unpublished observations, 1985.

114. **Fricke, R. F.,** unpublished observations, 1985.

115. **Raflo, G. T., Wangensteen, S. L., Glenn, T. M., and Lefer, A. M.,** Mechanism of the protective effects of prostaglandins E_1 and F_{2alpha} in canine endotoxin shock, *Eur. J. Pharmacol.,* 24, 86, 1973.

116. **Machiedo, G. W., Brown, C. S., Lavigne, J. E., and Rush, B. F.,** Beneficial effect of prostaglandin E_1 in experimental hemorrhagic shock, *Surg. Gynecol. Obstet.,* 143, 433, 1976.

117. **Cosgriff, T. M., Bunner, D. P., Wannemacher, R. W., Jr., Hodgson, L. A., and Dinterman, R. E.,** The hemostatic derangement produced by T-2 toxin in guinea pigs, *Toxicol. Appl. Pharmacol.,* 76, 454, 1984.

118. **Chang, I. M., Mar, W., Kim. J. H., and Kalantari Gotvandi, H. N., and Zong, M.,** Potential antidotes for T-2 toxin poisoning, *Chem. Abst.,* 104, 225, 1986.

119. **Gyongyossy-Issa, M. I. C., Khanna, V., and Khachatourians, G. G.,** Characterization or hemolysis induced by T-2 toxin, *Biochim. Biophys. Acta,* 838, 252, 1985.

120. **Cannon, M., Smith, K. E., and Carter, J.,** Prevention by ribosome-bound nascent polyphenylalanine chains, of the functional interaction of T-2 toxin with its receptor site, *Biochem. J.,* 156, 189.

121. **Tate, W. P. and Caskey, C. T.,** Peptidyltransferase inhibition by trichodermin, *J. Biol. Chem.,* 248, 7970, 1973.

122. **Feuerstein, G., Powell, J. A., Knower, A. T., and Hunter, K. W., Jr.,** Monoclonal antibodies to T-2 toxin: *in vitro* neutralization of protein synthesis inhibition and protection of rats against lethal toxemia, *J. Clin. Invest.,* 76, 2134, 1985.

Chapter 8

CONCLUSIONS AND FUTURE DIRECTIONS FOR RESEARCH

Val R. Beasley, David L. Bunner, and Robert H. Poppenga

TABLE OF CONTENTS

I. INTRODUCTION

In recent years, our understanding of the effects of trichothecene mycotoxins has been vastly expanded, in part because of emerging recognition of the importance of the compounds as naturally occurring contaminants of grains and forages, and of late as agents allegedly used for chemical warfare. It is hoped that it will be useful to summarize some of what we believe to be the major dysfunctions involved in trichothecene toxicosis. Nevertheless, it is clear that additional investigations will be needed before we thoroughly understand the complex pathophysiology that comprises trichothecene mycotoxicosis. Indeed, one of the goals of this chapter is to illustrate some of the many gaps in our present knowledge.

II. COMPOUNDS CURRENTLY MOST IMPLICATED IN TOXICOSES

The trichothecenes comprise a large group of naturally occurring and synthetically altered compounds. The naturally occurring toxins are produced by a variety of fungi, the most widely important of which are members of the genus *Fusarium*. As analytical capability has extended to various regions of the world, so has recognition of the occurrence of trichothecene mycotoxins. The trichothecenes that have been most commonly implicated in widespread outbreaks of toxicosis include: deoxynivalenol or DON (most often produced by *F. graminearum*, recognized especially in grains of the U.S., Canada, Europe, and Japan), nivalenol (produced by *F. graminearum*, most widely recognized in Japan), and T-2 toxin (based on retrospective studies using *F. sporotrichioides* isolated in the U.S.S.R. during outbreaks of human alimentary toxic aleukia or ATA, a disease experimentally reproduced in most respects using the domestic feline as a model animal). In addition, diacetoxyscirpenol (DAS), a toxin quite similar to T-2, has been implicated in a limited number of outbreaks of livestock poisoning. Satratoxins, macrocyclic trichothecenes principally identified in straw and forages and produced by *Stachybotrys atra*, have caused serious outbreaks of stachybotryotoxicosis, especially affecting the livestock of eastern Europe. An atypical but significant trichothecene toxicosis affecting livestock of Brazil results from consumption of macrocyclic toxins. At this time it is uncertain whether the toxins are produced by *Myrothecium* fungi associated with South American plants of the *Baccharis* genus or by the plants themselves. Detailed information reflecting our current (limited) knowledge of the whereabouts of these toxins is presented in the chapter "The Natural Occurrence of Trichothecenes".

III. HUMAN EXPOSURES

Considerable retrospective evidence has linked the trichothecene mycotoxins, T-2 toxin (in particular), to the occurrence of ATA in the U.S.S.R. during the 1940s. Specific etiologic diagnosis of ATA was not possible at that time; however, the ingestion of spoiled over-wintered grain, usually over periods of weeks, was linked to the severe bone marrow depression and death that often resulted from sepsis. Diffuse vascular injury was also characteristic of the toxicosis. Some deaths probably occurred within hours to a few days from unusually high levels of exposure. Although many treatments were administered to the affected patients, long-term withdrawal from exposure to spoiled grain was of the greatest overall importance for recovery.

More recently, acute i.v. exposure of man has been described as a result of the experimental use of DAS (anguidine) as an anticancer agent. The most commonly reported manifestations of toxicosis included nausea, vomiting, hypotension, confusion, and flushing of the skin. The antitumor effect was unfortunately weak, as discussed in the chapter entitled "Anticancer Effects of Trichothecenes".

It has been suggested that long-term environmental exposure to certain *Fusaria* might be associated with human chronic illness and cancer. Carcinogenesis, however, has not been supported in most animal studies, and, for the most part, the trichothecenes appear to be only weakly mutagenic.

Samples obtained in the late 1970s and early 1980s and alleged to be the chemical warfare agent "yellow rain" were found to contain the trichothecene mycotoxins, T-2 toxin, DAS, DON, and another *Fusarium* metabolite, zearalenone. Trichothecene toxins were also found in tissues of victims of these attacks, but definitive proof that the exposures were not environmental in nature has not been produced.

A case of apparent toxicosis in humans chronically exposed to a building highly contaminated by an aerosol of mold spores bearing macrocyclic trichothecenes was recently reported in the U.S. Signs and symptoms included skin rash, hair loss, malaise, fatigue, diarrhea, and sore throat.

To our knowledge, adverse effects of recent exposures of man to trichothecene-containing foods have not been reported, but the much improved ability to detect the trichothecenes should help to clarify this risk. Ingestion of mold-damaged grain as well as dust inhalation by grain workers should be considered as potential risks. Improved clinical awareness in human medicine of the potential manifestations of trichothecene mycotoxicoses is essential. This, together with specific and sensitive assays for the trichothecene toxins, will eventually help clarify the role that these compounds play as contaminants of foods and of certain workplace and residential environments.

IV. RELATIVE TOXICITY AMONG TRICHOTHECENES

Clearly the toxicity of the trichothecene mycotoxins is widely variable whether measured by protein synthesis inhibition or lethality. The trichothecene group contains extremely toxic compounds such as some of the macrocyclic compounds, including verrucarin A and roridin A. Some of the group A toxins, such as T-2 toxin and DAS are only slightly less toxic, whereas certain trichothecenes of group A, such as trichodermin, are of low toxicity. The group B toxins, which includes DON, nivalenol, and fusarenon-X also vary widely in toxicity. For reasons not fully explained at this time, different trichothecenes inhibit different stages of peptide synthesis (as discussed in the chapter "Biochemical Mechanism of Action of Trichothecene Mycotoxins").

Structure activity studies make it clear that the epoxide in the 12,13 position is essential for both protein synthesis inhibition and whole animal toxicity, and the double bond in the 9,10 position is also important. Interestingly, in screening trichothecenes in mice for their potential as antineoplastic agents, macrocyclic trichothecenes with an epoxide at the 9,10 position were among those with the most favorable anticancer: mouse toxicity ratio. Substitution with R-groups at carbons 3 and 15 produce the most potent "initiation-like inhibiting" protein synthesis inhibitors, while substitution at carbon 4 causes the formation of somewhat less potent toxins that act as elongation or termination inhibitors. The differences in toxicity among the trichothecenes are clearly affected by the solubility and three-dimensional structure of the various compounds. Undoubtedly, the characteristics of trichothecene mycotoxins that cause variation in distribution (among organs, tissues, cells, and organelles) and metabolism deserve additional investigation in an effort to better understand the relative toxicity of these compounds.

V. NEED FOR IMPROVED SCREENING METHODS

A. Natural Exposure

It has been difficult in the past to correlate the severity of toxicosis in farm animals with the specific quantitative presence of a given trichothecene toxin. Pathways of trichothecene biosynthesis have been studied and, as one would expect, they illustrate that the toxins do not suddenly appear, but they occur as members of synthetic and degradative processes that lead to and from the individual toxins included in most assays. Unidentified toxin combinations may therefore frequently occur in trichothecene-containing materials. It has been suggested that greater than additive effects may occur when more than one trichothecene is involved; limited testing in laboratory animals has raised this question as well. Thus, one would not anticipate identical effects from a single purified trichothecene mycotoxin added to an otherwise unmodified diet, as those that occur under conditions of natural exposure that involve the same toxin coexisting with a mixture of other trichothecenes. Variation in response to these different conditions of exposure is also a likely result of other nontrichothecene mold metabolites, depletion of nutritive value of the feed as a result of mold metabolism, and other stresses related to environmental conditions. In addition, nutritional balance, infectious disease, and physiologic state are also important. Therefore, correct assessment of the spectrum of toxins present, rather than values for just one or two toxins, is essential.

There is a continuing need for both the development and increased utilization of more efficient methods to screen agricultural commodities for trichothecene mycotoxins. Undoubtedly, trichothecene metabolites and other toxins often go unrecognized when present at concentrations below the limit of detection, or when standards for the given compound are not used. One can be certain that as more sensitive methods for trichothecene screening are utilized, contamination by these compounds will be recognized much more often. As analytical methodologies improve, and as the interactions between trichothecenes are better characterized, more reliable assessment of the toxicity and hazard of naturally contaminated foodstuffs will become possible. The authors are concerned with regard to conclusive assessments of the hazards of naturally contaminated foodstuffs on the basis of analysis for one or only a few trichothecenes. Similarly, because of the interactive effects of more than one metabolite at low concentrations, the setting of detection limits of an assay at a higher than necessary level (believed by laboratory personnel to reflect an approximate minimum toxic concentration for a single compound) may ultimately result in a greater degree of confusion than reporting out a positive but low degree of trichothecene contamination. Of importance is the fact that essentially all naturally occurring trichothecenes are comparatively toxic.

An example of the value of improved analytical methodology was the recent discovery of trichothecene contamination in soybeans at the University of Illinois. The new method, developed for screening feedstuffs for trichothecenes, relied upon conversion of the toxins and their acetylated and deacetylated derivatives to their parent alcohols. When all of the closely related derivatives are converted to their fully hydroxylated form, the single parent alcohol is quantified and thereafter termed "toxin equivalents".[1] Using this technique, *Fusarium*-contaminated soybeans (from the 1986 crop in an area of the midwestern U.S.) were found to contain unexpectedly high concentrations of "T-2 toxin-equivalents" (T-2 toxin + metabolites), small amounts of "DON-equivalents", and traces of "DAS-equivalents". In addition, zearalenone and zearalenol were present. The associated soybean meal contained up to 1.4 ppm of T-2 toxin-equivalents. In the soybean hulls, which contained the greatest amount of pink discoloration, there was up to 4.6 ppm of T-2 toxin-equivalents. The T-2 toxin-equivalents were subsequently found to result primarily from HT-2 toxin contamination of the soybeans. These observations were relayed to the soybean industry so that the probability of formulation of human foods and animal feeds with toxic amounts of the contaminated beans would be reduced.

Direct and indirect competitive-type enzyme-linked immunosorbent assays (ELISA) have been developed recently for various mycotoxins, including T-2 toxin and DON.[2,3] Certain of these methods can be applied to field screening applications for rapid assessment of the hazards of naturally contaminated feeds. The above-mentioned concerns with regard to being too narrow in the spectrum of toxins detected will probably force the continued development of ELISA methods that detect more compounds. In the foreseeable future, the efficiency of these methods should be so high that they or similar technologies will be quite widely employed in the grain industry. Much will depend upon the economics and perception of need.

VI. TRICHOTHECENE FATE IN ANIMAL TISSUES

As discussed in the chapter "The Absorption, Distribution, Metabolism, and Excretion of Trichothecene Mycotoxins", toxin fate depends upon the compound(s) involved, the species of animal exposed (and the structure of its digestive system), the microorganisms that comprise the digestive tract flora, and the diet. In addition, the adequacy of liver function and interactions with other xenobiotics that influence liver metabolism are involved.

In general, the toxins appear to be slowly absorbed from the stomach, rapidly absorbed from the small intestine, and, depending in part upon polarity, are either rapidly metabolized and excreted by the liver into the bile or excreted somewhat more slowly by the kidney. Structurally simple, relatively polar compounds such as DON are excretable in significant measure without alteration or after bacterial deepoxidation, but more complex molecules, such as T-2 toxin are eliminated in only negligible amounts as parent compound. Often ester side groups are replaced with hydroxyls. Most studies suggest that as hydroxylation proceeds toxicity is eventually reduced. In the case of T-2 toxin and certain of its derivatives, P-450-mediated hydroxylation of the 3' position of the isovaleryl group is common. The toxicologic assessment of metabolites indicates that the unaltered T-2 toxin is generally at least as toxic or more toxic than metabolized forms, although initial products of esterase and P-450 enzymes tend to be almost as harmful as their parent compounds. The reader is cautioned that there is considerable variability among trichothecenes with regard to *in vivo* and *in vitro* potency, and there are notable differences in metabolic pathways for the different toxins. In certain instances, extrapolation from comparative *in vitro* assays to assumptions of relative *in vivo* toxicity can lead to erroneous conclusions.

One reason for the substantial capacity of the liver to metabolize the trichothecenes may be an increase in blood flow through the liver in the presence of these toxins. The increase in hepatic blood flow has been documented for trichothecene dosed swine as discussed in more detail in the chapter "Effects on the Digestive System and Energy Metabolism". Some species utilize hepatic glucuronide conjugation to make T-2 toxin and its derivatives more polar and thus more readily excreted. Conversely, there is evidence suggesting that glucuronide deconjugation, apparently catalyzed principally by intestinal microbes, can result in the liberation of free toxin and other epoxide-bearing (and thus still toxic) T-2 toxin metabolites. Another significant aspect is the fact that ruminal microflora, as well as the intestinal flora of some other species, are sometimes adept at causing hydrolysis of the 12,13-epoxide group which results in effective detoxification. Ultimately, the vast majority of administered toxin can be accounted for by parent compound and metabolites still bearing the trichothecene skeleton in the feces and urine.

Transmission of naturally occurring trichothecene mycotoxins into milk or meat appears unlikely to result in a toxicologically significant hazard. Caution is still advised with regard to consumption of meat, milk, or eggs from livestock or poultry that have experienced high dose exposures, at least until recovery of the animals. The presence of preexistent liver disease or mixed function oxidase inhibitors tends to increase persistence of and susceptibility to the more highly toxic trichothecenes.

Generally speaking, one would not expect to detect nonradiolabeled trichothecene metabolites in animal tissues after a few days following the last oral exposure to the toxin. Dilution of toxin in the animals' tissues in itself is likely to be very protective. Absorption of trichothecenes from the skin is considerably slower than with other routes, and local metabolism is limited.

VII. TOXIC EFFECTS

A. Interpretation of Trichothecene Effects from the Literature

In reading any paper on the trichothecenes, as well as this book, one must ask whether the study represents effects unique to the laboratory, effects that occur only under conditions of massive exposure, or effects that occur only after prolonged exposure to chronically tolerated doses. Most studies do represent one of these three extremes and often they may not reflect accurately on the others. Some of the *in vitro* concentrations probably cannot be extrapolated to any likely circumstance of exposure, while other studies using *in vitro* and *in vivo* methods may be of value in understanding massive exposure. There are studies, of course, in which the *in vitro* or *in vivo* concentrations of toxins reflect those that occur naturally, and effects have been identified, some of which are likely to be of major importance even in subclinical toxicoses.

Caution is required when comparing the effects of single doses with research involving repeated exposures (such as feeding studies) since the net effects may be quite different. Generally speaking, acute, life-threatening toxicoses as a result of single naturally occurring exposures to trichothecenes is extremely rare, although it probably did happen in the worst outbreaks of ATA, and has been reported in a minority of stachybotryotoxicosis cases in the horse.

B. Mechanism of Action Studies

Careful comparison of *in vitro* and *in vivo* data with information on fate of the trichothecene is needed to arrive at the most relevant primary mechanisms of action for the cell systems being exposed. Table 1 illustrates that low ppb concentrations of T-2 toxin are capable of significantly inhibiting protein and DNA syntheses. As discussed in the chapter ''Biochemical Mechanism of Action of Trichothecenes'', it appears that inhibition of the ribosomal enzyme, peptidyl transferase, is responsible at least in part for cessation of protein synthesis, and it has been suggested that the earliest, most sensitive cellular effect is protein synthesis inhibition. Recent studies of T-2 toxin exposed L-6 myoblasts, however, have shown identical times of onset for protein and DNA synthesis inhibition, as well as inhibition of cellular uptake of amino acids, glucose, and calcium. These effects occur in minutes at extremely low (0.0004 to 0.004 μg/ml) concentrations and support the possibility that T-2 toxin may have several parallel mechanisms of action.[4] At later time points DNA synthesis could be reduced by depletion of enzymes resulting from protein synthesis inhibition, but earlier impairment could (perhaps) be due to impaired precursor uptake or even direct nuclear effects. T-2 toxin, macrocyclic trichothecenes, and presumably other highly toxic members of the group may also *directly* affect cardiac structure and/or function (as discussed in the chapter ''Effects on the Circulatory System''). A concentration of T-2 toxin of 1 ppm reduced the amplitude of contraction of papillary muscles *in vitro*; however, in contrast to the inhibition of protein and nucleic acid syntheses and the reductions in nutrient uptake induced by T-2 toxin at ppb concentrations, and the effects on the myocardium at 1 ppm, a level of 100 ppm was necessary to cause an increase in hemolysis or changes in erythrocyte morphology.

Unlike trichothecene-sensitive ribosomal peptidyl transferase, massive concentrations (generally >1000 ppm) of T-2 toxin are required to directly inhibit most other enzymes tested to date. Thus, the toxic effects of trichothecenes may depend upon more than one mechanism of action at low doses, and additional sites may become involved as doses or *in vitro* concentrations are increased.

Table 1

Effect of interest	Authors	Cell system	T-2 (µg/ml)	Incubation time	Results
Protein synthesis inhibition in intact cell systems	Rosenstein and LaFarge-Frayssinet 1983[14]	Rat hepatoma cells Murine splenic lymphocytes	0.005	27 h 72 h	> 50% inhibition of protein synthesis
	Ueno et al., 1973[15]	Rabbit reticulocytes	0.03	N/A[a]	ID$_{50}$ for protein synthesis
		Guinea pig reticulocytes	0.007		
	Gyongyossy-Issa and Khachatourians, 1985[16]	Murine splenic lymphocytes	0.0125 or higher	24 or 48 h	Rapid and nearly complete inhibition of protein synthesis
	Trusal, 1985[17]	Chinese hamster ovary (CHO) cells or African green monkey (VERO) cells	0.01 or 1.0	1 or 12 h	> 50% inhibition of protein synthesis at both toxin concentrations in VERO cells, > 50% inhibition at 1.0 µg/ml in CHO cells
	Oldham et al., 1980[20]	Human fibroblasts	0.5	Up to 4 h	100% inhibition of protein synthesis
DNA synthesis inhibition and susceptibility to damage by T-2 toxin	Rosenstein and LaFarge-Frayssinet, 1983[13]	Rat hepatoma cell culture Murine splenic lymphocyte culture	0.005	27 h 72h	47% inhibition of DNA synthesis 99% inhibition of DNA synthesis
	Lafarge-Frayssinet et al., 1981[21]	Murine splenic cell culture	0.0005	2 or 72 h	Significant damage at both 2- and 72-h incubation times
		Murine thymic cell culture		72 h	Single strand breaks at 72 h
		Rat primary hepatocyte culture		3 h	No effect
	Munsch and Muller, 1980[22]	Human Molt$_4$ cell culture Murine Nu$_8$ cell culture	0.0005	3 d	100% inhibition of DNA synthesis-significant declines in activity of enzymes associated with DNA synthesis
	Gyongyossy-Issa and Khachatourians, 1985	Murine splenic lymphocytes	0.0125 or greater	24 — 72 h	Decrease in DNA synthesis in both PHA stimulated and nonstimulated lymphocytes
	Agrelo and Schoental, 1980[23]	Human fibroblasts	0.032 or above	1 h	> 50% inhibition of DNA synthesis
	Oldham et al., 1980[20]	Human fibroblasts	0.5	Up to 4 h	100% inhibition of DNA synthesis
Cell membrane interactions.	Tsuchida et al., 1984[24]	Rat liver microsomes	0 to 40	N/A[a]	No stimulation of enzymatic lipid peroxidation
	DeLoach et al., 1986[25]	Bovine and rat erythrocytes	20	0 — 4 h	No occurrence of "holes" in plasma membrane
			100	Up to 4 h	No hemolysis of bovine erythrocytes, whereas 30% of rat erythrocytes were hemolyzed

Table 1 (continued)

Effect of interest	Authors	Cell system	T-2 (µg/ml)	Incubation time	Results
	Gyongyossy-Issa et al., 1985[16]	Guinea pig erythrocytes	200	6 h	100% lysis by 6 h after a 2-h lag period
			800	1 h	Occurrence of "holes" in plasma membrane
	Gyongyossy-Issa et al., 1986[26]	Guinea pig erythrocytes	176 — 300	> 20 min	Increase in hemolysis
	Segal et al., 1983[27]	Rat erythrocytes	2,330	~150 min	Hemolysis of 50% of erythrocytes
			177 — 466	45 min — 4 h	No significant evidence of lipid peroxidation
	Yarom et al., 1984[28]	Human platelets	10 — 50 µg/ 10^9 cells	30 min	Cell membrane permeability changes
	Bunner and Morris 1988[4]	L-6 myoblasts	4 pg—ng/ml	10 min	Decreased uptake of calcium, potassium, glucose, and amino acids
Cell morphology	Hsia et al., 1983[29]	Human fetal esophageal epithelial tissue	0.0002 — 0.0012	4 — 6 d	Vacuolation and degeneration of rough endoplasmic reticulum and mitochondria
	Trusal, 1985[17]	CHO or VERO cells	0.01 or 1.0	1 or 12 h	CHO cells—surface blebbing, disaggregation of polysomes, mitochondrial degeneration; VERO cells—no surface blebbing, otherwise as for CHO cells
	Trusal and O'Brien, 1986[18]	Cultured rat hepatocytes	0.01 or 1.0	1 or 12 h	Degranulation of rough endoplasmic reticulum and at 1.0 µg/ml for 12 h mitochondrial degeneration
	Yarom et al., 1983[30]	Isolated perfused rat hearts	2.5	20 — 30 min perfusion	Surface blebbing or empty sarcolemmal areas, hypercontracted sarcomeres, plasma membrane damage, mitochondrial degeneration
	Yarom et al., 1984[28]	Human platelets	10 — 50/10^9 cells	20 min	Increase in number of electron opaque bodies — otherwise no changes noted
	DeLoach et al., 1986[25]	Bovine erythrocytes	100	4 h	No pathomorphologic shape changes
		Rat erythrocytes			Stomatocyte-echinocyte shape indicative of impending hemolysis

Table 1 (continued)

Effect of interest	Authors	Cell system	T-2 (µg/ml)	Incubation time	Results
	Gyongyossy-Issa et al., 1986[26]	Guinea pig erythrocytes	200	2 — 320 min	Increase in erythrocyte size—increase in number of echinocytes between 2 and 60 min incubation; after 320 min incubation, there was an increase in number of large biconcave cells
	Yarom et al., 1986[31]	Cultured rat myocardial cells	500 µg/ml perfusate	10—30 min perfusion	1 h after perfusion, cells rounded and swollen with blebbing and fragmentation
Platelet interactions	Chan and Gentry, 1984[32]	Bovine platelets	190 or greater	1 — 30 min	> 50% inhibition of platelet aggregation (inhibition was dose dependent) following stimulation by ADP or collagen
			466	6 — 7 min	> 50% inhibition of thromboxane A_2 release from platelets
	Yarom et al., 1984[28]	Human platelets	50 — 300/10⁹ cells	10 — 30 min	T-2 toxin at all concentrations inhibited aggregation stimulated by collagen, epinephrine, and arachidonate; there were no changes in intracellular Ca^{2+} content or thromboxane A_2 production
Mitochondrial electron transport	Pace, 1983[33]	Rat liver mitochondria	1,030	2 — 3 min	Toxin affected mitochondrial respiration at 1 or more sites
Enzyme interactions	Oldham et al., 1980[20]	Human fibroblasts	0.5	Up to 4 h	No effect on electrophoretic banding patterns of cytoplasmic or membrane associated proteins
	Nakamura et al., 1977[34]	Rat liver epoxide hydrolase	~7500	15 min	No inhibition of enzyme activity occurred
		Glutathione-S-transferase	~1850	3 h	No inhibition of enzyme activity occurred
	Ueno and Matsumoto, 1975[35]	Rabbit muscle creatinine phosphokinase and lactate dehydrogenase	4,700 — 14,000	N/A	When enzymes were incubated with T-2 toxin prior to addition of enzyme substrate, there was a marked decrease in enzyme activity at both concentrations
		Yeast alcohol dehydrogenase		10 min	

Table 1 (continued)

Effect of interest	Authors	Cell system	T-2 (µg/ml)	Incubation time	Results
Vasoactive actions	Bubien and Woods, 1986[36]	Isolated canine false tendon preparation including papillary muscle cells and interventricular septum cells	1	60 min suffusion	Action potential alterations which were reversible when high energy phosphate source (ATP) was added to suffusate
	Bubien and Woods, 1986[36]	Isolated perfused canine atria	30	2 h perfusion	Atrial cells showed action potential changes and sinus node cells exhibited a significant increase in cycle length; perfusion produced a reversible bradycardia
	Yarom et al., 1986[31]	Cultured rat myocardial cells	100 — 500 µg/ml perfusate	3 — 10 min perfusion	> 50% cells nonbeating 30 min after 10 min perfusion; slowing of beat rate and decrease in amplitude
			2.5 or 5	24 h	Attenuated inotropic response following addition of calcium
	Yarom et al., 1983[30]	Isolated perfused rat hearts	Concentration not given; total dose of T-2 toxin perfused = 0.5 — 0.7 mg	15 — 30 min perfusion	Decline in contractile force and amplitude; premature ventricular contractions noted
	Wilson and Gentry, 1985[6]	Bovine ear perfusion system	4.6 — 4,660	Less than 3 h	Dose-dependent increase in perfusion pressure within 1 min of start of perfusion; no change in response when receptor blockers perfused first; impairment in response of vasculature to subsequent histamine or norepinephrine perfusion

[a]   N/A: not available.

C. Effects on Energy Metabolism

As described in the chapter ''Effects on the Digestive System and Energy Metabolism'', evidence of trichothecene effects on energy metabolism is not abundant. It is clear, however, that energy utilization is impaired, at least secondarily to other biochemical or pathophysiologic effects. In acute toxicosis, shock and the associated ischemia of peripheral tissues are bound to result in decreased delivery of oxygen and nutrients, reducing energy utilization in those areas.

Glucose malabsorption and increased hepatic glucose utilization seem to take place and these may be associated with lowered blood glucose. Of course, in reviewing certain of these reports, it is important to remember that unless blood samples are collected using tubes containing an enzyme inhibitor (such as sodium fluoride), glucose concentrations may fall after withdrawal (artificially) due to ongoing metabolism by white blood cells — even if the serum has been rapidly separated.

It is plausible that some of the effects on energy metabolism may result from depletion of necessary enzymes, such as amylophosphorylase, which functions in the synthesis of glycogen. Oxygen consumption by T-2 toxin-dosed animals may increase, perhaps in response to stress, but in tissues taken from such animals, such as liver or muscle, oxygen consumption may actually decrease. Oxygen consumption in liver tissue from rats dosed with T-2 toxin was reduced when several substrates were provided, and the reduction was greatest when glucose was used. With regard to the hyperoxemia reported for T-2 toxin-dosed rats, however, recent reevaluation of the data has suggested that at least in some studies, this finding was probably an artifact induced by low core body temperature and inadequate correction of the extrapolated value of pO_2 to normal body temperature.

Although glucocorticoids are released during trichothecene toxicosis, their normal effects on energy stores seem to be disrupted. The reduction in glucose utilization by tissues requiring insulin and not in tissues independent of the hormone suggest that altered insulin concentrations or function may be involved in the defective energy metabolism by induced trichothecenes.

The appearance of creatinuria and increased serum concentrations of inorganic phosphorus may indicate depletion of tissue ATP concentrations in T-2-dosed animals. In addition, provision of ATP alleviates *in vitro* effects of T-2 toxin on the myocardium. The reduced myocardial action potentials observed may be a result of a (energy dependent) reversible decline in slow inward calcium channel conductance due to ATP depletion. After administration of a trichothecene, the metabolic rates of fasted animals declined more rapidly than in nonfasted animals; fasting clearly increases susceptibility to the toxin.

D. Sensitivity of Various Species to Trichothecenes

As discussed in some detail in the chapter "Lethal Toxicity and Nonspecific Effects", different organisms vary widely in their susceptibility to trichothecenes. Bacteria are generally only mildly susceptible to trichothecenes. There is, however, evidence of marked changes in the microflora of the GI tracts of trichothecene-exposed animals. This factor should be considered in future studies that attempt to provide an understanding of the *in vivo* capability of GI flora to metabolize these toxins. Moreover, changes in the flora, along with stress, have been suggested as possible contributors to the overall adverse effects of the toxins.[5] With regard to the systemically absorbed trichothecenes, however, it appears that any weak antibacterial effect is likely to be overshadowed by immunotoxicity and, to date, no clinically useful antibiotics have been identified from among the group. In addition, antiviral effects have been found, but unfortunately, these seem to be attributable to toxic effects on the host cells. Fungi vary in sensitivity to trichothecenes.

Arthropods and fish are susceptible to trichothecenes. The most highly studied animal species, however, are poultry, laboratory rodents, and swine. Nevertheless, all species of mammals and birds tested are susceptible at sufficient doses.

In considering differences in susceptibility, it is essential to recognize many of the inherent differences among species with regard to organ-system structure and physiology. Among domestic mammals, cattle appear to be comparatively resistant to trichothecene effects and, among the more common species of domestic poultry, chickens being raised for meat are somewhat more tolerant. Parenterally dosed ruminants appear to be somewhat more sensitive than their orally dosed counterparts. These factors probably reflect dilution in the rumen of orally exposed animals which delays absorption, as well as the above-mentioned detoxification functions of ruminal and intestinal microorganisms. No reason for the comparatively high sensitivity of pigs, horses, dogs, and cats is known other than the fact that they have a simple stomach. Similarly, no explanation is available for the higher sensitivity of turkeys when compared to chickens. Reasons for the high susceptibility of geese may be related to the esophageal effects that probably occur because of the absence of a crop and myocardial sensitivity. One contributing factor (discussed in the chapter "Effects on Hemostasis and Red Cell Production") for the tendency of mice to experience anemia after repeated exposure to T-2 toxin is the comparatively short 20 to 65 d life span of mouse erythrocytes, as compared to more than 100 d in several other species. This is not likely to be the only factor, however, and the susceptibility among erythroid cells of different species should be compared *in vitro*.

Germ-free or specific pathogen-free rabbits and guinea pigs appear to be at increased risk for T-2 toxin-induced lethality. The uniformity of dose-response in such animals, however, often tends to be greater than in other animals of the same species. Of course, the degree of uniformity in the test groups can influence the likelihood of detecting toxin effects in the experimental setting, which is a particular concern when the number of animals to be tested is small.

In summary, at this time, comparatively little information has been uncovered to explain the variation in sensitivity to trichothecenes of different species and strains of animals.

E. Effects on Appetite and the Digestive Tract

The presence of dietary contamination with toxic concentrations of trichothecene mycotoxins generally results in reduced feed intake, but usually does not cause complete feed refusal. Swine given large doses of DON commonly vomit. Under natural conditions, however, only a small fraction, if any, of the pigs of an exposed group exhibit this effect, so that the term "vomitoxin" is truly a misleading name for this compound. Animals exposed to the less toxic trichothecenes, including DON, often show little other than reduced feed intake and, perhaps, failure to thrive.

The effects of trichothecenes on appetite are likely to be due to both the central nervous system (see the chapter "Effects of Trichothecenes on the Nervous System") and local alimentary (see the chapter "Effects on the Digestive System and Energy Metabolism") effects. Calves given T-2 toxin by capsule refused grain but continued to eat hay, a reversal in usual food preference, despite the fact that no palatability problem could be involved. By contrast, feeding studies with grains contaminated by *Fusarium graminearum* have shown that after washing (and presumptive removal of DON), animals immediately began to consume grain previously refused. This seems to indicate a direct palatability effect of type B trichothecenes or some other water-soluble *Fusarium* metabolite. Other work has indicated that animals offered DON-contaminated grain initially consumed it and reductions in intake were delayed, suggesting a "learned response". At this time it is unknown whether this response was due to primary and/or secondary (perhaps in response to pharyngeal, esophageal, or abdominal discomfort) central nervous system reactions. Direct application of trichothecenes to the brain can cause a rapid reduction in feed intake. It is difficult to interpret such data, however, because of a lack of information permitting comparison to concentrations that reach the same cells in the brain under conditions of natural exposure.

With the more highly toxic trichothecenes, such as T-2 toxin, and the (macrocyclic) satratoxins, oral and pharyngeal necrosis, sometimes with significant bacterial colonization, has been observed in a range of mammalian and avian species. These oral and pharyngeal lesions as well as the GI tract hemorrhage, mucosal damage, and local lymphoid necrosis are likely to greatly diminish an animal's tendency to eat.

Since DON often causes a reduction in feed intake, but almost never causes severe GI lesions under conditions of natural exposure, some mechanisms affecting appetite probably vary among animals poisoned by different trichothecenes. In swine, which appear to be quite sensitive to the anorexic effects of DON, the only lesion that has been documented in response to this toxin with any consistency whatsoever, under conditions resembling natural exposure, is mild hyperkeratosis of the esophageal portion of the stomach.

One of the major economic manifestations of trichothecene mycotoxin exposure is reduced weight gain. This is, in part, a result of the above-mentioned reduction in feed intake and, at sufficient doses, actual weight loss may occur. Changes in feed conversion are more variable: sometimes a reduction occurs, but in other instances, no changes have been detected despite reduced intake and growth rate. Animals sometimes develop a degree of tolerance with prolonged exposure, but replacement of the contaminated feed with clean feed is indicated for all clinically or subclinically poisoned animals. Supplementation with additional protein is also warranted in view of studies indicating increased tolerance of laboratory animals given additional protein.

GI upset, vomiting, and diarrhea are often observed in acute trichothecene toxicosis. As discussed in the chapter "Effects on the Digestive System and Energy Metabolism," there is no convincing evidence of a direct local effect of the toxins on GI motility and the viscera seems to retain the ability to respond to agonists. Diarrhea, which is frequently observed in acutely poisoned animals, may be the result of the combined effects of mucosal damage, fluid loss into the gut, and altered motility. Effects on GI blood flow are also likely to be of importance in acute toxicosis as described below and in the chapter "Effects on the Circulatory System".

F. Nervous System Effects

As discussed in the chapter "Effects of Trichothecene Mycotoxins on the Nervous System", numerous manifestations potentially associated with the nervous system have been observed in trichothecene-exposed humans and other animals; however, such clinical signs and symptoms as ataxia, apparent weakness, headache, confusion, and hallucinations could be secondary to hypotension, disruption of energy metabolism, hemorrhage into the brain, or even sepsis. Hypothesized effects on thermoregulation remain to be proven. Hypothermia sometimes observed in acute trichothecene toxicosis could be a result of shock, and the occasional hyperthermia could be due to agitation or compensatory responses (exaggerated respiration in an attempt to compensate for acidosis) of the test animal or bacterial invasion from the damaged intestinal tract.

Recent work with animals experiencing acute T-2 toxicosis has indicated that central nervous system involvement is significant, as reflected in part by the associated sympathoadrenal activation. In addition, increased production of PGE_2 in the brain may occur in trichothecene toxicosis and this may be related to the observed autonomic effects in both the digestive (altered motility, etc.) and circulatory (vasoconstriction, accelerated heart rate) systems.

G. Effects on the Circulatory System

Sufficient local concentrations of trichothecene mycotoxins are capable of causing vascular damage. Of course, parenchymal damage in an organ may secondarily impede blood flow or even result in destruction of the associated vascular beds. In view of some of the studies involving trypan blue dye and some of the reports of vascular damage in T-2-dosed laboratory animals, however, it appears likely that vascular damage may make a significant contribution to trichothecene-associated tissue damage and even hemorrhage. Indeed, vascular necrosis seems to predate necrosis of other cells in skin topically exposed to T-2 toxin. A study by Wilson and Gentry[6] also suggested direct vascular constriction as well as interference with responses to normal vascular control mechanisms. Moreover, if direct vascular damage or dysfunction is a predominant effect of trichothecenes, this may help to explain the release of certain prostaglandins, and the association of gastric, pancreatic, and splenic damage with local deprivation of blood flow. Recent data[37] indicate an absence of alterations in vascular permeability in the brains of trichothecene-dosed animals when evaluated by a similar serum protein-bound dye technique. Certainly, further investigation of direct trichothecene-induced vs. secondary vascular damage is called for.

The hemodynamic effects of high doses of trichothecenes are well documented. In acute trichothecene toxicoses, shock occurs, and the associated reductions in cardiac output and aortic pressure are accompanied by the elaboration of catecholamines. Blood is shunted away from the periphery and toward the brain, heart, liver, and intestine. Increased vagal tone (perhaps due to stimulation of the chemoreceptor trigger zone and secondarily the emetic center) may be associated with vomiting, but this remains to be conclusively proven. What role, if any, that increased vagal tone may play in the hypotension often seen in acute trichothecene toxicosis remains to be investigated. Clearly, the heart retains some responsiveness to adrenergic stimulation until late in the acute toxic syndrome.

Episodes of acute toxicosis are capable of damaging the myocardium. The relative significance of direct myotoxicity-, local vascular-, and shock-associated effects remains speculative, but trichothecenes do not appear to be concentrated to a great degree in the myocardium. As discussed previously, some of the adverse effects of trichothecenes on the heart may be a result of depletion of ATP and an associated reduction in calcium channel conductance. For the most part, doses that produce cardiac lesions *in vivo* are lower than concentrations producing dysfunction or damage *in vitro*. This suggests the need to study trichothecene $\pm$ catecholamines $\pm$ other products of circulatory shock (lactic acid, thromboxane, prostacyclin, other prostanoids, myocardial depressant factor, etc.) in an attempt to understand the pathogenesis of the myocardial lesions. The reason for the apparently great sensitivity of the goose to trichothecene-induced cardiotoxicity also deserves to be investigated.

H. Immunomodulatory Effects of Trichothecenes

The importance of the trichothecenes as immunosuppressive agents in many instances of exposure is difficult to judge. Laboratory studies (see the chapter "The Immunotoxicity of Trichothecene Mycotoxins") indicate that, in many experimental settings, immune parameters are depressed, but occasionally (as in the case of doses that damage T-suppressor cells) immune responses are stimulated. Nevertheless, under conditions of natural exposure and in several studies involving simultaneous exposure of animals to trichothecenes and pathogens, it appears that immunosuppression, and not immunostimulation, is of primary importance. The best documented immunosuppressive effects of naturally occurring trichothecene exposure are those that were associated epidemiologically with ATA of humans. Indeed, in ATA, sepsis was a major cause of death. In view of the relative susceptibility of cells of the immune system to trichothecenes, and studies indicating enhanced lethality from simultaneous exposure to infectious agents, this effect is likely to be a major factor in many instances of chronic, subclinical toxicosis due to the more toxic membranes of this group. Immunosuppression as a result of exposure to DON has not been adequately investigated, but it is likely to be a less potent immunomodulatory agent than T-2 toxin. One aspect of trichothecene mycotoxicosis that has often been ignored and that may deserve additional consideration is immunosuppression that results, not from the primary effects of trichothecenes themselves, but from the endogenous production of corticosteroids secondary to tissue damage.

I. Effects on Coagulation of Blood

It seems that the ability of trichothecenes to cause hemorrhage has been debated more than virtually any of the other effects of these toxins. It is clear, however, that T-2 toxin does reduce the activities of clotting proteins and interferes with platelet functions as well. In addition, the toxins can, at least in some species, cause bone marrow suppression and platelet depletion, as observed in cats given T-2 toxin and humans experiencing ATA. In addition, hemorrhage has been observed in animals with experimental trichothecene toxicosis. Despite the failure of some studies to reproduce the hemorrhagic syndrome associated with exposure of livestock to the more highly toxic trichothecenes, the authors are of the opinion that naturally occurring cases of toxicosis are likely to be accompanied by hemorrhage from time to time. Also, it is common for research scientists to have difficulty reproducing all the conditions that contribute to any disease manifestation observed in the field. The experimental failure to induce hemorrhage in livestock may be analogous to the therapeutic use of anticoagulants in human patients in which hemorrhage is avoided, although clotting is nevertheless impaired. On the whole, the authors suggest that when hemorrhage occurs, it is not likely to be the only manifestation of T-2 toxin toxicosis in livestock, and other clinical effects will often be noted in the clinical picture.

In cases of peracute administration of single, life-threatening doses of trichothecenes, the actual mechanism for the hemorrhage sometimes observed remains speculative. It appears that the tendency for trichothecene toxicosis to cause hemorrhage varies widely as a result of major differences between toxins and between the species of animals exposed. The more highly toxic trichothecenes are more likely to induce hemorrhage than are less toxic members of the group, and the more susceptible species of animals appear to include humans, cats, and mice.

J. Effects on the Skin

The chapter entitled "Effects on the Integumentary System" describes the dermal manifestations of the trichothecenes after both local and systemic administration. When applied to the skin, the toxins cause "irritation". This has led to several animal-based bioassay techniques using skin reactions after topical application. Distinct differences exist between species with regard to the ability to produce systemic effects after topical application. Humans are clearly sensitive to the local effects of concentrated solutions of trichothecenes, as indicated by numerous reports pertaining to laboratory accidents. *In vitro* studies suggest that human epidermis is not a particularly effective barrier to T-2 toxin and is comparable to several rodent animal models. Using rodent-based systems, excellent correlation has been found between *in vitro* and *in vivo* models of dermal absorption. Laboratory animals experience much more severe systemic reactions than pigs, and this is apparently related to more rapid penetration of the skin.

Cutaneous and mucous membrane reactions can be of value diagnostically in those areas (i.e., perioral, oral, pharyngeal) which are exposed to either contaminated foodstuffs or bedding straw containing the more highly toxic trichothecenes. Such lesions are not, however, encountered in all instances of trichothecene toxicosis, even with the more acutely toxic members of the group. With DON, such lesions are not likely under conditions of natural exposure.

After topical administration, the skin is a site of gradual esterase metabolism of trichothecenes. In addition, the underlying dermis and fat may serve as a depot after absorption. It appears that mediators of inflammation, such as histamine from mast cells, are involved in the cutaneous reaction to trichothecenes. Ongoing studies will help to confirm whether the initial toxic effect of T-2 toxin occurs in the vasculature of the skin with secondary effects on other structures vs. primary necrosis of the adjacent structures with secondary damage to the vasculature. As mentioned above, this consideration deserves to be investigated with regard to certain other trichothecene-sensitive tissues.

After systemic administration of sufficient doses, abnormalities in the integument, such as "rough hair coat" in mammals and abnormal feathers in birds may sometimes be observed.

K. Depression of Red Blood Cell Production

T-2 toxin has been studied for its effects on red blood cell production since anemia not attributable to hemorrhage has been observed in exposed animals and in human victims of ATA. This effect, much like that of platelet depletion, is somewhat species specific. Perhaps partially because of the short erythrocyte life span (mentioned above), mice are one of the more consistently susceptible animals to trichothecene-associated anemia, and young mice are more sensitive than mature individuals. Despite the continued intake of T-2 toxin, with time, both mice and cats have demonstrated the ability to resume hematopoiesis. At least in the mice, recovery coincided with hepatic enlargement, which was a probable manifestation of associated enzyme induction and accelerated detoxification of the T-2 toxin. The bone marrow of dogs appears to be quite sensitive to acutely toxic doses of DAS.

L. Effects on Reproduction

The reproductive toxicity of the trichothecenes cannot be ignored (as described in the chapter "Reproductive Toxicology of Trichothecenes"). Egg production may be reduced in birds exposed to the more highly toxic trichothecenes and fertility and hatchability of laid eggs may decline. Reversibility of the adverse reproductive effects seems to vary. Female chickens and turkeys have demonstrated the ability to recover function. Female swine may remain fertile after a single abortifacient dose, but become sterile after repeated exposure to a diet highly contaminated with T-2 toxin. In some instances, there has been atrophy of the reproductive tracts of female swine. In other studies, the reproductive effects of trichothecenes have been life-threatening, as in the case of female mice that appeared to die as a result of placental hemorrhage.

Trichothecenes at sufficient doses can cause damage to the testicles of male turkeys. Similarly, laboratory rodents have experienced sterility and degeneration of the spermatogenic cells of the seminiferous tubules after exposure to trichothecenes.

Pups born of DON-exposed rats grew at a slower rate than unexposed controls and cross fostering did not alleviate the effect, indicating a lasting manifestation of *in utero* exposure. Because of the widespread occurrence of DON, further study of this manifestation, using food animal species, is needed. Maternally toxic doses may also be embryotoxic and malformations may occur in animals exposed *in utero*, particularly with regard to the brain and skeletal system. Although confirmatory studies are called for, generally speaking, sterility, embryotoxicity, and teratogenesis caused by the trichothecenes would not be expected to be a major problem unless toxic effects are also observed in the parent stock.

M. Effects on the Respiratory Tract

As discussed in the chapter "Acute Respiratory Tract Toxicity of the Trichothecene Mycotoxin, T-2 Toxin", victims of ATA developed lesions not only of the fingers and mouth, but also of the nose. In addition, naturally occurring dusts containing *Stachybotrys* organisms have been associated with burning of the nasal passages, bloody nasal discharges, coughing, and a variety of other complaints.[7,8] These effects have never been regarded as the predominant manifestations of trichothecenes and, therefore, have not been seriously investigated in the laboratory. Allegations of human exposure to trichothecenes in the form of a chemical-warfare agent have, however, resulted in some recent investigations of inhalation toxicity.

It appears that at least in small laboratory animals, the respiratory tract toxicity of T-2 toxin is quite concentration-dependent. Of note was the finding, with rats, mice, and guinea pigs, that lethal toxicity by the respiratory route was 2 to 20 times of that after parenteral exposure. Perhaps because of a longer residence time in the lung, a saline suspension of T-2 toxin by inhalation was approximately twice as toxic as an equivalent inhaled dose of the toxin in ethanol. Death was also much more rapid after aerosol administration of the saline suspension (2 h as opposed to 8 to 12 h after parenteral dosing). At higher doses, T-2 toxin in ethanol was also capable of causing death within 2 h. Even though exposure of the lower respiratory tract to a high T-2 toxin burden was followed by a much more rapid onset of death, there was no evidence of altered blood gas exchange and blood oxygen levels remained normal. The lower toxin burden presumably permits redistribution to the rest of the body and was associated with lesser toxicity; when it occurred, death took place at later times (similar in onset to that after systemic administration). Despite the trends in response with regard to lethality, pulmonary lesions were not marked regardless of the manner of administration, and lesions in other tissues were similar to those after i.v. dosing. In other studies, assessment of rat pulmonary macrophages exposed to T-2 toxin *in vitro* indicated that both protein synthesis and phagocytic activity were quite sensitive to 10^{-7} *M* (46.25 ppb) concentrations of the toxin.[9]

When swine were exposed to T-2 toxin via nebulization of an ethanol solution with the addition of sufficient dilution air to result in inhalation of respirable particles of crystalline T-2 toxin, the effects again most closely resemble systemic administration. Considering the estimated retained dose, the toxicity after inhalation exposure was similar to that after p.o. or i.v. administration. Lung lesions were mild and pulmonary failure did not occur even when swine succumbed to lethal toxicoses after inhalation exposure. The exposure protocol, however, did not involve administration of extremely high mass concentrations of aerosol, so that we did not determine whether more rapid death would result as with the rodents. After inhalation administration of a sublethal dose of the toxin, swine experienced mild, patchy to diffuse, interstitial pneumonia and a degree of decreased systemic and pulmonary immune function. The edema, fibrin deposition, and debris in the affected areas of the lung were indicative of both vascular and alveolar damage.

N. Trichothecenes as Potential Anticancer Drugs

DAS was selected for clinical anticancer trials because it was effective in screening tests against leukemia using the mouse P388 model system. More recently, a great many trichothecene derivatives have been synthesized and tested in the laboratory for use as potential anticancer drugs (as detailed in the chapter "Anticancer Properties of Trichothecenes"). Although some have shown promise, relatively few have had substantive benefit *in vivo*, in part because of the inherent toxicity of many of the trichothecenes. When the prototype (naturally occurring) compound, DAS (anguidine), was given to human cancer patients, toxic (and sometimes lethal) effects clearly outweighed any benefit. Cancers caused by (lymphoid) cell types, which are likely to be among the most sensitive to trichothecenes, were not chosen for these studies, and cell types not known to be particularly sensitive, were studied in some detail. Some of the more recently synthesized compounds have improved efficacy and safety in laboratory animals as compared to DAS, and these and other compounds may deserve additional trials in test animals. Perhaps of much greater importance in the foreseeable future is the possibility that the inherently potent toxicity of some of the 12,13-epoxytrichothecenes could be exploited in combination with antibodies against cancer cell components, to create so-called "magic bullet" chemotherapeutic agents.

O. Similarities to and Differences from Radiation Injury

The term "radiomimetic" has been used a great deal with regard to the effects of trichothecene mycotoxins. Clearly, there are some important similarities between radiation- and trichothecene-induced injury. Perhaps the most radiosensitive of cells are the lymphocytes,[10] and at least after acutely toxic doses, the lymphocytes are among those cells most sensitive to trichothecene mycotoxins. In T-2 toxin-dosed pigs, lymphoid necrosis has been observed as early as 1 h postdosing; similarly, radiation can cause lymphoid necrosis within 1 h.[11] Moreover, in our work with swine, as in radiation damage,[11] the proportion of fragmented to intact lymphocytes was far less in the thymus than in other lymphoid tissues. Further, the precursors of granulocytes and erythrocytes and cells of the gut mucosae are more resistant than lymphoid cells, but are still sensitive to both radiation and trichothecene poisoning.

Many of the clinical manifestations of acute radiation toxicosis are similar to those induced by highly toxic doses of trichothecene mycotoxins. These include: tremors, vomiting, repeated evacuation of the bowel, watery diarrhea, and agitation alternating with apathetic behavior, ataxia, and coma. Also, some of the prolonged effects of radiation injury resemble the effects of *repeated* exposure to the more highly toxic trichothecene mycotoxins. Included are pharyngitis, immunosuppression, thrombocytopenia, and anemia.

Some *key differences* between the *syndromes* induced by radiation and those caused by trichothecenes also exist. Convulsive seizures, reported with severe radiation poisoning, are extremely rare with trichothecene toxicosis. Also, in our T-2 toxin-dosed pigs, both germinal cells and mature GI epithelial cells were often damaged, whereas with radiation, the germinal cells are consistently most sensitive to injury. In addition, unlike radiation, trichothecene mycotoxins are not consistently mutagenic (as described in the chapter "Mutagenicity and Carcinogenicity of T-2 Toxin"), which is in agreement with our knowledge of the differences in sites of action.

Another distinct difference between the manifestations of T-2 toxicosis and those attributable to radiation injury is revealed by the fact that radiation poisoning is commonly evaluated in terms of 30-d LD_{50} doses.[10-12] Obviously, therefore, death after single doses of radiation may occur instantaneously or occur after a prolonged delay. In contrast, the administration of a single dose of a trichothecene mycotoxin is almost always followed either by death or relatively complete recovery within several days.

P. Proposed Association with Leukoencephalomalacia

Although a recent report has alleged that both fescue foot of cattle and leukoencephalomalacia of horses[13] are manifestations of T-2 toxicosis, we remain skeptical. To our knowledge, neither disease has been reproduced using trichothecenes in the laboratory, and in the case of the former, ergot alkaloid-like compounds are more plausible and have been found in endophyte-infected fescue. Also, cattle repeatedly given either oral or parenteral doses of T-2 toxin failed to display any lesions similar to fescue foot. In addition, leukoencephalomalacia has been reproduced by workers[38] who have reported that the implicated organisms (strains of *Fusarium moniliforme*) do not produce T-2 toxin.

VIII. THERAPY FOR TRICHOTHECENE MYCOTOXICOSIS

Therapy for trichothecene mycotoxicosis has been, until recently, limited to symptomatic measures. Probably because of bone marrow suppression and immunosuppression, victims of ATA sometimes appeared to benefit from blood transfusions and antibacterials. Vitamins and calcium were also given but were not proven to be of benefit. For chronic trichothecene exposure in any species, provision of a highly nutritious diet may be of value and is supported by the increased lethality associated with fasting. Termination of exposure is perhaps the most essential aspect of dealing with an outbreak of naturally occurring trichothecene toxicosis.

Animals with increased activity of mixed function oxidase enzymes are more tolerant of T-2 toxin, while those with inhibited activity are more susceptible. These findings are compatible with the known pathways of metabolism of this toxin. Pretreatment of mice with agents that induce epoxide hydrolase also induced a degree of resistance.

After oral exposure to acutely toxic doses of trichothecenes, the use of adsorbents such as activated charcoal or certain resins is of value. If the administration of activated charcoal is delayed over a period of hours, its benefit is gradually diminished. Activated charcoal appears to be of significant therapeutic value even after parenteral exposure to T-2 toxin. Overall, these observations are compatible with evidence indicating that T-2 toxin is comparatively slowly adsorbed from the stomach, that it undergoes enterohepatic recycling, and that it has an affinity for the adsorbents. Limiting dermal exposure by washing with soap or a detergent, or adsorption onto activated charcoal is also warranted.

The primary emphasis of recent therapeutic investigations has been in the screening of drugs to alleviate acute toxicosis due to the trichothecenes. To date, glucocorticosteroids have proven to be the agents most consistently beneficial in alleviation of the life-threatening systemic effects of *absorbed* trichothecenes. Whether these drugs act principally by virtue of stabilization of lysosomal membranes, by improving energy metabolism, by enhancement of circulation in the microvasculature, or by other effects is unclear at this time. Recent data[39] have indicated that at least some of the organs (stomach and spleen) are less damaged by T-2 toxin when the animals are given a corticosteroid, while others (gut) experience no apparent benefit. This may be compatible with a glucocorticoid-induced improvement in vascular integrity in (and perfusion of) organs otherwise deprived of blood supply during T-2 toxicosis.

One or two pharmacologic doses of a potent glucocorticosteroid seem to be more effective than multiple doses. Nonsteroidal anti-inflammatory drugs should not be used as a substitute for the glucocorticosteroids. It is important to recognize that there are no data to indicate that anti-inflammatory drugs of any kind are indicated in subacute or chronic toxicosis. In view of the immunosuppressive effects of both the more highly toxic trichothecenes and the glucocorticoids, additive or synergistic toxicity appears likely.

In addressing a patient with acute trichothecene toxicosis, it also makes sense to provide support in the form of correction of the metabolic acidosis and i.v. fluids, perhaps including dextrans, to lessen hypotension. Humans who had been given anguidine and developed hypotension were treated with apparent success with i.v. fluids and dopamine.

Glutathione prodrugs may be of some value for trichothecene-exposed animals. Benefit from the use of antioxidants has been inconsistent. Vitamin C seems to be efficacious in mice but not rats and vitamin E, but not a water-soluble analog, has been effective as a pretreatment. Butylated hydroxytoluene is also effective as a pretreatment, but as with vitamin E, it does not appear to be of great benefit when administered after the T-2 toxin exposure.

Monoclonal antibodies to T-2 toxin are an effective experimental therapy, although the spectrum of trichothecenes to which the antibodies bind is thus far limited to this toxin and closely related derivatives.

Practically speaking, the approaches to a subacutely or chronically exposed individual are quite different from that needed for an acutely poisoned victim. For chronically exposed animals, the usual approach should include a change to a highly nutritious diet which is free from significant concentrations of trichothecenes or other mycotoxins, minimization of stresses, and control of any infectious diseases. For humans, in addition to the above measures, anemia should also be treated as needed by means of blood transfusions. For acutely poisoned individuals, oral activated charcoal, i.v.-administered glucocorticosteroids, and supportive therapy for shock and metabolic acidosis should be instituted. If available, specific monoclonal antibody therapy should be used.

IX. DIRECTIONS FOR FUTURE RESEARCH

The role that trichothecenes might play in agriculture and the occurrence and epidemiology of intoxications in both veterinary and human medicine can now be explored more easily using readily available analytical chemistry and immunologic methods to detect not only the principle trichothecene toxins, but certain of their metabolites as well. The considerable difficulties in unraveling the mechanisms of *in vivo* toxicosis should be aided by careful study of known *in vitro* actions with focused *in vivo* models.

Present data suggest the possibility of multiple simultaneous effects on many cellular processes, including not only protein synthesis inhibition but impaired RNA and DNA synthesis and impaired cell membrane transport of calcium, potassium, glucose, and amino acids. Direct and indirect cardiovascular effects may also occur, and some of the latter reflect central nervous system reactions.

Depletion of specific important proteins may play an important role in the toxicity of trichothecenes *in vivo*, but this concept needs documentation. Certainly coagulation factor activities are reduced within hours, but actual quantification of the proteins (rather than activity alone) has not been accomplished.

Mechanisms of action in different species and at different doses may also vary. Chronic exposure with bone marrow suppression, for example, probably results from a different direct mechanism of action than that causing hypotension after acute high dose exposure. The relationships between dose, timing of exposure, specific mechanisms of action, and the time course of toxicosis need to be studied in concert to appreciate *in vivo* interrelationships. Such efforts are likely to present a continuing challenge for the foreseeable future.

REFERENCES

1. **Rood, H. D., Buck, W. B., and Swanson, S. P.,** Gas chromatographic screening method for T-2 toxin, diacetoxyscirpenol, deoxyvalenol and related trichothecenes in feeds, *J. Assoc. Off. Anal. Chem.,* 71, 493, 1988.
2. **Gendloff, E. H., Pestka, J. J., Swanson, S. P., and Hart, L. P.,** Detection of T-2 toxin in *Fusarium sporotrichiodes*-infected corn by enzyme-linked immunosorbent assay, *Appl. Environ. Microbiol.,* 47, 1161, 1984.
3. **Warner, R., Ram, B. P., Hart, C. P., and Pestka, J. J.,** Screening for zearalenone in corn by competitive direct enzyme-linked immunosorbent assay, *J. Agric. Food Chem.,* 34, 714, 1986.
4. **Bunner, D. L., and Morris, E. R.,** Alteration of multiple cell membrane functions in L-6 myoblasts by T-2 toxin: an important mechanism of action, *Toxicol. Appl. Pharmacol.,* 92, 113, 1988.
5. **Tenk, I., Fodor, E., and Szathmary, C. S.,** The effect of pure *Fusarium* toxins (T-2, F-2, DAS) on the microflora of the gut and on plasma glucocorticoid levels in rat and swine, *Zentralbl. Bakteriol. Hyg., I. Abt. Orig. A,* 252, 384, 1982.
6. **Wilson, D. J. and Gentry, P. A.,** T-2 toxin can cause vasoconstriction in an *in vitro* bovine ear perfusion system, *Toxicol. Appl. Pharmacol.,* 70, 159, 1985.
7. **Andrassy, K., Horvath, I., Lakos, T., and Toke, Z.,** Mass incidence of mycotoxicoses in Hajdu-Bihar county, *Mykosen,* 23, 130, 1979.
8. **Croft, W. A., Jarvis, B. B., and Yatawara, C. S.,** Airborne outbreak of trichothecene toxicosis, *Atmos. Environ.,* 20, 549, 1986.
9. **Sorenson, W. G., Gerberick, G. F., Lewis, D. M., and Castranova, V.,** Toxicity of mycotoxins for the rat pulmonary macrophage *in vitro*, Environ. Health Perspect., 66, 45, 1986.
10. **Alexander, P.,** *Atomic Radiation and Life,* Penguin Books, Baltimore, 1965.
11. **Yoffey, J. M. and Courtice, F. C.,** *Lymphatics, Lymph and Lymphoid Tissue,* Harvard University Press, Cambridge, MA, 1956, 510.
12. **Pizzarello, D. J. and Witcovski, R. L.,** *Basic Radiation Biology,* Lea & Febiger, Philadelphia, 1967, 301.
13. **Gabal, M. A., Awad, Y. L., Morcos, M. B., Barakat, A. M., and Malik G.,** Fusariotoxicoses of farm animals and mycotoxic leukoencephalomalacia of the equine associated with the finding of trichothecenes in feedstuffs, *Vet. Hum. Toxicol.,* 28, 207, 1986.
14. **Rosenstein, Y. and Lafarge-Frayssinet, C.,** Inhibitory effect of *Fusarium* T-2 toxin on lymphoid DNA and protein synthesis, *Toxicol. Appl. Pharmacol.,* 70, 283, 1983.
15. **Ueno, Y., Nakajima, M., Sakai, K., Ishii, K., Sato, N., and Shimada, N.,** Comparative toxicology of trichothec mycotoxins: inhibition of protein synthesis in animal cells, *J. Biochem.,* 74, 285, 1973.
16. **Gyongyossy-Issa, M. I. C. and Khachatourians, G. G.,** Interaction of T-2 toxin and murine lymphocytes and the demonstration of a threshold effect on macromolecular synthesis, *Biochim. Biophys. Acta,* 844, 167, 1985.
17. **Trusal, L. R.,** Morphological changes in CHO and VERO cells treated with T-2 mycotoxin: correlation with inhibition of protein synthesis, *Cell Biochem. Funct.,* 3, 205, 1985.
18. **Trusal, L. R. and O'Brien, J. C.,** Ultrastructural effects of T-2 mycotoxin on rat hepatocytes *in vitro*, *Toxicon,* 24, 481, 1986.
19. **Cundliffe, E. and Davies, J. E.,** Inhibition of initiation, elongation, and termination of eukaryotic protein synthesis by trichothecene fungal toxins, *Antimicrob. Agents Chemother.,* 11, 491, 1977.

20. **Oldham, J. W., Allred, L. E., Milo, G. E., Kindig, O., and Capen, C. C.,** The toxicological evaluation of the mycotoxins T-2 and T-2 tetraol using normal human fibroblasts *in vitro, Toxicol. Appl. Pharmacol.,* 52, 159, 1980.
21. **LaFarge-Frayssinet, C., DeCloitre, F., Mousset, S., Martin, M., and Frayssinet, C.,** Induction of DNA single-strand breaks by T-2 toxin, a trichothecene metabolite of *Fusarium, Mutat. Res.,* 88, 115, 1981.
22. **Munsch, N. and Muller, W. E. G.,** Effects of T-2 toxin on DNA polymerases and terminal deoxynucleotidyl transferse of Molt$_4$ and Nu$_8$ cell lines, *Immunopharmacology,* 2, 313, 1980.
23. **Agrelo, C. G. and Schoental, R.,** Synthesis of DNA in human fibroblasts treated with T-2 toxin and HT-2 toxin (the trichothecene metabolites of *Fusarium* species) and the effects of hydroxyurea, *Toxicol. Lett.,* 5, 155, 1980.
24. **Tsuchida, M., Miura, T., Shimizu, T., and Albara, K.,** Elevation of thiobarbituric acid values in the liver intoxicated by T-2 toxin, *Biochem. Med.,* 31, 147, 1984.
25. **DeLoach, J. R., Andrews, K., and Naqi, A.,** Interaction of T-2 toxin with bovine carrier erythrocytes: effects on cell lysis, permeability, and entrapment, *Toxicol. Appl. Pharmacol.,* 88, 123, 1986.
26. **Gyongyossy-Issa, M. I. C., Khanna, V., and Khachatourians, G. G.,** Changes induced by T-2 toxin in the erythrocyte membrane, *Food Chem. Toxicol.,* 24, 311, 1986.
27. **Segal, R., Milo-Goldzweig, I., Joffe, A. Z., and Yagen, B.,** Trichothecene-induced hemolysis. I. The hemolytic activity of T-2 toxin, *Toxicol. Appl. Pharmacol.,* 70, 343, 1983.
28. **Yarom, R., More, R., Eldor, A., and Yagen, B.,** The effect of T-2 toxin on human platelets, *Toxicol. Appl. Pharmacol.,* 73, 210, 1984.
29. **Hsia, C., Tzian, B., and Harris, C. C.,** Proliferative and cytotoxic effects of *Fusarium* T-2 toxin on cultured human fetal esophagus, *Carcinogenesis,* 4, 1101, 1983.
30. **Yarom, R., More, R., Raz, S., Shimoni, Y., Sarel, O., and Yagen, B.,** T-2 toxin effect on isolated perfused rat hearts, *Basic Res. Cardiol.,* 78, 623, 1983.
31. **Yarom, R., Hasin, Y., Raz, S., Shimoni, Y., Fixler, R., and Yagen, B.,** T-2 toxin effect on cultured myocardial cells, *Toxicol. Lett.,* 31, 1, 1986.
32. **Chan, P. K.-C. and Gentry, P. A.,** Inhibition of bovine platelet function by T-2 toxin, HT-2 toxin, diacetoxyscirpenol and deoxynivalenol, *Food Cosmet. Toxicol.,* 22, 643, 1984.
33. **Pace, J. G.,** Effect of T-2 mycotoxin on rat liver mitochondria electron transport system, *Toxicon,* 21, 675, 1983.
34. **Nakamura, Y., Ohta, M,. and Ueno, Y.,** Reactivity of 12,13-epoxytrichothecenes with epoxide hydrolase, glutathione-s-transferase and glutathione, *Chem. Pharm. Bull.,* 25, 3410, 1977.
35. **Ueno, Y. and Matsumoto, H.,** Inactivation of some thiolenzymes by trichothecene mycotoxins from *Fusarium* species, *Chem. Pharm. Bull.,* 23, 2439, 1975.
36. **Bubien, J. K. and Woods, W. T.,** Differential effects of trichothecenes on the canine cardiac action potential, *Toxicon,* 24, 467, 1986.
37. **Feuerstein, G. et al.,** unpublished observations.
38. **Marasas, W. F. O.,** personal communication.
39. **Poppenga, R. H. et al.,** unpublished observation.

INDEX